# GABA

# GABA

Edited by

**S. J. Enna**
Department of Molecular and Integrative Physiology
Department of Pharmacology, Toxicology, and Therapeutics
University of Kansas Medical Center
Kansas City, Kansas 66160, USA

ADVANCES IN
**PHARMACOLOGY**

VOLUME 54

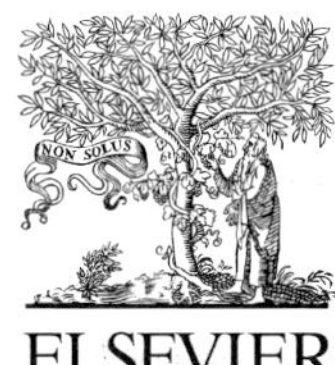


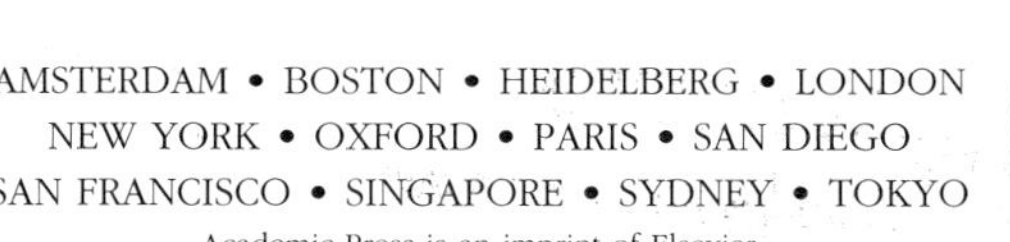
AMSTERDAM • BOSTON • HEIDELBERG • LONDON
NEW YORK • OXFORD • PARIS • SAN DIEGO
SAN FRANCISCO • SINGAPORE • SYDNEY • TOKYO
Academic Press is an imprint of Elsevier

Academic Press is an imprint of Elsevier
525 B Street, Suite 1900, San Diego, California 92101-4495, USA
84 Theobald's Road, London WC1X 8RR, UK

This book is printed on acid-free paper. 

For information on all Academic Press publications visit our Web site at www.books.elsevier.com

ISBN-13: 978-0-12-032957-1
ISBN-10: 0-12-032957-3

PRINTED IN THE UNITED STATES OF AMERICA
06 07 08 09 9 8 7 6 5 4 3 2 1

# Contents

## $GABA_A$ Agonists and Partial Agonists: THIP (Gaboxadol) as a Non-Opioid Analgesic and a Novel Type of Hypnotic

(This is a revised and updated version of an article entitled "$GABA_A$ agonists and partial agonists: THIP (Gaboxadol) as a non-opioid analgesic and a novel type of hypnotic" that appeared in *Biochem. Pharmacol.* **68**, 1573–1580 (2004).)

Povl Krogsgaard-Larsen, Bente Frølund, and Tommy Liljefors



## Rat Modeling for GABA Defects in Schizophrenia

Francine M. Benes and Barbara Gisabella



## Epigenetic Targets in GABAergic Neurons to Treat Schizophrenia

E. Costa, E. Dong, D. R. Grayson, W. B. Ruzicka, M. V. Simonini, M. Veldic, and A. Guidotti

## From Gene to Behavior and Back Again: New Perspectives on GABA$_A$ Receptor Subunit Selectivity of Alcohol Actions

(This is a revised and updated version of an article entitled "γ-Aminobutyric Acid A Receptor Subunit Mutant Mice: New Perspectives on Alcohol Actions" that appeared in *Biochem. Pharmacol.* **68,** 1581–1602 (2004).)

Stephen L. Boehm II, Igor Ponomarev, Yuri A. Blednov, and R. Adron Harris



## A Role for GABA in Alcohol Dependence

(This is a revised and updated version of an article entitled "A role for GABA mechanisms in the motivational effects of alcohol" that appeared in *Biochem. Pharmacol.* **68,** 1515–1525 (2004).)

George F. Koob

# Abbreviations

[(3)H]FLU: [(3)H]flunitrazepam
[(3)H]MUS: [(3)H]muscimol
AD: Anterodorsal thalamic nucleus
AM: Anteromedial thalamic nucleus
*APC*/EBP: *Aplysia* CCAAT/enhancer-binding protein
ApoER: Apolipoprotein E receptor
AV: Anteroventral thalamic nucleus
BDNF: Brain-derived nerve growth factor
bHLH: Basic helix-loop-helix transcription factor
CBP: Cyclic AMP response element binding protein (CREB)-binding protein
CL: Centrolateral thalamic nucleus
CM: Centromedial thalamic nucleus
CNS: Central nervous system
DAB1: Mouse disabled-1
dLGN: Dorsolateral geniculate nucleus
DNMT1: DNA methyltransferase 1
ERK: Extracellular signal regulated kinase
GABA: $\gamma$-Aminobutyric acid
$GABA_A$: $\gamma$-Aminobutyric acid receptor A
$GABA_{B(1a)}$: $\gamma$-Aminobutyric acid receptor B, subunit 1a
$GABA_{B(1b)}$: $\gamma$-Aminobutyric acid receptor B, subunit 1b
$GABA_{B(1c)}$: $\gamma$-Aminobutyric acid receptor B, subunit 1c
$GABA_B$: $\gamma$-Aminobutyric acid receptor B
$GABA_{B1}$: $\gamma$-Aminobutyric acid receptor B, subunit 1
$GABA_{B2}$: $\gamma$-Aminobutyric acid receptor B, subunit 2
$GABA_C$: $\gamma$-Aminobutyric acid receptor C
GABAergic: $\gamma$-Aminobutyric acidergic
GAD: Glutamic acid decarboxylase
$GAD_{67}$: Glutamic acid $decarboxylase_{67}$

GD: Gestational day
GPCR: G-protein–coupled receptors
HAT: Histone acetyl transferase
HDAC: Histone deacetylases
IMD: Intermediodorsal thalamic nucleus
LD: Laterodorsal thalamic nucleus
LG: Lateral geniculate body
LGN: Lateral geniculate nucleus
LP: Lateroposterior thalamic nucleus
LP-Pul: Lateroposterior pulvinar complex
LTD: Long-term depression
LTP: Long-term potentiation
MBD: Methyl binding domain
MD: Mediodorsal thalamic nucleus
MET: Methionine
MG: Medial geniculate nuclear complex
MGN: Medial geniculate nucleus
MS-275: 2′-Aminophenyl benzamide
NMDA: *N*-Methyl-D-aspartate
NMR2A: Methyl-D-aspartate receptor subunit $2_A$
NPS: Nonpsychiatric subjects
P: Postnatal day
PC: Paracentral thalamic nucleus
Pf: Parafascicular thalamic nucleus
Po: Posterior thalamic nucleus
Pul: Pulvinar nucleus
PV: Paraventricular thalamic nucleus
PVP: Posterior paraventricular thalamic nucleus
Re: Reuniens thalamic nucleus
Rh: Rhomboid thalamic nucleus
Rt: Reticular thalamic nucleus
SAHA: Suberoylanilide hydroxamic acid
SAM: *S*-Adenosyl methionine
Sm: Submedius thalamic nucleus
SZ: Schizophrenia
THIP: 4,5,6,7-Tetrahydroisothiazolo-[5,4-c]pyridine-3-ol or 4,5,6,7-Tetrahydroisoxazolo[5,4-c]pyridine-3-ol
TSA: Trichostatin A
VA: Ventral anterior thalamic nucleus
VB: Ventrobasal complex
VL: Ventrolateral thalamic nucleus
VLDLR: Very low-density lipoprotein receptor
vLGN: Ventrolateral geniculate nucleus
VM: Ventromedial thalamic nucleus
VP: Ventroposterior thalamic nuclei
VPA: Valproic acid
VPI: Ventroposteroinferior thalamic nucleus
VPL: Ventroposterolateral thalamic nucleus
VPM: Ventroposteromedial thalamic nucleus

# Contributors

*Numbers in parentheses indicate the pages on which the authors' contributions begin.*

*R. Adron Harris* (171) Waggoner Center for Alcohol and Addiction Research, University of Texas at Austin, Texas 78712

*Francine M. Benes* (73) Program in Structural and Molecular Neuroscience, McLean Hospital, Belmont, Massachusetts

*Yuri A. Blednov* (171) Waggoner Center for Alcohol and Addiction Research, University of Texas at Austin, Texas 78712

*Stephen L. Boehm* II (171) Department of Psychology, State University of New York at Binghamton, New York 13902

*José M. Castro-Lopes* (29) Institute of Histology and Embryology, Faculty of Medicine of Porto and IBMC, 4200-319 Porto, Portugal

*Mary Chebib* (285) Faculty of Pharmacy, The University of Sydney, NSW, 2006, Australia

*E. Costa* (95) Department of Psychiatry, Psychiatric Institute, University of Illinois at Chicago, Chicago, Illinois 60612

*E. Dong* (95) Department of Psychiatry, Psychiatric Institute, University of Illinois at Chicago, Chicago, Illinois 60612

*Rujee K. Duke* (285) Department of Pharmacology, The University of Sydney, NSW, 2006, Australia

*S. J. Enna* (1) Department of Molecular and Integrative Physiology, and Department of Pharmacology, Toxicology, and Therapeutics, University of Kansas Medical Center, Kansas City, Kansas 66160

*Hua-Jun Feng* (147) Department of Neurology, Vanderbilt University, Nashville, Tennessee 37232

*Joana Ferreira-Gomes* (29) Institute of Histology and Embryology, Faculty of Medicine of Porto and IBMC, 4200-319 Porto, Portugal

*Bente Frølund* (53, 265) Department of Medicinal Chemistry, The Danish University of Pharmaceutical Sciences, 2 Universitetsparken, DK-2100 Copenhagen, Denmark

*Martin J. Gallagher* (147) Department of Neurology, Vanderbilt University, Nashville, Tennessee 37232

*Barbara Gisabella* (73) Program in Neuroscience and Department of Psychiatry, Harvard Medical School, Belmont, Massachusetts

*D. R. Grayson* (95) Department of Psychiatry, Psychiatric Institute, University of Illinois at Chicago, Chicago, Illinois 60612

*A. Guidotti* (95) Department of Psychiatry, Psychiatric Institute, University of Illinois at Chicago, Chicago, Illinois 60612

*Jane R. Hanrahan* (285) Faculty of Pharmacy, The University of Sydney, NSW, 2006, Australia

*Graham A. R. Johnston* (285) Department of Pharmacology, The University of Sydney, NSW, 2006, Australia

*Jing-Qiong Kang* (147) Department of Neurology, Vanderbilt University, Nashville, Tennessee 37232

*George F. Koob* (205) Molecular and Integrative Neurosciences Department, The Scripps Research Institute, La Jolla, California

*Povl Krogsgaard-Larsen* (53, 265) Department of Medicinal Chemistry, The Danish University of Pharmaceutical Sciences, 2 Universitetsparken, DK-2100 Copenhagen, Denmark

*Orla Miller Larsson* (265) Department of Pharmacology and Pharmacotherapy, The Danish University of Pharmaceutical Sciences, DK-2100 Copenhagen, Denmark

*Tommy Liljefors* (53) Department of Medicinal Chemistry, The Danish University of Pharmaceutical Sciences, 2 Universitetsparken, DK-2100 Copenhagen, Denmark

*Robert L. Macdonald* (147) Department of Neurology, Department of Molecular Physiology, and Department of Biophysics and Pharmacology, Vanderbilt University, Nashville, Tennessee 37232

*Karsten Madsen* (265) Department of Pharmacology and Pharmacotherapy, The Danish University of Pharmaceutical Sciences, DK-2100 Copenhagen, Denmark

*Kenneth E. McCarson* (1) Department of Pharmacology, Toxicology, and Therapeutics, University of Kansas Medical Center, Kansas City, Kansas 66160

*Kenneth N. Mewett* (285) Department of Pharmacology, The University of Sydney, NSW, 2006, Australia

*Fani L. Neto* (29) Institute of Histology and Embryology, Faculty of Medicine of Porto and IBMC, 4200-319 Porto, Portugal

*Igor Ponomarev* (171) Waggoner Center for Alcohol and Addiction Research, University of Texas at Austin, Texas 78712

*Rasmus Prætorius Clausen* (265) Department of Medicinal Chemistry, The Danish University of Pharmaceutical Sciences, 2 Universitetsparken, DK-2100 Copenhagen, Denmark

*Eugene Roberts* (119) Director, Department of Neurobiochemistry, Emeritus, Beckman Research Institute, City of Hope Medical Center, Duarte, California 91010

*W. B. Ruzicka* (95) Department of Psychiatry, Psychiatric Institute, University of Illinois at Chicago, Chicago, Illinois 60612

*Arne Schousboe* (265) Department of Pharmacology and Pharmacotherapy, The Danish University of Pharmaceutical Sciences, DK-2100 Copenhagen, Denmark

*Werner Sieghart* (231) Division of Biochemistry and Molecular Biology, Center for Brain Research, and Section of Biochemical Psychiatry, University Clinic for Psychiatry, Medical University Vienna, Austria

*M. V. Simonini* (95) Department of Psychiatry, Psychiatric Institute, University of Illinois at Chicago, Chicago, Illinois 60612

*M. Veldic* (95) Department of Psychiatry, Psychiatric Institute, University of Illinois at Chicago, Chicago, Illinois 60612

**S. J. Enna*,† and Kenneth E. McCarson†**

*Department of Molecular and Integrative Physiology, University of Kansas Medical Center, Kansas City, Kansas 66160

†Department of Pharmacology, Toxicology, and Therapeutics, University of Kansas Medical Center, Kansas City, Kansas 66160

# The Role of GABA in the Mediation and Perception of Pain

## I. Chapter Overview

For nearly three decades efforts have been made to define the role of GABAergic transmission in the mediation and perception of pain. The anatomical distribution of GABA neurons and receptors, as well as the antinociceptive responses to $GABA_A$ and $GABA_B$ receptor agonists, is consistent with the notion that manipulation of this transmitter system may be of clinical benefit in the treatment of acute, inflammatory, and neuropathic pain. Contained in this report is a review of the data in support of this proposition, a discussion of disparate and contradictory findings, and a description of theories used to explain variation in the antinociceptive responses to GABAergic drugs. Particular emphasis is placed on interpreting the results in the context of the anatomical localization and function of GABA neurons as well as the molecular and pharmacological properties of GABA receptor subtypes. Included is a discussion of evidence suggesting

*Advances in Pharmacology, Volume 54*

1054-3589/06 $35.00
DOI: 10.1016/S1054-3589(06)54001-3

that GABA receptor expression and function, and therefore the antinociceptive responses to GABA agonists, vary as a function of the duration and intensity of a painful stimulus and of drug therapy. Such findings may facilitate the identification of pain syndromes that are particularly responsive to manipulation of GABAergic transmission.

## II. Introduction

As the primary inhibitory neurotransmitter in the central nervous system, γ-aminobutyric acid (GABA) is widely distributed throughout the neuraxis. Given its ubiquity, and relatively high concentrations in brain and spinal cord, it is likely that GABA plays a major role in mediating or modulating most, if not all, central nervous system functions. Evidence for this is provided by the fact that GABA receptor agonists and antagonists display a wide variety of pharmacological effects such as anxiolysis, hypnosis, muscle relaxation, amnesia, cognitive enhancement, stimulant, and anticonvulsant activities (Bowery and Enna, 2000; Enna, 1997; Möhler, 2001). Thus, manipulation of GABAergic transmission has proved to be of benefit in the treatment of a host of neurological and psychiatric disorders.

While it has been known for decades that GABA receptor agonists, as well as inhibitors of GABA uptake and metabolism, display significant antinociceptive activity in animal models of acute, inflammatory, and neuropathic pain (Kendall *et al.*, 1982; Levy and Proudfit, 1977; Malan *et al.*, 2002; Sands *et al.*, 2003; Shafizadeh *et al.*, 1997; Smith *et al.*, 1994; Thomas *et al.*, 1996; Vaught *et al.*, 1985; Zorn and Enna, 1985a), these findings have yet to yield novel drugs for the routine management of these conditions. Some reasons for this are the side effects, particularly sedation, associated with such agents, and the development of tolerance to their antinociceptive actions (Enna *et al.*, 1998; Malcangio *et al.*, 1995). However, thanks to advances in defining their structural, molecular, and biochemical properties, it may soon be possible to identify and target the GABA receptor and transporter subtypes that are most intimately involved in regulating pain threshold. This could result in the development of agents with fewer side effects than those associated with nonselective GABA receptor agonists and GABA uptake inhibitors. Moreover, evidence is accumulating that GABA receptor expression and function, and therefore the antinociceptive responses to drugs, vary as a function of the duration and intensity of a painful stimulus (Hama and Borsook, 2005). Such findings may make it possible to identify pain syndromes that are particularly responsive to manipulation of GABAergic transmission.

Reviewed in this report are selected publications describing the antinociceptive actions of drugs and chemicals known to influence GABAergic transmission. Particular emphasis is placed on interpreting the results in the context of what is known about the anatomical location and function of GABA neurons and with respect to the molecular and pharmacological properties of GABA receptors and receptor subtypes. These reports reveal that GABA receptor systems are found in peripheral and spinal cord pathways important for the origination and transmission of pain impulses, and in brain regions crucial for interpreting and responding to these signals. It is also established that agents known to modify GABA transmission display antinociceptive properties and that pain itself, as well as analgesics or antinociceptive agents, alters GABAergic transmission. Taken together, these studies support the notion that GABA plays a crucial role in nociceptive processing and agents that modify the function of this transmitter system could be useful analgesics.

## III. Molecular and Anatomical Considerations

### A. Receptor Subtypes

#### *1. GABA$_A$*

There are two major classes of GABA receptors: ionotropic GABA$_A$ and metabotropic GABA$_B$ (Alger and Le Beau, 2001). The GABA$_A$ receptor is a pentameric structure (Fig. 1), activation of which increases the neuronal concentration of chloride ion, hyperpolarizing the cell. As with other ligand-gated ion channels, GABA$_A$ receptor function is subject to modulation by drugs acting at sites on individual subunits or subunit combinations (Möhler *et al.*, 1997). This includes the benzodiazepines, such as diazepam, the barbiturates, such as phenobarbital, and the convulsant picrotoxin. Agonists and antagonists for the GABA$_A$ receptor recognition site include muscimol and bicuculline, respectively.

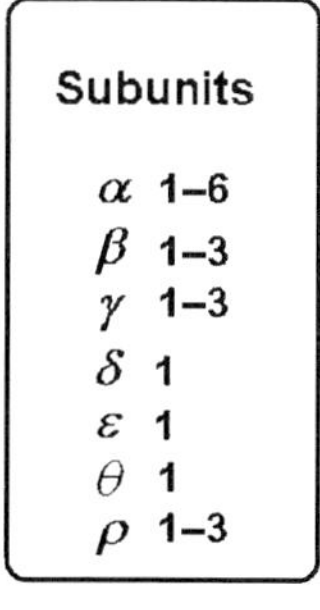


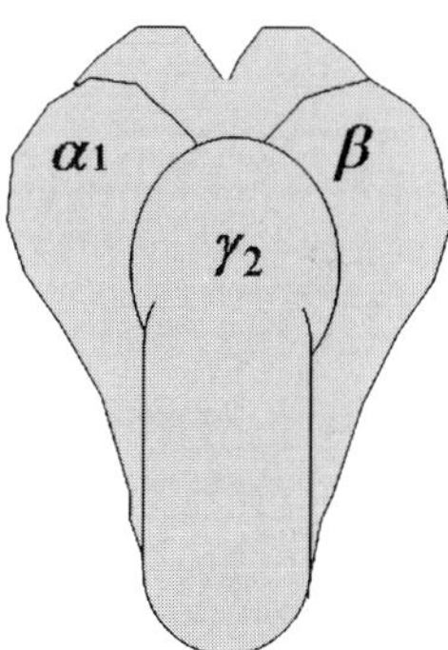


**FIGURE 1** Schematic representation of the GABA$_A$ receptor. Listed in the inset are the different GABA$_A$ receptor subunits. Adapted from Möhler *et al.*, 2004 (with permission).

At least 18 $GABA_A$ receptor subunits, along with a number of splice variants, have been identified in mammalian tissue (Fig. 1) (Möhler *et al.*, 2004; see also W. Sieghart, this volume). Given the pentameric nature of the site and the number of subunits, there are potentially thousands of molecularly distinct $GABA_A$ receptors. However, as only certain subunit combinations yield a response to GABA, it is estimated that the number of different $GABA_A$ receptors in the mammalian central nervous system is probably less than 100 and possibly as few as two dozen (Möhler *et al.*, 1997).

While the precise stoichiometry of native $GABA_A$ receptors is unknown, subunit-labeling studies suggest the majority of these sites are composed of $\alpha 1$, $\alpha 2$, $\gamma 2$, and $\beta$ subunits (Fig. 1). Subunit composition is of critical importance in evaluating the response to drugs since it determines the sensitivity of a particular $GABA_A$ receptor to individual agonists, antagonists, or modulators (Möhler *et al.*, 2004). For example, the $\alpha 1$ or $\alpha 2$, $\gamma 2\beta$ combination responds to benzodiazepine and nonbenzodiazepine anxiolytics and hypnotics. In contrast, receptors lacking the $\gamma$ subunit, or that possess $\gamma$ subunits in combination with $\alpha 4$ or $\alpha 6$ subunits, are generally insensitive to the benzodiazepines and related drugs (Möhler *et al.*, 1997). Thus, subunit composition undoubtedly plays an important role with respect to antinociceptive responses to agents acting at $GABA_A$ receptor sites.

## 2. $GABA_B$

$GABA_B$ receptors are class III, metabotropic, heterodimeric, G-protein–coupled sites (Fig. 2) (Binet *et al.*, 2004; Kubo and Tateyama, 2005). While numerous $GABA_B$ receptor subunit isoforms have been identified, initial studies indicated that fully functional $GABA_B$ receptors must be composed of a $GABA_{B1}$ and a $GABA_{B2}$ protein (Fig. 2) (Chronwall *et al.*, 2001; Enna, 2001a; Jones *et al.*, 1998; Kaupmann *et al.*, 1998). However, more recent findings suggest that $GABA_{B1}$ alone or $GABA_{B1}$ homodimers may display some activity as well (Gassmann *et al.*, 2004). Activation of $GABA_B$ receptors, which are located both pre- and postsynaptically throughout the central nervous system, decreases $Ca^{2+}$ and increases $K^+$ membrane conductance, leading to cellular hyperpolarization. Since $GABA_B$ receptors are coupled to $G_i$ or $G_o$ proteins, their activation can lead to either an increase or a decrease in cyclic AMP accumulation, depending upon the types of adenylyl cyclase in the cell and the presence or absence of $G\alpha s$ subunits (Bowery and Enna, 2000; Enna, 2001a,b). Stimulation of presynaptic $GABA_B$ receptors inhibits neurotransmitter release from nerve endings (Bowery, 2001; Brenowitz *et al.*, 1998).

While the possibility of pharmacologically and molecularly distinct $GABA_B$ receptors has been proposed (Cunningham and Enna, 1996; Enna, 2001a), the limited number of subunits (Fig. 2), the obligatory heterodimeric structure, and the conserved nature of the recognition site make this unlikely. Thus, it appears that direct-acting agonists, such as baclofen, and

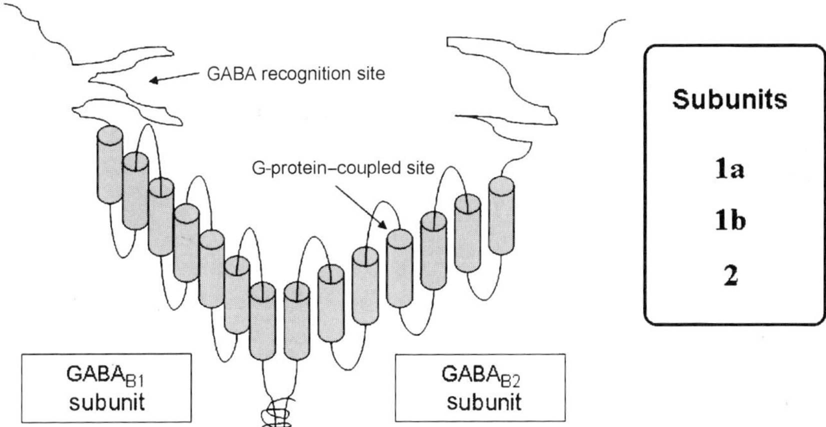


**FIGURE 2** Schematic representation of the GABA$_B$ receptor. Listed in the insert are the predominant GABA$_B$ receptor subunits. Adapted from cover figure of *Biochemical Pharmacology* 68(8), 2004 (with permission).

antagonists, such as CGP 27492, interact with all GABA$_B$ sites, although allosteric modulators may able to discriminate among this receptor population (Binet *et al.*, 2004; Urwyler *et al.*, 2003). Nevertheless, the weight of evidence suggests that agents acting directly on the GABA$_B$ receptor recognition site yield similar pharmacological profiles, including effects on nociception.

## B. Sensory Pathways and GABA

The transmission and perception of pain are complex processes involving both the central and peripheral nervous systems. In general, pain impulses are generated, propagated, and sustained by the liberation of various autocoids, ions, and neurotransmitters at various points between the site of tissue damage, along the afferent sensory fibers, and within the spinal cord and brain. Some endogenous agents, including adenosine and a variety of neuropeptides, are responsible for initiating, amplifying, and transmitting the pain impulse, whereas others, such as opioids, tend to be mitigating. Given the widespread distribution of GABAergic neurons, activation of this transmitter system may either enhance or reduce the propagation of pain impulses.

Nociceptive primary afferent neurons, in particular A-$\delta$ and C fibers, are responsible for transmitting the pain impulse from peripheral structures to the spinal cord. Damage due to thermal, mechanical, or chemical injury causes the release of various substances from the traumatized tissue including proteolytic enzymes responsible for liberating bradykinin from gamma globulins. Adenosine, potassium, and bradykinin stimulate chemosensitive nociceptors, initiating the pain impulse and inducing the release of substance P and prostaglandins from these nerve endings and nearby tissues. Substance P, in turn, causes the liberation of histamine from mast cells in the affected area. Similar to bradykinin, histamine and some prostaglandins, such as $PGE_2$, are pronociceptive agents that can directly stimulate or sensitize C fibers. Hyperalgesia occurs with the continued presence of these pain-producing substances in the vicinity of the nociceptive afferent terminals.

The afferent peripheral nociceptors, which are located in the lateral portion of the dorsal root, enter the spinal cord and synapse in the marginal zone and substantia gelatinosa of the dorsal horn. These regions contain cell bodies of the secondary neurons that project to higher levels (Eisenach, 1999) (Fig. 3). Glutamic acid and substance P are the two major excitatory neurotransmitters released at this synapse. At this level, the pain impulse

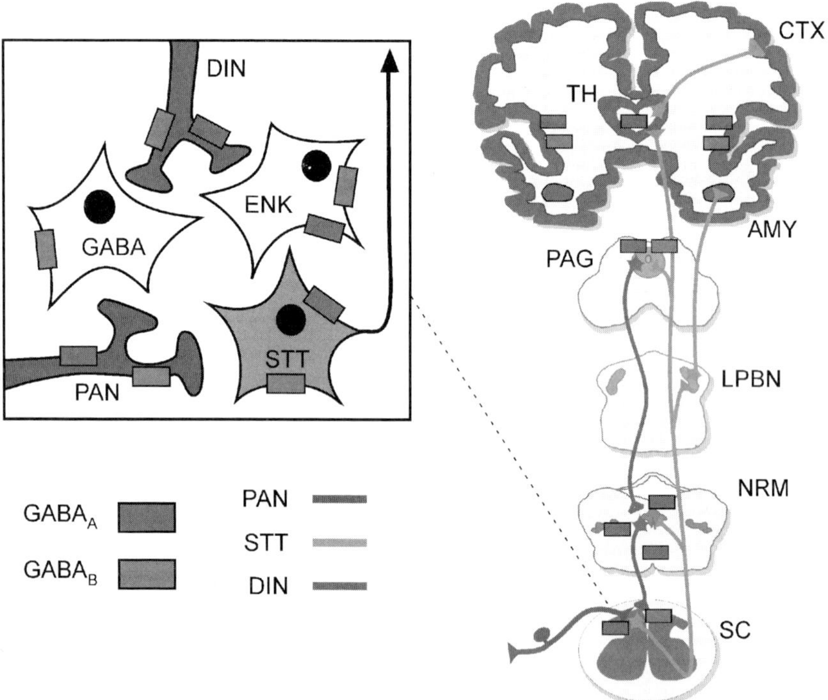


**FIGURE 3** Anatomical localization of GABA receptors in the central and peripheral nervous systems. Depicted in the inset is the circuitry within the dorsal horn of the spinal cord. Abbreviations: CTX, primary sensory cortex; TH, thalamus; AMY, amygdala; PAG, periaqueductal gray; LPBN, lateral parabrachial nucleus; NRM, medullary raphe nucleus; SC, spinal cord; PAN, primary afferent nociceptor C and A-$\delta$ fibers; DIN, descending inhibitory neuron; GABA, GABAergic interneuron; ENK, enkaphalinergic interneuron; STT, spinothalamic tract projection; $GABA_A$, $GABA_A$ receptor; $GABA_B$, $GABA_B$ receptor. (See Color Insert.)

traveling along afferent C and A-$\delta$ fibers predominantly activates spinothalamic neurons that compose the anterolateral component of the somatosensory projection system. The neospinothalamic tract portion of this projection targets the ventroposterior thalamus and the primary sensory cortex, providing the major discriminative and sensory aspects of pain sensation. Paleospinothalamic projections, in contrast, diffusely target a number of brain regions, including the lateral reticular formation, the superior colliculus, the periaqueductal gray, the pons, and the amygdala (Fig. 3). These influences on higher brain centers are responsible for many of the autonomic, motivational, and affective responses to pain.

Besides receiving input from the afferent limb of the anterolateral system, the periaqueductal gray of the midbrain and the periventricular gray of the thalamus receive efferent inputs from both the hypothalamus and cerebral cortex. Neurons from the periaqueductal gray and periventricular gray project to the medullary raphe nucleus that, in turn, sends descending serotonergic projections to the dorsal horn of the spinal cord (Eisenach, 1999) (Fig. 3). Other bulbospinal projections include a noradrenergic pathway that arises in the pons. Both descending serotonergic and noradrenergic neurons, which travel as part of the dorsolateral funiculus, inhibit or facilitate pain transmission at the level of the dorsal horn.

GABAergic neurons, as well as $GABA_A$ and $GABA_B$ receptors, are present in spinal cord and brain areas associated with the mediation and perception of pain (Fig. 3). With regard to higher brain regions, there is evidence that activation of $GABA_A$ receptors in the parafasiculus thalami induces an antinociceptive response (Reyes-Vazquez *et al.*, 1986). Moreover, there are GABAergic projections from the ventral tegmental area and substantia nigra to the ventrolateral periaqueductal gray and dorsal medullary raphe nucleus that regulate the behavioral and physiological responses to pain (Kirouac *et al.*, 2004). There are also data indicating that $GABA_A$ receptors are located on inhibitory neurons projecting from the rostral ventral medulla to the dorsal horn (Gilbert and Franklin, 2001). Local injection of a GABA agonist into this region facilitates transmission of a pain impulse through the spinal cord. In contrast, an increase in overall GABAergic activity in the rostral agranular insular cortex induces analgesia by enhancing the descending inhibition of spinal cord nociceptive neurons (Jasmin *et al.*, 2003). However, selective activation of $GABA_B$ receptors in the same area produces hyperalgesia, perhaps by way of projections to the amygdala (Jasmin *et al.*, 2003).

In the spinal cord there are GABA receptors located in the dorsal horn on pre- and postsynaptic sites in the region of the A-$\delta$ and C fiber synapses (Yang *et al.*, 2002) (Fig. 3). $GABA_B$ receptors are located on laminae I and II of the dorsal horn, the site of the first synapse in the pain pathway encompassing the terminal beds of small diameter, nociceptive-specific primary afferent neurons (Hokfelt *et al.*, 1975; Price *et al.*, 1984). Activation of presynaptic $GABA_B$ receptors on substance P or glutamate, containing neurons tends to enhance the pain threshold by inhibiting the release of these transmitters (Malcangio and Bowery, 1994). Thus, stimulation of $GABA_B$ receptors located presynaptically on the descending inhibitory serotonergic or noradrenergic terminals may lower the pain threshold by diminishing the release of transmitter from these cells (Yang *et al.*, 2002). Likewise, direct $GABA_A$ or $GABA_B$ receptor-mediated inhibition of opioid-containing neurons tends to facilitate pain transmission by reducing the release of this endogenous analgesic (Mahmoudi and Zarrindast, 2002). It is also possible that activation of some GABA receptors indirectly influences the transmission of pain by causing hyperpolarization of inhibitory neurons thereby releasing a brake on afferent or efferent cells critical for transmitting or attenuating the impulse.

Both types of GABA receptors have been identified on primary afferent A-$\delta$ and C fibers (Carlton *et al.*, 1999; Desarmenien *et al.*, 1984). Activation of the $GABA_A$ sites causes depolarization, whereas stimulation of the $GABA_B$ axonal receptors shortens the calcium component of the action potential. While the physiological role of these receptors is unclear, they may be of pharmacological importance by contributing to the overall response to systemically administered GABA receptor agonists.

Although activation of GABA receptors in localized regions of the brain and spinal cord can have variable effects on the pain threshold, generalized activation of either $GABA_A$ or $GABA_B$ receptors typically yields an antinociceptive response (Kendall *et al.*, 1982; Levy and Proudfit, 1977; Malan *et al.*, 2002; Sands *et al.*, 2003; Shafizadeh *et al.*, 1997; Smith *et al.*, 1994; Thomas *et al.*, 1996; Vaught *et al.*, 1985; Zorn and Enna, 1985a). This suggests that, on balance, GABA receptor systems tend to inhibit the propagation of pain impulses. Further evidence for this is provided by the loss of GABA-containing neurons, GABA transporters, and GABAergic activity in the spinal cord in animal models of neuropathic pain or following spinal cord injury (Drew *et al.*, 2004; Ibuki *et al.*, 1997; Miletic *et al.*, 2003; Moore *et al.*, 2002; Somers and Clemente, 2002). While it has been speculated that this decline in GABAergic function is responsible, in part, for the persistent pain and allodynia seen in these conditions, others suggest this may not be the case (Polgar *et al.*, 2003).

Taken together, these reports indicate that GABAergic neurons and receptors are located in regions of the central nervous system that are critical for transmitting and perceiving many aspects of pain. Given its widespread distribution, GABAergic transmission facilitates the transmission of pain impulses in some areas and inhibits it in others. Inasmuch as the sensitivity of pain pathways is altered over time through the process of central sensitization (Attal and Bouhassira, 1999; Ossipov *et al.*, 2000), it is likely that the response to GABAergic agents may vary as a function of when they are administered relative to the initial insult.

## IV. Pharmacological Studies

### A. $GABA_A$ Receptor Agents

The most definitive data supporting a role for GABA in the transmission and perception of pain are derived from pharmacological studies. In general, both clinical and preclinical experiments indicate that agents known to enhance GABAergic transmission display antinociceptive activity (Bowery and Enna, 2000; Dirig and Yaksh, 1995; Hill *et al.*, 1981; Johnston, 1992; Kaneko and Hammond, 1997; Kendall *et al.*, 1982; Kjaer and Nielsen, 1983; Malan *et al.*, 2002; Rode *et al.*, 2005; Vaught *et al.*, 1985; Zorn and Enna, 1985a,b). However, the response to such compounds and to GABA receptor antagonists varies as a function of dose, route and site of administration, and the nature, intensity, and duration of the pain stimulus (Vaught *et al.*, 1985; Zambotti *et al.*, Zorn and Enna, 1987).

With regard to the $GABA_A$ receptor system, direct-acting agonists examined as antinociceptive agents include muscimol, 4,5,6,7-tetrahydroisoxazolo[5,4-c]pyridine-3-ol (THIP), isoguvacine, and kojic amine, along with benzodiazepines, such as diazepam and midazolam, which are allosteric modulators at this site. Bicuculline and picrotoxin are $GABA_A$ receptor antagonists often employed for examining the relationship between GABA receptors and pain.

Systemically administered direct-acting GABA receptor agonists display analgesic activity in tail immersion and hot-plate assays (Andree *et al.*, 1983; Grognet *et al.*, 1983; Hammond and Drower, 1984; Kendall *et al.*, 1982; Pelley and Vaught, 1987; Vaught *et al.*, 1985; Zorn and Enna, 1985a,b, 1987). Moreover, intrathecal administration of muscimol or isoguvacine is effective in diminishing, and bicuculline in enhancing, inflammatory pain, especially during the late phase response (Green and Dickenson, 1997; Kaneko and Hammond, 1997). These findings suggest that the GABAergic tone regulating nociceptive transmission in the spinal cord is normally quite low, increasing in response to a persistent painful stimulus.

Numerous studies have been performed to examine the effect of $GABA_A$ receptor agonists and antagonists on the pain associated with nerve injury. The weight of evidence indicates that $GABA_A$ receptor agonists display analgesic activity in most animal models of neuropathic pain with, for example, subcutaneous administration of THIP, or subcutaneous or intrathecal administration of muscimol, reversing mechanical allodynia associated with nerve injury (Hwang and Yaksh, 1997; Malan *et al.*, 2002; Rode *et al.*, 2005). Further evidence of a role for GABA in modulating the symptoms of neuropathy is provided by the finding that both bicuculline and picrotoxin, $GABA_A$ receptor antagonists, cause allodynia when administered intrathecally (Loomis *et al.*, 2001). It has also been reported that neuropathic thermal hyperalgesia and mechanical allodynia are permanently reversed by intrathecal injection of GABA (Eaton *et al.*, 1999). However, as this effect is not observed if the neurotransmitter is administered later than 2–3 weeks following nerve injury, it appears a decline in spinal GABA levels contributes to the induction, but not the maintenance, of chronic neuropathic pain. This suggests that $GABA_A$ agonists may be most effective as a treatment for neuropathic pain if they are administered soon after the nerve injury.

While benzodiazepines are not generally considered analgesics, and are ineffective in treating the pain associated with inflammation (Dirig and Yaksh, 1995) or nerve injury, under certain circumstances they can be shown to induce antinociceptive responses (Nadeson *et al.*, 1996; Zambotti *et al.*, 1991). For example, while intrathecal administration of either midazolam or diazepam increases thermal tail flick latencies in rat, diazepam is much less effective, or even ineffective, in this test if it is injected intraperitoneally or intracerebroventricularly. This suggests the $GABA_A$ receptors that mediate benzodiazepine-induced antinociception are concentrated in the spinal cord. These findings also support the notion of low basal activity in these pathways since benzodiazepines are incapable of enhancing $GABA_A$ receptor function in the absence of released neurotransmitter. Alternatively, these results may indicate that most of the $GABA_A$ receptors responsible for regulating pain threshold have a subunit composition that is unresponsive to benzodiazepines.

Gene deletion and point mutation studies indicate that the anesthetic, sedative, hypnotic, anticonvulsant, anxiolytic, and antinociceptive responses to a variety of agents vary with the subunit composition of $GABA_A$ receptors (Rudolph and Möhler, 2004; Ugarte *et al.*, 1999). For example, deletion of the gene expressing the $\rho$ subunit, which is a component of $GABA_A$ receptors located in the spinal cord and dorsal root ganglia, decreases the pain threshold in mice (Zheng *et al.*, 2003). It has also been found that THIP is selective for extrasynaptic $GABA_A$ receptors composed of $\alpha4\beta3\delta$ subunits, the combination of which is unresponsive to benzodiazepines (Brown *et al.*, 2002; Krogsgaard-Larsen *et al.*, 2004; Shen *et al.*, 2005). Moreover, gene deletion studies reveal that $GABA_A$ ($\beta3^{-/-}$) mice are hyperalgesic with regard to both thermal and tactile stimuli, display a decreased responsiveness to GABA in the dorsal root ganglia, and are unresponsive to THIP (Krasowski *et al.*, 1998; Ugarte *et al.*, 1999). Even though THIP is not absolutely specific for $\alpha4\beta3\delta$-containing $GABA_A$ receptors, with some of its hypnotic effects mediated by sites containing $\alpha1$ or $\beta2$ subunits (Blednov *et al.*, 2003a), these results suggest that the antinociceptive response to $GABA_A$ receptor activation is mediated primarily by receptors devoid of a benzodiazepine binding component, explaining the general lack of antinociceptive activity of this drug class.

Like the benzodiazepines, other central nervous system depressants, such as barbiturates and propofol, lack analgesic activity when administered systemically. Indeed, their use is often accompanied by hyperalgesia (Yokoro *et al.*, 2001). Studies have revealed that the response to these agents may be determined, in part, by the route of administration. For example, intrathecal injection of phenobarbital induces analgesia in the tail-flick assay, but intracerebroventricular injection causes hyperalgesia (Yokoro *et al.*, 2001). Since the effects of propofol and phenobarbital on pain threshold are blocked by bicuculline, it appears this action is mediated by enhancement of $GABA_A$ receptors in select regions of the central nervous system (Wang *et al.*, 2004; Yokoro *et al.*, 2001). Likewise, the antinociceptive responses to sevoflurane or halothane are blocked by the intrathecal administration of bicuculline, indicating they are due to a general anesthetic-induced enhancement of spinal cord $GABA_A$ receptor activity (Mason *et al.*, 1996; Wang *et al.*, 2005). These data indicate that regulation of GABAergic activity in the brain and spinal cord contributes to the hyper- and hypoalgesic effects of various pharmacological agents.

The antinociceptive responses to agents that activate GABAergic transmission are mediated, in part, through the cholinergic muscarinic system. Thus, the antinociceptive effects of THIP and kojic amine in the mouse tail-flick assay are reduced by administration of atropine whereas the sedative effects are not (Grognet *et al.*, 1983; Kendall *et al.*, 1982; Pelley and Vaught, 1987; Vaught *et al.*, 1985; Zorn and Enna, 1987). There is a synergistic interaction between intrathecal neostigmine, a cholinesterase inhibitor, and muscimol with respect to their antiallodynic effects in an animal model of neuropathic pain (Hwang *et al.*, 2001). In contrast, it has been reported that a relatively high dose of THIP (15 mg/kg) administered intraperitoneally fails to induce an antinociceptive response in rats and blocks the antinociceptive action of a cholinesterase inhibitor (Zorn and Enna, 1987). These reports indicate that activation of $GABA_A$ receptors results in disinhibition of cholinergic neurons, which contributes to the antinociceptive response to the GABAergic agents. The findings with THIP are consistent with reports that it is a partial agonist at some $GABA_A$ receptors and, as such, may reduce GABAergic tone at higher doses (Krogsgaard-Larsen *et al.*, 2004).

Whereas facilitation of GABAergic transmission in the spinal cord generally raises nociceptive thresholds, the opposite appears true following activation of supraspinal $GABA_A$ receptors. For example, microinjection of THIP into the medullary raphe nucleus and the nucleus reticularis gigantocellularis pars alpha produces hyperalgesia while injection of bicuculline into the same regions causes hypoalgesia, as measured by tail-flick latency to a noxious thermal stimulus (Drower and Hammond, 1988; Hama *et al.*, 1998). This implies the GABAergic system, by way of $GABA_A$ receptors, inhibits the descending serotonergic pathways that regulate nociceptive transmission in the dorsal horn. Likewise, GABAergic neurons appear to be inhibitory on descending noradrenergic projections since intracerebroventricular injection of muscimol attenuates the antinociceptive effects of clonidine (Nguyen *et al.*, 1997). It has also been found that microinjection of either muscimol, a $GABA_A$ receptor agonist, or naloxone, an opioid receptor antagonist, into the periaqueductal gray inhibits c-Fos expression in the pontine nuclei, suggesting inhibition of noradrenergic outflow to the spinal cord (Ohashi *et al.*, 2003; Orii *et al.*, 2003). Furthermore, it has been found that the intracerebroventricular injection of muscimol or the microinjection of THIP into the periaqueductal gray matter blocks an opioid-induced increase in tail-flick latency (Depaulis *et al.*, 1987). Conversely, administration of picrotoxin, a $GABA_A$ receptor antagonist, into this brain region enhances the opioid-induced effect (Hough *et al.*, 2001). These findings suggest the GABAergic system, through $GABA_A$ receptors, tonically inhibits the antinociceptive descending spinal inhibition output from the periaqueductal gray matter. It is speculated that opioids disinhibit these pathways by reducing GABAergic tone in this brain region. A positive relationship between the $GABA_A$ and opioid systems is further suggested by the discovery of cross-tolerance to the antinociceptive effects of THIP, muscimol, and morphine following the continuous administration of any one of these agents (Andree *et al.*, 1983; Murray *et al.*, 1983; Srinivasan *et al.*, 1991). Thus, there appears to be a reciprocal interaction between these two systems with $GABA_A$ receptor activation enhancing opioid activity in some cases and opioids enhancing GABAergic tone in others.

In summary, generalized stimulation of $GABA_A$ receptors both enhances and reduces the transmission of pain. Which of these responses predominates depends on the basal tone of the system and the sensitivities of the various spinal and supraspinal $GABA_A$ receptors at the time of drug administration. Also of importance is the state of cholinergic and opioid pathways that mediate, in part, the anti- and pronociceptive responses to $GABA_A$ receptor agents.

## B. $GABA_B$ Receptor Agents

The effects of $GABA_B$ receptor agonists and antagonists on nociception are similar to those reported for agents that act at the $GABA_A$ site. Direct-acting $GABA_B$ receptor agonists employed for these studies include baclofen and CGP 44532. Baclofen is particularly popular since it is the prototypical $GABA_B$ receptor agonist and is used clinically as a treatment for spasticity and as an adjuvant therapy for managing certain types of pain (Fromm, 1994; Lind *et al.*, 2004; Loubser and Akman, 1996; Sindrup and Jensen, 2002; Slonimski *et al.*, 2004; Yaksh, 1999). Its effectiveness as an analgesic, although limited, provides proof of a role for GABA in regulating pain thresholds in humans. While it has been proposed that gabapentin, a GABA analog employed as an antiepileptic and for the treatment of neuropathic pain (Dworkin *et al.*, 2003; Karceski *et al.*, 2005; Sabatowski *et al.*, 2004), is a subtype-selective $GABA_B$ receptor agonist (Ng *et al.*, 2001), the weight of evidence does not support this conclusion (Cheng *et al.*, 2004;

Lanneau *et al.*, 2001). Rather, gabapentin and pregabalin, a structural analog, appear to influence neuronal activity by binding selectively to the $\alpha2\delta$ subunit of a calcium channel (Gee *et al.*, 1996). $GABA_B$ receptor antagonists commonly utilized for pain studies include phaclofen, 2-hydroxysaclofen, CGP 35348, and CGP 55845.

As is the case with $GABA_A$ receptor agonists, $GABA_B$ agonists, when administered either systemically or intrathecally, are effective in attenuating acute nociceptive responses to thermal stimuli or the persistent nociception associated with inflammation (Dirig and Yaksh, 1995; Enna *et al.*, 1998; Green and Dickenson, 1997; Hammond and Drower, 1984; Sands *et al.*, 2003; Vaught *et al.*, 1985; Zorn and Enna, 1985b). The antinociceptive response to $GABA_B$ agonists is thought to be related, at least in part, to their ability to inhibit presynaptically the release of tachykinins, glutamate, and other spinal neurotransmitters responsible for propagating nociceptive impulses (Enna *et al.*, 1998; Li *et al.*, 2002; Riley *et al.*, 2001). It has also been noted that many antinociceptive agents interact with G-protein–coupled receptors, such as $GABA_B$ sites, that regulate inwardly rectifying potassium channels (Blednov *et al.*, 2003b). Further evidence that enhanced GABAergic activity helps mitigate inflammatory pain is provided by the finding that administration of CGP 35348, a $GABA_B$ receptor antagonist, prolongs the duration of the late phase of formalin-induced nociceptive responses in rat (Green and Dickenson, 1997). Furthermore, not only does tolerance develop to the antinociceptive and sedative effects of baclofen following prolonged administration but also baclofen-tolerant animals are hyperalgesic with regard to formalin-induced inflammatory nociception (Enna *et al.*, 1998; Sands *et al.*, 2003). Unlike baclofen, antinociceptive tolerance does not appear to develop to long-term administration of CGP 44532, a more potent $GABA_B$ receptor agonist (Enna *et al.*, 1998). The reason for this difference between baclofen and CGP 44532 is unknown.

Baclofen displays antinociceptive activity in animal models of neuropathic pain whether administered intrathecally, intraperitoneally, intracerebroventricularly, or subcutaneously (Deseure *et al.*, 2003; Franek *et al.*, 2004; Hwang and Yaksh, 1997; Hwang *et al.*, 2001; Smith *et al.*, 1994; von Heijne *et al.*, 2001; Zarrindast and Mahmoudi, 2001; Zarrindast *et al.*, 2000). Moreover, the intrathecal administration of baclofen enhances the antiallodynic response to spinal cord stimulation, and intracerebroventricular administration of CGP 35348, a $GABA_B$ receptor antagonist, blocks the antinociceptive response to imipramine, a tricyclic antidepressant used for the treatment of neuropathic pain (Cui *et al.*, 1996; Zarrindast *et al.*, 2000). Unlike baclofen, CGP 35024, a $GABA_B$ receptor agonist, reduces hyperalgesia in a neuropathic pain model at doses that do not produce sedation, suggesting it may be possible to improve the side-effect profile of $GABA_B$ receptor agonists as treatments for pain (Patel *et al.*, 2001).

Baclofen is reported to be effective in reducing mechanical allodynia in an animal model of trigeminal pain whether it is administered during or after the development of the syndrome, suggesting no change in the sensitivity of the relevant $GABA_B$ receptors in this condition (Deseure *et al.*, 2003). In contrast, the antinociceptive effects of baclofen in the sciatic nerve ligation model of neuropathic pain declines in the ipsilateral but not contralateral limb, indicating a change in responsiveness over time (Franek *et al.*, 2004). These contradictory conclusions may arise from differences in the animal models or the route of administration of baclofen with constant infusion being employed in the trigeminal pain study and daily subcutaneous injections in the sciatic nerve model.

Discrepant results have also been found with $GABA_B$ receptor antagonists. For example, while intrathecal administration of baclofen diminishes allodynia associated with the Chung model of neuropathic pain, intrathecal infusion or microinjection into the ventromedial medulla of CGP 35348, a $GABA_B$ receptor antagonist, has no effect on normal pain threshold or on tactile allodynia (Hwang and Yaksh, 1997; Thomas *et al.*, 1996). This suggests that spinal cord $GABA_B$ receptor tone is low in regions associated with the transmission of pain impulses, both under basal conditions and after the development of tactile allodynia. In contrast, it has been reported that intrathecal administration of phaclofen, a $GABA_B$ receptor antagonist, to normal animals produces tactile allodynia and hyperalgesia, suggesting GABAergic tone in the spinal cord is important for maintaining nociceptive thresholds (Malan *et al.*, 2002). In addition, gene deletion studies reveal that selective elimination of either the $GABA_{B1}$ or $GABA_{B2}$ subunit results in hyperalgesia (Gassmann *et al.*, 2004; Schuler *et al.*, 2001; Vacher and Bettler, 2003), making it appear that an endogenous $GABA_B$ receptor tone contributes to maintaining pain thresholds. It has been reported that inactivation of the gene expressing the $\beta 3$ subunit of the $GABA_A$ receptor not only reduces the pain threshold and the response to THIP, a $GABA_A$ receptor agonist, but also attenuates the antinociceptive response to baclofen (Ugarte *et al.*, 1999). This suggests an ongoing, endogenous GABA receptor tone with respect to nociception and an interaction between $GABA_A$ and $GABA_B$ receptor systems in mediating the antinociceptive response to $GABA_B$ agonists. Alternatively, it is possible that a non-GABAergic neurotransmitter system important for mediating the antinociceptive response to baclofen is affected by the deletion of the $\beta 3$ subunit gene (Rudolph and Möhler, 2004).

Thus, the results of pharmacological studies have yielded some uncertainty about the extent to which the $GABA_B$ receptor system contributes to maintaining nociceptive threshold in the absence of a painful stimulus. While the apparently disparate results are difficult to reconcile, they may reflect the fact that the responses to drugs known to be effective in the treatment of neuropathic pain vary over time (Hama and Borsook, 2005). This indicates that a change in the sensitivity of critical pathways could alter the responsiveness to certain therapies. Thus, pro- and antinociceptive responses to $GABA_B$ agonists and antagonists are likely to vary depending upon when they are administered relative to the induction of neuropathy. The results of gene deletion experiments strongly suggest that endogenous GABA, interacting with $GABA_B$ receptors, is an important component in the ongoing regulation of the pain threshold.

Antinociceptive responses to $GABA_B$ receptor agonists and antagonists are dependent on dose and route of administration (Thomas *et al.*, 1995). Thus, microinjection of low doses of baclofen into certain supraspinal regions of the rat brain, such as the medullary raphe nucleus and the nucleus reticularis gigantocellularis pars alpha, increases tail-flick latencies (hypoalgesia) to a nociceptive stimulus, whereas higher doses decrease latencies (hyperalgesia). It is speculated low doses of baclofen disinhibit outflow neurons in these brain regions by attenuating the release of GABA or norepinephrine, with higher doses reducing the release of excitatory neurotransmitters, such as glutamate, or directly hyperpolarizing these efferent neurons (Thomas *et al.*, 1995). It has also been found that the antinociceptive response to subcutaneously administered baclofen is blocked by the intrathecal, but not supraspinal (ventromedial medulla), administration of CGP 35348, a selective $GABA_B$ receptor antagonist, suggesting the antinociceptive action of baclofen is mediated primarily by activation of spinal cord $GABA_B$ receptor systems (Thomas *et al.*, 1996).

Variability in the antinociceptive properties of $GABA_B$ agonists may also be related to the fact that other transmitter systems are involved in mediating the effects of these agents. As reported for the $GABA_A$ receptor agonist muscimol, intracerebroventricular administration of baclofen inhibits clonidine-induced antinociceptive responses, indicating that $GABA_B$ receptor activation in certain supraspinal regions results in inhibition of efferent noradrenergic pathways that modulate pain transmission in the spinal cord (Nguyen *et al.*, 1997). Moreover, the antinociceptive response to baclofen in a mouse hot-plate test is blocked by atropine, a cholinergic muscarinic receptor antagonist but not by mecamylamine, a nicotinic receptor antagonist (Vaught *et al.*, 1985). Conversely, it has been reported that intrathecal administration of CGP 55845, a $GABA_B$ receptor antagonist, attenuates the antiallodynic effects of intrathecally administered muscarine or neostigmine (Chen and Pan, 2003). These reports suggest that the antinociceptive response to the $GABA_B$ receptor antagonist is secondary to a disinhibition of cholinergic activity.

Intrathecal injection of CGP 35348, a $GABA_B$ receptor antagonist, blocks the antinociception induced by direct application of opioids into the medullary raphe nucleus, indicating an interaction between the $GABA_B$ and opioid systems (Hurley *et al.*, 2003). It has been reported that SR 141716A, a cannabinoid receptor antagonist, blocks the antinociceptive effects of intrathecally administered baclofen in a model of inflammatory pain (Naderi *et al.*, 2005). Based on this finding, it is speculated that the antinociceptive effects of $GABA_B$ receptor agonists are due to endocannabinoid release in the spinal cord. These results are undoubtedly a reflection of the widespread distribution of $GABA_B$ receptors throughout the neuraxis. Because of this, the response to their activation is, in part, the net result of the attenuation or stimulation of neurotransmitter release in various regions of the brain and spinal cord. Thus, the antinociceptive action of $GABA_B$ agonists depends upon not only the sensitivity of this receptor system but on the capacity of other neuronal pathways to respond appropriately to $GABA_B$ receptor activation.

The plasticity of the $GABA_B$ receptor system, which may contribute to variability in the response to $GABA_B$ receptor agonists and antagonists, is illustrated by studies aimed at examining the effects of pain and/or drug administration on $GABA_B$ receptor function and subunit expression. Thus, it has been demonstrated that persistent mechanical stimulation or inflammatory pain increases the number of $GABA_B$-containing neurons in the brainstem while decreasing the number of $GABA_B$ receptors and increasing the production of $GABA_{B1}$ and $GABA_{B2}$ subunit proteins in the spinal cord (Malcangio and Bowery, 1994; Malcangio *et al.*, 1995; McCarson and Enna, 1999; Pinto *et al.*, 2003; Sands *et al.*, 2003; Smith *et al.*, 1994). Likewise, partial sciatic nerve ligation, an animal model of neuropathic pain, increases spinal cord $GABA_B$ receptor sensitivity and $GABA_B$ receptor subunit expression at a time when there is a decrease in thermal and mechanical pain thresholds (McCarson *et al.*, 2005). These observations suggest the development of neuropathic pain may be associated with a decline in spinal cord GABAergic activity. It has also been reported that prolonged systemic administration of baclofen results in tolerance to its antinociceptive effects, a decrease in the functional activity $GABA_B$ receptors, and an attenuation of pain-induced increases in spinal neurokinin receptor gene expression (Enna *et al.*, 1998; McCarson and Enna, 1996; Sands *et al.*, 2003). These findings indicate the responsiveness of the $GABA_B$ receptor system is modified by persistent nociception and by the continuous administration of $GABA_B$ agonists. They also illustrate a lack of concordance between $GABA_B$ receptor function and subunit expression, suggesting nongenomic mechanisms for regulating receptor sensitivity, and possibly alternative functions for $GABA_B$ subunit proteins (McCarson *et al.*, 2005; Sands *et al.*, 2003).

Further evidence supporting an involvement of the spinal cord $GABA_B$ receptor system in neuropathic pain is provided by studies aimed at examining the effect of drugs used to treat this condition. For example, continuous administration of the tricyclic antidepressants desipramine or amitriptyline, or of fluoxetine, a selective serotonin reuptake inhibitor, attenuates the thermal hypersensitivity that develops as a result of sciatic nerve ligation and modifies the changes in spinal cord $GABA_B$ receptor function and subunit expression that occur in this model of neuropathy (McCarson *et al.*, 2005, 2006; Sands *et al.*, 2004). Such discoveries make it appear that the efficacy of these agents as treatments for neuropathic pain may be related to an ability to maintain spinal cord $GABA_B$ receptor function. They also suggest that drug-induced changes in the expression of $GABA_B$ subunit genes in rat may predict clinical efficacy for the treatment of this condition. Since the $GABA_B$ receptor system is modified by pain and drug treatments, exposure to either may contribute to variations in the antinociceptive effects of $GABA_B$ agonists.

## C. Inhibitors of GABA Uptake and Metabolism

Inhibition of GABA uptake or metabolism is another strategy for enhancing GABAergic transmission. The utility of this approach is demonstrated by the successful development of such agents for the treatment of epilepsy and neuropathic pain (Bialer *et al.*, 2004; Kinloch and Cox, 2005; Novak *et al.*, 2001; Solaro and Tanganelli, 2004; Todorov *et al.*, 2005). Compounds in this category include γ-vinyl GABA (vigabatrin), a GABA transaminase inhibitor, and the GABA uptake inhibitors SKF 89976A, nipecotic acid ethyl ester, and tiagabine, an R-nipecotic acid derivative that selectively inhibits the GAT-1 GABA transporter (Borden *et al.*, 1994; Krogsgaard-Larsen *et al.*, 2000; Soudijn and van Wijngaarden, 2000). Given the antinociceptive properties of direct-acting $GABA_A$ and $GABA_B$ receptor agonists, it is not surprising that inhibitors of GABA uptake and metabolism share this property since they nonselectively activate both sites. All of these agents display thermal antinociceptive properties when administered systemically or intrathecally and are efficacious in reducing inflammatory nociception (Costa *et al.*, 1982; Laughlin *et al.*, 2002; Zorn and Enna, 1985a). SKF 89976A, a GABA uptake inhibitor, is reported to be more efficacious in a test of thermal nociception than direct-acting GABA receptor agonists or inhibitors of GABA metabolism (Zorn and Enna, 1986). In addition, inhibitors of GABA uptake or metabolism are efficacious in reducing thermal hyperalgesia and mechanical allodynia that develop in animal models of neuropathic pain (Alves *et al.*, 1999; Zhu *et al.*, 2005).

As is true for $GABA_A$ and $GABA_B$ receptor agonists, the antinociceptive effects of inhibitors of GABA uptake or metabolism are blocked by atropine, a cholinergic muscarinic receptor antagonist (Costa *et al.*, 1982; Kendall *et al.*, 1982; Zorn and Enna, 1985a). In addition, the antinociceptive effects of γ-vinyl GABA are inhibited by bicuculline, a $GABA_A$ receptor antagonist, and the responses to tiagabine by saclofen, a $GABA_B$ receptor antagonist (Jasmin *et al.*, 2003; Laughlin *et al.*, 2002). The results with atropine, bicuculline, and saclofen demonstrate that the antinociceptive responses to inhibitors of GABA uptake or metabolism are mediated by activation of GABA receptors.

The clinical effectiveness of inhibitors of GABA uptake or metabolism demonstrates a role for GABA in the regulation of seizure and pain thresholds. However, as is the case with direct-acting GABA receptor agonists, their use as antinociceptive agents is limited by side effects, particularly sedation.

## V. Summary and Conclusions

A great deal of effort has been expended in attempting to define the role of GABA in mediating the transmission and perception of pain. Pursuit of this question has been stimulated by the fact that GABAergic neurons are widely distributed throughout the central nervous system, including regions of the spinal cord dorsal horn known to be important for transmitting pain impulses to the brain. In addition, GABA neurons and receptors are found in supraspinal sites known to coordinate the perception and response to painful stimuli and this neurotransmitter system has been shown to regulate control of sensory information processing in the spinal cord. The discovery that GABA receptor agonists display antinociceptive properties in a variety of animal models of pain has provided an impetus for developing such agents for this purpose. It has been shown that GABA receptor agonists, as well as inhibitors of GABA uptake or metabolism, are clinically effective in treating this symptom. However, even with an enhanced understanding of the relationship between GABAergic transmission and pain, it has proven difficult to exploit these findings in designing novel analgesics that can be employed for the routine management of pain.

Work in this area has revealed a host of reasons why GABAergic drugs have, to date, been of limited utility in the management of pain. Chief among these are the side effects associated with such agents, in particular sedation. These limitations are likely due to the simultaneous activation of GABA receptors throughout the neuraxis, most of which are not involved in the transmission or perception of pain. This makes it difficult to fully exploit the antinociceptive properties of GABAergic drugs before untoward effects intervene. The discovery of molecularly and pharmacologically distinct $GABA_A$ receptors may open the way to developing subtype selective agents that target those receptors most intimately involved in the transmission and perception of pain. The more limited repertoire of $GABA_B$ receptor subunits makes it more difficult to develop subtype selective agents for this site. Nonetheless, a $GABA_B$ agonist, CGP 35024, has been identified that induces antinociceptive responses at doses well below those that cause sedation (Patel *et al.*, 2001). It has also been reported that, unlike baclofen, tolerance to antinociceptive responses is not observed with CGP 44532, a more potent $GABA_B$ receptor agonist (Enna *et al.*, 1998). While the reasons for these differences in responses to members of the same class remain unknown, these findings suggest it may be possible to design a $GABA_B$ agonist with a superior clinical profile than existing agents.

Besides the challenges associated with identifying subtype selective $GABA_A$ and $GABA_B$ receptor agonists, the development of GABA analgesics has been hindered by the fact that the responsiveness of these receptor systems appear to vary with the type and duration of pain being treated and the mode of drug administration. Further studies are necessary to more precisely define the types of pain most amenable to treatment with GABAergic drugs. Inasmuch as the antinociceptive responses to these agents in laboratory animals are mediated, at least in part, through activation or inhibition of other neurotransmitter and neuromodulator systems, it is conceivable that GABA agonists will be most efficacious as analgesics when administered in combination with other agents.

The results of anatomical, biochemical, molecular, and pharmacological studies support the notion that generalized activation of GABA receptor systems dampens the response to painful stimuli. The data leave little doubt that, under certain circumstances, stimulation of neuroanatomically discreet GABA receptor sites could be of benefit in the management of pain. Continued research in this area is warranted given the limited choices, and clinical difficulties, associated with conventional analgesics.

## Acknowledgments

Preparation of this review was made possible, in part, by a grant from the Lied Foundation (SJE). We thank Ms. Lynn LeCount and Ms. Jerri Rook for their editorial assistance.

## References

Alger, B. E., and Le Beau, F. E. N. (2001). Physiology of the GABA and glycine systems. *In* "Pharmacology of GABA and Glycine Neurotransmission" (H. Möhler, Ed.), pp. 3–76. Springer-Verlag, Berlin.

Alves, N. D., de Castro-Costa, C. M., de Carvalho, A. M., Santos, F. J., and Silveira, D. G. (1999). Possible analgesic effect of vigabatrin in animal experimental chronic neuropathic pain. *Arq. Neuropsiquiatr.* **57**, 916–920.

Andree, T., Kendall, D. A., and Enna, S. J. (1983). THIP analgesia: Cross tolerance with morphine. *Life Sci.* **32**, 2265–2272.

Attal, N., and Bouhassira, D. (1999). Mechanisms of pain in peripheral neuropathy. *Acta Neurol. Scand. Suppl.* **173**, 12–24.

Bialer, M., Johannessen, S. I., Kupferberg, H. J., Levy, R. H., Perucca, E., and Tomson, T. (2004). Progress report on new antiepileptic drugs: A summary of the Seventh Eilat Conference (EILAT VII). *Epilepsy Res.* **61**, 1–48.

Binet, V., Goudet, C., Brajon, C., Le Corre, L., Archer, F., Pin, J.-P., and Prezeau, L. (2004). Molecular mechanisms of action of $GABA_B$ receptor activation: New insights from the mechanism of action of CGP7930, a positive allosteric modulator. *Biochem. Soc. Trans.* **32**, 871–872.

Blednov, Y. A., Jung, S., Alva, H., Wallace, D., Rosahl, T., Whiting, P. J., and Harris, R. A. (2003a). Deletion of the alpha1 or beta2 subunit of $GABA_A$ receptors reduces actions of alcohol and other drugs. *J. Pharmacol. Exp. Ther.* **304**, 30–36.

Blednov, Y. A., Stoffel, M., Alva, H., and Harris, R. A. (2003b). A pervasive mechanism for analgesia: Activation of GIRK2 channels. *Proc. Natl. Acad. Sci. USA* **100**, 277–282.

Borden, L. A., Murali Dhar, T. G., Smith, K. E., Weinshank, R. L., Branchek, T. A., and Gluchowski, C. (1994). Tiagabine, SK&F 89976-A, CI-966, and NC-711 are selective for the cloned GABA transporter GAT-1. *Eur. J. Pharmacol.* **269**, 219–224.

Bowery, N. G. (2001). Pharmacology of $GABA_B$ receptors. *In* "Pharmacology of GABA and Glycine Neurotransmission" (H. Möhler, Ed.), pp. 311–328. Springer-Verlag, Berlin.

Bowery, N. G., and Enna, S. J. (2000). Gamma-aminobutyric acid (B) receptors: First of the functional metabotropic heterodimers. *J. Pharmacol. Exp. Ther.* **293**, 2–7.

Brenowitz, S., David, J., and Trussell, L. (1998). Enhancement of synaptic efficacy by presynaptic $GABA_B$ receptors. *Neuron* **20**, 135–141.

Brown, N., Kerby, J., Bonnert, T. P., Whiting, P. J., and Wafford, K. A. (2002). Pharmacological characterization of a novel cell line expressing human alpha(4)beta(3)delta GABA(A) receptors. *Br. J. Pharmacol.* **136**, 965–974.

Carlton, S. M., Zhou, S., and Coggeshall, R. E. (1999). Peripheral GABA(A) receptors: Evidence for peripheral primary afferent depolarization. *Neuroscience* **93**, 713–722.

Chen, S. R., and Pan, H. L. (2003). Spinal GABAB receptors mediate antinociceptive actions of cholinergic agents in normal and diabetic rats. *Brain Res.* **965**, 67–74.

Cheng, J. K., Lee, S. Z., Yang, J. R., Wang, C. H., Liao, Y. Y., Chen, C. C., and Chiou, L. C. (2004). Does gabapentin act as an agonist at native GABA(B) receptors. *J. Biomed. Sci.* **11**, 346–355.

Chronwall, B. M., Davis, T. D., Severidt, M. W., Wolfe, S. E., McCarson, K. E., Beatty, D. M., Low, M. J., Morris, S. J., and Enna, S. J. (2001). Constitutive expression of $GABA_B$ receptors in mIL-tsA58 cells requires both $GABA_{B1}$ and $GABA_{B2}$ genes. *J. Neurochem.* **77**, 1237–1247.

Costa, L. G., Doctor, S. V., and Murphy, S. D. (1982). Antinociceptive and hypothermic effects of trimethyltin. *Life Sci.* **31**, 1093–1102.

Cui, J. G., Linderoth, B., and Meyerson, B. A. (1996). Effects of spinal cord stimulation on touch-evoked allodynia involve GABAergic mechanisms. An experimental study in the mononeuropathic rat. *Pain* **66**, 287–295.

Cunningham, M. D., and Enna, S. J. (1996). Evidence for pharmacologically distinct $GABA_B$ receptors associated with cAMP production in rat brain. *Brain Res.* **720**, 220–224.

Depaulis, A., Morgan, M. M., and Liebeskind, J. C. (1987). GABAergic modulation of the analgesic effects of morphine microinjected in the ventral periaqueductal gray matter of the rat. *Brain Res.* **436**, 223–228.

Desarmenien, M., Feltz, P., Occhipinti, G., Santangelo, F., and Schlichter, R. (1984). Coexistence of $GABA_A$ and $GABA_B$ receptors on A delta and C primary afferents. *Br. J. Pharmacol.* **81**, 327–333.

Deseure, K., Koek, W., Adriaensen, H., and Colpaert, F. C. (2003). Continuous administration of the 5-hydroxytryptamine1A agonist (3-chloro-4-fluoro-phenyl0-[4-fluoro-4-[[5-methyl-pyridin-2-ylmethyl)-amino]-methyl]piperidin-1-yl]-methadone (F 13640) attenuates allodynia-like behavior in a rat model of trigeminal neuropathic pain. *J. Pharmacol. Exp. Ther.* **306**, 505–514.

Dirig, D. M., and Yaksh, T. L. (1995). Intrathecal baclofen and muscimol, but not midazolam, are antinociceptive using the rat-formalin model. *J. Pharmacol. Exp. Ther.* **275**, 219–227.

Drew, G. M., Siddall, P. J., and Duggan, A. W. (2004). Mechanical allodynia following contusion injury of the rat spinal cord is associated with loss of GABAergic inhibition in the dorsal horn. *Pain* **109**, 379–388.

Drower, E. J., and Hammond, D. L. (1988). GABAergic modulation of nociceptive threshold: Effects of THIP and bicuculline microinjected in the ventral medulla of the rat. *Brain Res.* **450**, 316–324.

Dworkin, R. H., Corbin, A. E., Young, J. P., Sharma, U., LaMoreaux, L., Bockbrader, H., Garofalo, E. A., and Poole, R. M. (2003). Pregabalin for the treatment of postherpetic neuralgia: A randomized, placebo-controlled trial. *Neurology* **60**, 1274–1283.

Eaton, M. J., Martinez, M. A., and Karmally, S. (1999). A single intrathecal injection of GABA permanently reverses neuropathic pain after nerve injury. *Brain Res.* **835**, 334–339.

Eisenach, J. C. (Ed.) (1999). "Textbook of Pain,"4th edn. Churchill Livingstone, London.

Enna, S. J. (1997). $GABA_B$ receptor agonists and antagonists: Pharmacological properties and therapeutic possibilities. *Expert Opin. Investig. Drugs* **6**, 1319–1325.

Enna, S. J. (2001a). A $GABA_B$ mystery: The search for pharmacologically distinct $GABA_B$ receptors. *Mol. Interv.* **1**, 208–218.

Enna, S. J. (2001b). $GABA_B$ receptor signaling pathways. *In* "Pharmacology of GABA and Glycine Neurotransmission" (H. Möhler, Ed.), pp. 329–342. Springer-Verlag, Berlin.

Enna, S. J., Harstad, E. B., and McCarson, K. E. (1998). Regulation of neurokinin-1 receptor expression by $GABA_B$ receptor agonists. *Life Sci.* **62**, 1525–1530.

Franek, M., Vaculin, S., and Rokyta, R. (2004). $GABA_B$ receptor agonist baclofen has non-specific antinociceptive effect in the model of peripheral neuropathy in the rat. *Physiol. Res.* **53**, 351–355.

Fromm, G. H. (1994). Baclofen as an adjuvant analgesic. *J. Pain Symptom Manage.* **9**, 500–509.

Gassmann, M., Shaban, H., Vigot, R., Sansig, G., Haller, C., Barbieri, S., Hameau, Y., Schuler, V., Muller, M., Kinzel, B., Klebs, K., Schmutz, M., *et al.* (2004). Redistribution of $GABA_B(1)$ protein and atypical GABAB responses in GABAB(2)-deficient mice. *J. Neurosci.* **24**, 6086–6097.

Gee, N. S., Brown, J. P., Dissanayake, V. U., Offord, J., Thurlow, R., and Woodruff, G. N. (1996). The novel anticonvulsant drug, gabapentin (Neurontin), binds to the $\alpha_2\delta$ subunit of a calcium channel. *J. Biol. Chem.* **271**, 5768–5776.

Gilbert, A. K., and Franklin, K. B. (2001). GABAergic modulation of descending inhibitory systems from the rostral ventromedial medulla (RVM). Dose-response analysis of nociception and neurological deficits. *Pain* **90**, 25–36.

Green, G. M., and Dickenson, A. (1997). GABA-receptor control of the amplitude and duration of the neuronal responses to formalin in the rat spinal cord. *Eur. J. Pain* **1**, 95–104.

Grognet, A., Hertz, F., and DeFeudis, F. V. (1983). Comparison of the analgesic actions of THIP and morphine. *Gen. Pharmacol.* **14**, 585–589.

Hama, A. T., and Borsook, D. (2005). The effect of antinociceptive drugs tested at different times after nerve injury in rats. *Anesth. Analg.* **101**, 175–179.

Hama, A. T., Fritschy, J.-M., and Hammond, D. L. (1998). Differential distribution of $GABA_A$ receptor subunits on bulbospinal serotonergic and nonserotonergic neurons of the ventromedial medulla of the rat. *J. Comp. Neurol.* **384**, 337–348.

Hammond, D. L., and Drower, E. J. (1984). Effects of intrathecally administered THIP, baclofen and muscimol on nociceptive threshold. *Eur. J. Pharmacol.* **103**, 121–125.

Hill, R. C., Maurer, R., Buescher, H. H., and Roemer, D. (1981). Analgesic properties of the GABA-mimetic THIP. *Eur. J. Pharmacol.* **69**, 221–224.

Hokfelt, T., Kellerth, J. O., Nilsson, G., and Pernow, B. (1975). Experimental immunohistochemical studies on the location and distribution of substance P in cat primary sensory neurons. *Brain Res.* **100**, 235–252.

Hough, L. B., Nalwalk, J. W., Leurs, R., Menge, W. M., and Timmerman, H. (2001). Significance of GABAergic systems in the action of improgan, a non-opioid analgesic. *Life Sci.* **68**, 2751–2757.

Hurley, R. W., Banfor, P., and Hammond, D. L. (2003). Spinal pharmacology of antinociception produced by microinjection of mu or delta opioid receptor agonists in the ventromedial medulla of the rat. *Neuroscience* **118**, 789–796.

Hwang, J. H., and Yaksh, T. L. (1997). The effect of spinal GABA receptor agonists on tactile allodynia in a surgically-induced neuropathic pain model in the rat. *Pain* **70**, 15–22.

Hwang, J. H., Hwang, K. S., Kim, J. U., Choi, I. C., Park, P. H., and Han, S. M. (2001). The interaction between intrathecal neostigmine and GABA receptor agonists in rats with nerve ligation injury. *Anesth. Analg.* **93**, 1297–1303.

Ibuki, T., Hama, A. T., Wang, X. T., Pappas, G. D., and Sagen, J. (1997). Loss of GABA-immunoreactivity in the spinal dorsal horn of rats with peripheral nerve injury and promotion of recovery by adrenal medullary grafts. *Neuroscience* **76**, 845–858.

Jasmin, L., Rabkin, S. D., Granato, A., Boudah, A., and O'Hara, P. T. (2003). Analgesia and hyperalgesia from GABA-mediated modulation of the cerebral cortex. *Nature* **424**, 316–320.

Johnston, G. A. (1992). $GABA_A$ agonists as targets for drug development. *Clin. Exp. Pharmacol. Physiol.* **19**, 73–78.

Jones, K. A., Borowsky, B., Tamm, J. A., Craig, D. A., Durkin, M. M., Dai, M., Yao, W. J., Johnson, M., Gunwaldsen, C., Huang, L. Y., Tang, C., Shen, Q., *et al.* (1998). $GABA_B$ receptors function as a heterodimeric assembly of the subunits of $GABA_BR1$ and $GABA_BR2$. *Nature* **396**, 674–679.

Kaneko, M., and Hammond, D. L. (1997). Role of spinal gamma-aminobutyric acid A receptors in formalin-induced nociception in the rat. *J. Pharmacol. Exp. Ther.* **282**, 928–938.

Karceski, S., Morrell, M. J., and Carpenter, D. (2005). Treatment of epilepsy in adults: Expert opinion, 2005. *Epilepsy Behav.* **7**, 1–64.

Kaupmann, K., Malitschek, B., Schuler, V., Heid, J., Froestl, W., Beck, P., Mosbacher, J., Bischoff, S., Kulik, A., Shigemoto, R., Karschin, A., and Bettler, B. (1998). GABA-B receptor subtypes assemble into functional heterodimeric complexes. *Nature* **396**, 683–687.

Kendall, D. A., Browner, M., and Enna, S. J. (1982). Comparison of the antinociceptive effect of gamma-aminobutyric acid (GABA) agonists: Evidence for a cholinergic involvement. *J. Pharmacol. Exp. Ther.* **220**, 482–487.

Kinloch, R. A., and Cox, P. J. (2005). New targets for neuropathic pain therapeutics. *Expert Opin. Ther. Targets* **9**, 685–698.

Kirouac, G. J., Li, S., and Mabrouk, G. (2004). GABAergic projection from the ventral tegmental area and substantia nigra to the periaqueductal gray and the dorsal raphe nucleus. *J. Comp. Neurol.* **469**, 170–184.

Kjaer, M., and Nielsen, H. (1983). The analgesic effect of the GABA-agonist THIP in patients with chronic pain of malignant origin. A phase-1–2 study. *Br. J. Clin. Pharmacol.* **16**, 477–485.

Krasowski, M. D., Rick, C. E., Harrison, N. L., Firestone, L. L., and Homanics, G. E. (1998). A deficit of functional GABA(A) receptors in neurons of beta 3 subunit knockout mice. *Neurosci. Lett.* **240**, 81–84.

Krogsgaard-Larsen, P., Frolund, B., and Frydenvang, K. (2000). GABA uptake inhibitors. Design, molecular pharmacology and therapeutic aspects. *Curr. Pharm. Des.* **6**, 1193–1209.

Krogsgaard-Larsen, P., Frolund, B., Liljefors, T., and Ebert, B. (2004). GABA(A) agonists and partial agonists: THIP (Gaboxadol) as a non-opioid analgesic and novel type of hypnotic. *Biochem. Pharmacol.* **68**, 1573–1580.

Kubo, Y., and Tateyama, M. (2005). Towards a view of functioning dimeric metabotropic receptors. *Curr. Opin. Neurobiol.* **15**, 289–295.

Lanneau, C., Green, A., Hirst, W. D., Wise, A., Brown, J. T., Dennier, E., Charles, K. J., Wood, M., Davies, C. H., and Pangalos, M. N. (2001). Gabapentin is not a $GABA_B$ receptor agonist. *Neuropharmacology* **41**, 965–975.

Laughlin, T. M., Tram, K. V., Wilcox, G. L., and Birnbaum, A. K. (2002). Comparison of antiepileptic drugs tiagabine, lamotrigine, and gabapentin in mouse models of acute, prolonged, and chronic nociception. *J. Pharmacol. Exp. Ther.* **302**, 1168–1175.

Levy, R. A., and Proudfit, H. K. (1977). The analgesic action of baclofen [beta-(4-chlorophenyl)-gamma-aminobutyric acid]. *J. Pharmacol. Exp. Ther.* **202**, 437–445.

Li, D. P., Chen, S. R., Pan, Y. Z., Levey, A. I., and Pan, H. L. (2002). Role of presynaptic muscarinic and GABA(B) receptors in spinal glutamate release and cholinergic analgesia in rats. *J. Physiol.* **543**, 807–818.

Lind, G., Meyerson, B. A., Winter, J., and Linderoth, B. (2004). Intrathecal baclofen as adjuvant therapy to enhance the effect of spinal cord stimulation in neuropathic pain: A pilot study. *Eur. J. Pain* **8**, 377–383.

Loomis, C. W., Khandwala, H., Osmond, G., and Hefferan, M. P. (2001). Coadministration of intrathecal strychnine and bicuculline effects synergistic allodynia in the rat: An isobolographic analysis. *J. Pharmacol. Exp. Ther.* **296**, 756–761.

Loubser, P. G., and Akman, N. M. (1996). Effects of intrathecal baclofen on chronic spinal cord injury pain. *J. Pain Symptom Manage.* **12**, 241–247.

Mahmoudi, M., and Zarrindast, M. R. (2002). Effect of intracerebraoventricular injection of GABA receptor agents on morphine-induced antinociception in the formalin test. *J. Psychopharmacol.* **16**, 85–91.

Malan, T. P., Heriberto, H. P., and Poerreca, F. (2002). Spinal $GABA_A$ and $GABA_B$ receptor pharmacology in a rat model of neuropathic pain. *Anesthesiology* **96**, 1161–1167.

Malcangio, M., and Bowery, N. G. (1994). Spinal cord substance P release and hyperalgesia in monoarthritic rats: Involvement of $GABA_B$ receptor system. *Br. J. Pharmacol.* **113**, 1561–1566.

Malcangio, M., Libri, V., Teoh, H., Constanti, A., and Bowery, N. G. (1995). Chronic (-)-baclofen or CGP36742 alters $GABA_B$ receptor sensitivity in rat brain and spinal cord. *Neuroreport* **6**, 399–403.

Mason, P., Owens, C. A., and Hammond, D. L. (1996). Antagonism of the antinocifensive action of halothane by intrathecal administration of $GABA_A$ receptor antagonists. *Anesthesiology* **84**, 1205–1214.

McCarson, K. E., and Enna, S. J. (1996). Relationship between $GABA_B$ receptor activation and neurokinin receptor expression in spinal cord. *Pharmacol. Res. Commun.* **8**, 191–194.

McCarson, K. E., and Enna, S. J. (1999). Nociceptive regulation of $GABA_B$ receptor gene expression in rat spinal cord. *Neuropharmacology* **38**, 1767–1773.

McCarson, K. E., Ralya, A., Reisman, S. A., and Enna, S. J. (2005). Amitriptyline prevents thermal hyperalgesia and modifications in rat spinal cord $GABA_B$ receptor expression and function in an animal model of neuropathic pain. *Biochem. Pharmacol.* **71**, 196–2002.

McCarson, K. E., Duric, V., Reisman, S. A., Winter, M., and Enna, S. J. (2006). $GABA_B$ receptor function and subunit expression in the rat spinal cord as indicators of stress and the antinociceptive response to antidepressants. *Brain Res.* **1068**, 109–117.

Miletic, G., Draganic, P., Pankratz, M. T., and Miletic, V. (2003). Muscimol prevents long-lasting potentiation of dorsal horn field potentials in rats with chronic constriction injury exhibiting decreased levels of the GABA transporter GAT-1. *Pain* **105**, 347–353.

Möhler, H. (2001). Functions of $GABA_A$-receptor: Pharmacology and pathophysiology. *In* "Pharmacology of GABA and Glycine Neurotransmission" (H. Möhler, Ed.), pp. 101–116. Springer-Verlag, Berlin.

Möhler, H., Benke, J., Benson, B., Luscher, B., Rudolph, U., and Fritschy, J. M. (1997). Diversity in structure, pharmacology, and regulation of $GABA_A$ receptors. *In* "The GABA Receptors" (S. J. Enna and N. G. Bowery, Eds.), pp. 11–36. Humana Press, Totowa, New Jersey.

Möhler, H., Fritschy, J.-M., Crestani, F., Hensch, T., and Rudolph, U. (2004). Specific $GABA_A$ circuits in brain development and therapy. *Biochem. Pharmacol.* **68**, 1685–1690.

Moore, K. A., Kohno, T., Karchewski, L. A., Scholz, J., Baba, H., and Woolf, C. J. (2002). Partial peripheral nerve injury promotes a selective loss of GABAergic inhibition in the superficial dorsal horn of the spinal cord. *J. Neurosci.* **22**, 6724–6731.

Murray, T. F., McGill, W., and Cheney, D. L. (1983). A comparison of the analgesic activities of 4,5,6,7-tetrahydroisoxazolo[5,4-c]pyridine-3-ol (THIP) and 6-chloro-2[1-piperazinyl] pyrazine (MK 212). *Eur. J. Pharmacol.* **90**, 179–184.

Naderi, N., Shafaghi, B., Khodayar, M. J., and Zarindast, M. R. (2005). Interaction between gamma-aminobutyric acid GABAB and cannabinoid CB1 receptors in spinal pain pathways in rat. *Eur. J. Pharmacol.* **514**, 159–164.

Nadeson, R., Guo, Z., Porter, V., Gent, J. P., and Goodchild, C. S. (1996). Gamma-aminobutyric acid A receptors and spinally mediated antinociception in rats. *J. Pharmacol. Exp. Ther.* **278**, 620–626.

Ng, G. Y. K., Bertrand, S., Sullivan, R., Ethier, N., Wang, J., Yergey, J., Belley, M., Trimble, L., Bateman, K., Alder, L., Smith, A., McKernan, R., *et al.* (2001). $\gamma$-Aminobutyric acid type B receptors with specific heterodimer composition and postsynaptic actions in hippocampal neurons are targets of anticonvulsant gabapentin action. *Mol. Pharmacol.* **59**, 144–152.

Nguyen, T. T., Matsumoto, K., and Watanabe, H. (1997). Involvement of supraspinal GABA-ergic systems in clonidine-induced antinociception in the tail-pinch test in mice. *Life Sci.* **61**, 1097–1103.

Novak, V., Kanard, R., Kissel, J. T., and Mendell, J. R. (2001). Treatment of painful sensory neuropathy with tiagabine: A pilot study. *Clin. Auton. Res.* **11**, 357–361.

Ohashi, Y., Guo, T., Orii, R., Maze, M., and Fujinaga, M. (2003). Brain stem opioidergic and GABAergic neurons mediate the antinociceptive effect of nitrous oxide in Fischer rats. *Anesthesiology* **99**, 947–954.

Orii, R., Ohashi, Y., Halder, S., Giombini, M., Maze, M., and Fujinaga, M. (2003). GABAergic interneurons at supraspinal and spinal levels differentially modulate the antinociceptive effect of nitrous oxide in Fischer rats. *Anesthesiology* **98**, 1223–1230.

Ossipov, M. H., Lai, J., Malan, T. P., and Porreca, F. (2000). Spinal and supraspinal mechanisms of neuropathic pain. *Ann. NY Acad. Sci.* **909**, 12–24.

Patel, S., Naeem, S., Kesingland, A., Froestl, W., Capogna, M., Urban, L., and Fox, A. (2001). The effects of $GABA_B$ agonists and gabapentin on mechanical hyperalgesia in models of neuropathic and inflammatory pain in the rat. *Pain* **90**, 217–226.

Pelley, K. A., and Vaught, J. L. (1987). An antinociceptive profile of kojic amine: An analogue of gamma-aminobutyric acid (GABA). *Neuropharmacology* **26**, 301–307.

Pinto, M., Lima, D., Castro-Lopes, J., and Tavares, I. (2003). Noxious-evoked c-fos expression in brainstem neurons immunoreactive for $GABA_B$, $\mu$-opioid, and NK-1 receptors. *Eur. J. Neurosci.* **17**, 1393–1403.

Polgar, E., Hughes, D. I., Riddell, J. S., Maxwell, D. J., Puskar, Z., and Todd, A. J. (2003). Selective loss of spinal GABAergic or glycinergic neurons is not necessary for development of thermal hyperalgesia in the chronic constriction injury model of neuropathic pain. *Pain* **104**, 229–239.

Price, G. W., Wilkin, G. P., Turnbull, M. J., and Bowery, N. G. (1984). Are baclofen sensitive GABA-B receptors present on primary afferent terminals of the spinal cord? *Nature* **307**, 71–74.

Reyes-Vazquez, C., Enna, S. J., and Dafny, N. (1986). The parafasciculus thalami as a site for mediating the antinociceptive response to GABAergic drugs. *Brain Res.* **383**, 177–184.

Riley, R. C., Trafton, J. A., Chi, S. I., and Basbaum, A. I. (2001). Presynaptic regulation of spinal cord tachykinin signaling via $GABA_B$ but not $GABA_A$ receptor activation. *Neuroscience* **103**, 725–737.

Rode, F., Jensen, D. G., Blackburn-Munro, G., and Bjerrum, O. J. (2005). Centrally-mediated antinociceptive actions of $GABA_A$ receptor agonists in the rat spared nerve injury model of neuropathic pain. *Eur. J. Pharmacol.* **516**, 131–138.

Rudolph, U., and Möhler, H. (2004). Analysis of $GABA_A$ receptor function and dissection of the pharmacology of benzodiazepines and general anesthetics through mouse genetics. *Annu. Rev. Pharmacol. Toxicol.* **44**, 475–498.

Sabatowski, R., Galvez, R., Cherry, D. A., Jacquot, F., Vincent, E., Moisonobe, P., Versavel, M., and the 1008–045 Study Group (2004). Pregablin reduces pain and improves sleep and mood disturbances in patients with post-herpetic neuralgia: Results of a randomized, placebo-controlled clinical trial. *Pain* **109**, 26–35.

Sands, S. A., McCarson, K. E., and Enna, S. J. (2003). Differential regulation of $GABA_B$ receptor subunit expression and function. *J. Pharmacol. Exp. Ther.* **305**, 191–196.

Sands, S. A., McCarson, K. E., and Enna, S. J. (2004). Relationship between the antinociceptive response to disipramine and changes in GABAB receptor function and subunit expression in the dorsal horn of the rat spinal cord. *Biochem. Pharmacol.* **67**, 743–749.

Schuler, V., Luscher, C., Blanchet, C., Klix, N., Sansig, G., Klebs, K., Schmutz, M., Heid, J., Gentry, C., Urban, L., Fox, A., Spooren, W., *et al.* (2001). Epilepsy, hyperalgesia, impaired memory, and loss of pre- and postsynaptic $GABA_B$ responses in mice lacking $GABA_{B(1)}$. *Neuron* **31**, 47–58.

Shafizadeh, M., Semnanian, S., Zarrindast, M. R., and Hashemi, B. (1997). Involvement of GABA-B receptors in the antinociception induced by baclofen in the formalin test. *Gen. Pharmacol.* **28**, 611–615.

Shen, H., Gong, Q. H., Yuan, M., and Smith, S. S. (2005). Short-term steroid treatment increases delta GABA(A) receptor subunit expression in rat CA1 hippocampus: Pharmacological and behavioral effects. *Neuropharmacology* **49**, 573–586.

Sindrup, S. H., and Jensen, T. S. (2002). Pharmacology of trigeminal neuralgia. *Clin. J. Pain* **18**, 22–27.

Slonimski, M., Abram, S. E., and Zuniga, R. E. (2004). Intrathecal baclofen in pain management. *Reg. Anesth. Pain Med.* **29**, 269–276.

Smith, G. D., Harrison, S. M., Birch, P. J., Malcangio, M., and Bowery, N. G. (1994). Increased sensitivity to the antinociceptive activity of (+/−) baclofen in an animal model of chronic neuropathic, but not chronic inflammatory, hyperalgesia. *Neuropharmacology* **33**, 1103–1108.

Solaro, C., and Tanganelli, P. (2004). Tiagabine for treating painful tonic spasms in multiple sclerosis: A pilot study. *J. Neurol. Neurosurg. Psychiat.* **75**, 341.

Somers, D. L., and Clemente, F. R. (2002). Dorsal horn synaptosomal content of aspartate, glutamate, glycine and GABA are differentially altered following chronic constriction injury to the rat sciatic nerve. *Neurosci. Lett.* **323**, 171–174.

Soudijn, W., and van Wijngaarden, I. (2000). The GABA transporter and its inhibitors. *Curr. Med. Chem.* **7**, 1063–1079.

Srinivasan, D., Ramaswamy, S., Bapna, J. S., and Srinivasan, B. (1991). Tolerance pattern to GABAmimetic analgesics and their influence on morphine tolerance and dependence. *Fundam. Clin. Pharmacol.* **5**, 769–775.

Thomas, D. A., McGowan, M. K., and Hammond, D. L. (1995). Microinjection of baclofen in the ventromedial medulla of rats: Antinociception at low doses and hyperalgesia at high doses. *J. Pharmacol. Exp. Ther.* **275**, 274–284.

Thomas, D. A., Navarrete, I. M., Graham, B. A., McGowan, M. K., and Hammond, D. L. (1996). Antinociception produced by systemic R(+)-baclofen hydrochloride is attenuated by CGP35348 administered to the spinal cord or ventromedial medulla of rats. *Brain Res.* **718**, 129–137.

Todorov, A. A., Kolchev, C. B., and Todorov, A. B. (2005). Tiagabine and gabapentin for the management of chronic pain. *Clin. J. Pain* **21**, 358–361.

Ugarte, S. D., Homanics, G. E., Firestone, L. L., and Hammond, D. L. (1999). Sensory thresholds and the antinociceptive effects of GABA receptor agonists in mice lacking the $\beta_3$ subunit of the $GABA_A$ receptor. *Neuroscience* **95**, 795–806.

Urwyler, S., Pozza, M. F., Lingenhoehl, K., Mosbacher, J., Lampert, C., Froestl, W., Koller, M., and Kaupmann, K. (2003). N,N′-Dicyclopentyl-2-methylsulfanyl-5-nitro-pyrimidine-4,6-diamine (GS39783) and structurally related compounds: Novel allosteric enhancers of $\gamma$-aminobutyric $acid_B$ receptor function. *J. Pharmacol. Exp. Ther.* **307**, 322–330.

Vacher, C.-M., and Bettler, B. (2003). $GABA_B$ receptors as potential therapeutic targets. *Curr. Drug Target CNS Neurol. Disorders* **2**, 248–259.

Vaught, J. L., Pelley, K., Costa, L. G., Settler, P., and Enna, S. J. (1985). A comparison of the antinociceptive responses to the GABA receptor agonists THIP and baclofen. *Neuropharmacology* **24**, 211–216.

von Heijne, M., Hao, J. X., Sollevi, A., and Xu, X. J. (Heijne 2001). Effects of intrathecal morphine, baclofen, clonidine and R-PIA on the acute allodynia-like behaviours after spinal cord ischaemia in rats. *Eur. J. Pain* **5**, 1–10.

Wang, Q. Y., Cao, J. L., Zeng, Y. M., and Dai, T. J. (2004). $GABA_A$ receptor partially mediated propofol-induced hyperalgesia at superspinal level and analgesia at spinal cord level in rats. *Acta Pharmacol. Sin.* **25**, 1619–1625.

Wang, Y. W., Deng, X. M., You, X. M., Liu, S. X., and Zhao, Z. Q. (2005). Involvement of GABA and opioid peptide receptors in sevoflurane-induced antinociception in rat spinal cord. *Acta Pharmacol. Sin.* **26**, 1045–1048.

Yaksh, T. (1999). A drug has to do what a drug has to do. *Anesth. Analg.* **89**, 1075–1080.

Yang, K., Ma, W. L., Feng, Y. P., Dong, Y. X., and Li, Y. Q. (2002). Origins of GABA(B) receptor-like immunoreactive terminals in the rat spinal dorsal horn. *Brain Res. Bull.* **15**, 499–507.

Yokoro, C. M., Pesquero, S. M., Turchetti-Maia, R. M., Francischi, J. N., and Tatsuo, M. A. (2001). Acute phenobarbital administration induces hyperalgesia: Pharmacological evidence for the involvement of supraspinal GABA-A receptors. *Braz. J. Med. Biol. Res.* **34**, 397–405.

Zambotti, F., Zonta, N., Tammiso, R., Conci, F., Hafner, B., Zecca, L., Ferrario, P., and Montegazza, P. (1991). Effects of diazepam on nociception in rats. *Naunyn Schmiedebergs Arch. Pharmacol.* **344**, 84–89.

Zarrindast, M. R., and Mahmoudi, M. (2001). GABA mechanisms and antinociception in mice with ligated sciatic nerve. *Pharmacol. Toxicol.* **89**, 79–84.

Zarrindast, M.-R., Valizadeh, S., and Sahebgharani, M. (2000). $GABA_B$ receptor mechanism and imipramine-induced antinociception in ligated and non-ligated mice. *Eur. J. Pharmacol.* **407**, 65–72.

Zheng, W., Xie, W., Zhang, J., Strong, J. A., Wang, L., Yu, L., Xu, M., and Lu, L. (2003). Function of $\gamma$-aminobutyric acid receptor/channel $\rho_1$ subunits in spinal cord. *J. Biol. Chem.* **278**, 48321–48329.

Zhu, S. S., Zeng, Y. M., Wang, J. K., Yan, R., Nie, X., and Cao, J. L. (2005). Inhibition of thermal hyperalgesia and tactile allodynia by intrathecal administration of gamma-aminobutyric acid transporter-1 inhibitor NO-711 in rats with chronic constriction injury. *Sheng Li Xue Bao* **57**, 233–239.

Zorn, S. H., and Enna, S. J. (1985a). GABA uptake inhibitors produce a greater antinociceptive response in the mouse tail immersion assay than other types of GABAergic drugs. *Life Sci.* **37**, 1901–1912.

Zorn, S. H., and Enna, S. J. (1985b). The effect of mouse spinal cord transaction on the antinociceptive response to gamma-aminobutyric acid agonists THIP (4,5,6,-tetrahydroisoxazolo[5,4-c]pyridine-3-ol) and baclofen. *Brain Res.* **338**, 380–383.

Zorn, S. H., and Enna, S. J. (1986). GABA uptake inhibitors produce a greater antinociceptive response in the mouse tail-immersion assay than other types of GABAergic drugs. *Life Sci.* 37, 1901–1912.

Zorn, S. H., and Enna, S. J. (1987). The GABA agonist THIP, attenuates antinociception in the mouse by modifying central cholinergic transmission. *Neuropharmacology* **26**, 433–437.

**Fani L. Neto*, Joana Ferreira-Gomes*, and José M. Castro-Lopes**
Institute of Histology and Embryology
Faculty of Medicine of Porto and IBMC
4200-319 Porto, Portugal

# Distribution of GABA Receptors in the Thalamus and Their Involvement in Nociception

## I. Chapter Overview

GABA receptors are ubiquitously expressed in the central nervous system (CNS), including the thalamus. This region is an important target for sensory information, acting as a relay to several cortical areas. Moreover, nociceptive input is believed to be modulated in the thalamus by intrinsic inhibitory mechanisms. Since GABA mediates most inhibitory actions in the thalamus, the distribution of the three currently known receptor subtypes, $GABA_A$, $GABA_B$, and $GABA_C$, in particular nuclei of the thalamus, may give some clues on its involvement in the processing of nociceptive information. The present review aims at giving an overall picture of the distribution of GABA receptors subunits in the thalamus, both during development and

* F. L. Neto and J. Ferreira-Gomes contributed equally to this work.

*Advances in Pharmacology, Volume 54*

1054-3589/06 $35.00
DOI: 10.1016/S1054-3589(06)54002-5

adulthood, and also focuses on the reports that implicate thalamic GABA receptors in the modulation of nociceptive input.

## II. Introduction

In the mammalian, $\gamma$-aminobutyric acid (GABA) is present in more than 30% of the CNS neurons, being involved in regulating a widespread number of functions (Bloom and Iversen, 1971; Hendry *et al.*, 1987; Iversen and Bloom, 1972; Roberts, 1986). GABA transmission results in hyperpolarizing responses, which are mediated through three pharmacologically different receptor types. The first receptor discovered, named $GABA_A$, is formed by a pentamer of molecularly different subunits, which assemble to form an ion pore that conducts chloride ions across the cell membrane (Sieghart *et al.*, 1999; Steiger and Russek, 2004; Wafford, 2005). $GABA_A$ receptors have at least 19 different receptor subunits, which have been grouped according to their sequence similarity into 8 distinct families: $\alpha(1–6)$, $\beta(1–3)$, $\gamma(1–3)$, $\delta$, $\epsilon$, $\pi$, $\theta$, and $\rho(1–3)$ (Bonnert *et al.*, 1999; Rabow *et al.*, 1995; Steiger and Russek, 2004; Wilke *et al.*, 1997). However, the majority of $GABA_A$ receptor subtypes are believed to be formed by two $\alpha$, two $\beta$, and one $\gamma$ subunit (Steiger and Russek, 2004), whereas the $\rho(1–3)$ subunits are now believed to be the components of a third type of receptors termed $GABA_C$ (Bormann, 2000; Enz and Cutting, 1998) (see later). The subunit composition of $GABA_A$ receptors seems to differ across specific neuronal cell types and brain regions, deeply affecting the receptor pharmacology, sensitivity and function in different brain circuits (Steiger and Russek, 2004). In addition to GABA binding sites, the $GABA_A$ receptor complex contains binding sites for compounds that allosterically modify the activity of GABA such as benzodiazepines, $\beta$-carbolines, and barbiturates (Gardner *et al.*, 1993; Medina *et al.*, 1998; Sieghart, 1995).

A number of experiments have shown that GABA itself and a GABA analog termed baclofen were able to presynaptically inhibit neurotransmitter release and that classic antagonists, like picrotoxin and bicuculline, which are effective in blocking the $GABA_A$ ionotropic receptor, had no effect on this action (Bowery *et al.*, 1981, 2002; Hill and Bowery, 1981). This was the basis for the discovery of the second type of GABA receptors, named $GABA_B$. These are currently known to belong to the metabotropic G-protein–coupled receptors (GPCRs) family and consist of a heterodimer composed of 2 seven transmembrane proteins (Calver *et al.*, 2003; Kaupmann *et al.*, 1997). Only two subunits, $GABA_{B1}$ and $GABA_{B2}$, and two isoforms, $GABA_{B(1a)}$ and $GABA_{B(1b)}$, have been characterized so far, which are able to assemble into a functional receptor *in vivo* in the proportion $GABA_{B(1a/1b)}$: $GABA_{B2}$ (Kaupmann *et al.*, 1997, 1998a; Kuner *et al.*, 1999; Marshall *et al.*, 1999; White *et al.*, 1998). Other isoforms have been reported (Bowery *et al.*, 2002), but there is not any strong evidence that they can act as subunits of physiological receptors, except for a rat variant called $GABA_{B(1c)}$ that has been reported to yield functionality *in vitro* (Pfaff *et al.*, 1999). $GABA_B$ receptors induce slow and prolonged effects through the activation of downstream signaling cascades leading to inhibition of adenylyl cyclase, which causes inhibition of presynaptic calcium channels and activation of postsynaptic potassium channels (Gage, 1992; Kaupmann *et al.*, 1998b; Misgeld *et al.*, 1995; Wu and Saggau, 1997).

A third type of GABA receptor was discovered and referred to as $GABA_C$, which, as the $GABA_A$ receptor type, is insensitive to baclofen and consists of a pentameric transmembrane protein made up of different assemblies of monomers to form an ion pore (Bormann, 2000; Chebib, 2004; Enz, 2001) and is coupled to chloride channels generating a fast inhibitory response (Olsen and DeLorey, 1999). Several lines of evidence suggest that $GABA_C$ receptors are composed of three different $\rho(1–3)$ subunits in human, rat, and chicken (Albrecht and Darlison, 1995; Bormann, 2000; Cutting *et al.*, 1991, 1992; Enz and Cutting, 1998; Ogurusu and Shingai, 1996; Ogurusu *et al.*, 1995; Wegelius *et al.*, 1996; Zhang *et al.*, 1995) that share only 30–38% sequence homology with the $GABA_A$ receptor subunits and can assemble as homooligomers (Bormann, 2000). However, $GABA_C$ receptors are distinct from the $GABA_A$ receptors subtype in that, although being also blocked by picrotoxin, they are insensitive to bicuculline (Chebib, 2004; Chebib and Johnston, 2000).

GABA receptors' widespread distribution and broad effects made them important targets in the study of a wide number of disorders such as schizophrenia, epilepsy, asthma, depression, anxiety, drug addition, insomnia, and pain (Calver *et al.*, 2002; Coyle, 2004; Frolund *et al.*, 2002; Jasmin *et al.*, 2004; Lloyd *et al.*, 1987; Sanacora *et al.*, 2004; Wong *et al.*, 2003). In the thalamus, the majority of the studies implicate GABA receptors in epilepsy (Futatsugi and Riviello, 1998; Huguenard, 1999), but their involvement in processing of nociceptive input has also been reported by some authors (Ferreira-Gomes *et al.*, 2004; Ipponi *et al.*, 1999; Jia *et al.*, 2004; Oliveras and Montagne-Clavel, 1994; Rausell *et al.*, 1992; Reyes-Vazquez *et al.*, 1986). Inhibitory interaction in the thalamus seems to be mediated almost entirely by GABA, which is present in a number of synapses occurring at both proximal and distal dendritic sites (Duggan and McLennan, 1971; Ralston and Ralston, 1994; Roberts *et al.*, 1992; Rustioni *et al.*, 1983; Wang *et al.*, 2005). Moreover, although in rat most somatosensory and medial thalamic nuclei are devoid of intrinsic interneurons (Harris and Hendrickson, 1987; Oertel *et al.*, 1983; Ottersen and Storm-Mathisen, 1984; Saporta and Kruger, 1977), GABAergic terminals are found in these regions, as well as GABAergic neurons in the reticular nucleus of the thalamus (Rt) (Oertel *et al.*, 1983; Ottersen and Storm-Mathisen, 1984; Price, 1995; Wang *et al.*, 2005).

## III. GABA Receptors in the Thalamus

### A. Distribution in the Adult

#### 1. Binding Studies for $GABA_A$ and/or $GABA_B$

During 1980s and early 1990s, research on the distribution of GABA receptors employed essentially autoradiographic localization of receptor binding sites. The majority of these studies encompasses a large array of brain regions but do not give any particular detail as to specific thalamic nuclei. A large variety of different ligands were used, such as muscimol, bicuculline, flunitrazepam, $\gamma$-hydroxibutyrate, and baclofen, and most of these studies indicate the existence of $GABA_A$ and/or $GABA_B$ binding sites within the thalamus (Bowery *et al.*, 1987; Chu *et al.*, 1990; Heaulme *et al.*, 1987; Hechler *et al.*, 1992; Kultas-Ilinsky *et al.*, 1988; Montpied *et al.*, 1988; Olsen *et al.*, 1990; Palacios *et al.*, 1981; Shinotoh *et al.*, 1986; Vogt *et al.*, 1992). In rat, the levels of $GABA_A$ and $GABA_B$ receptor binding density are high but vary greatly between thalamic nuclei (Bowery *et al.*, 1987). Thus, moderate to high levels of $GABA_A$ and $GABA_B$ binding sites were found in the laterodorsal (LD), ventrolateral (VL), and ventromedial (VM) thalamic nuclei, as well as in the lateral geniculate body (LG), in contrast to the rhomboid thalamic nucleus (Rh) where less $GABA_B$ binding sites were observed (Bowery *et al.*, 1987). In the ventroposterior thalamic nuclei (VP), high densities of both receptor subtypes were detected, but fewer $GABA_A$ sites were detected in the medial portion (VPM) comparatively to $GABA_B$ while in the lateral part (VPL) the opposite occurred. Similarly, the lateroposterior thalamic nucleus (LP) showed a higher density of $GABA_B$ sites. In contrast, no significant binding levels of the two receptors were observed in the paraventricular (PV), reuniens (Re), and gelatinosus (or submedius [Sm]) thalamic nuclei (Bowery *et al.*, 1987). However, depending on the radioligand used, some mismatches across different studies were found in what concerns the binding sites of $GABA_B$ receptors, suggesting the existence of pharmacologically different $GABA_B$ receptor subtypes. Thus, binding studies using [3H]CGP54626 have shown very high to high density of $GABA_B$ receptors throughout most of the dorsal and medial thalamic nuclei, such as in the LD, intermediodorsal thalamic nucleus (IMD), dorsolateral and medial geniculate nuclei (dLGN and MGN, respectively), as well as in the posterior paraventricular thalamic nucleus (PVP) and in the Re. In contrast, the ventrolateral geniculate nuclei (vLGN) and the Rt exhibited low or very low levels of radioligand binding sites, respectively (Bischoff *et al.*, 1999).

In rhesus monkey, the normal distribution of the two $GABA_A$ receptor binding sites was studied by binding to [(3)H]muscimol ([(3)H]MUS) and to [(3)H]flunitrazepam ([(3)H]FLU) followed by quantitative autoradiography on cryostat sections of fresh frozen thalamic tissue, especially in motor-related nuclei (Ambardekar *et al.*, 2003). This study estimated that the concentration of benzodiazepine receptors (low-affinity $GABA_A$ binding sites) is substantial in some thalamic nuclei of the monkey. Thus, the mediodorsal nucleus (MD) had the highest density of [(3)H]FLU binding sites, followed by the anteroventral (AV) and the VL nuclei. In what respects to [(3)H] MUS binding, the AV, MD, and VL displayed high density (Ambardekar *et al.*, 2003), in agreement with a similar distribution found in rat and cat thalamus (Kultas-Ilinsky *et al.*, 1988; Palacios *et al.*, 1981). Also, in rabbit, muscimol binding to $GABA_A$ receptors was high in the AV, while it was moderate in the anterior dorsal and lateral nuclei (Vogt *et al.*, 1992). In what concerns $GABA_B$ binding sites, in the monkey, highest levels were found in the medial geniculate nuclear complex (MG) followed closely by the lateroposterior pulvinar complex (LP-Pul), MD, as well as the anteromedial–anteroventral nuclei (AM–AV) (Bowery *et al.*, 1999). In the ventral nuclei, the VPM showed the highest binding density, whereas in the intralaminar nuclei, the centromedial thalamic nucleus (CM) displayed significantly less binding sites with a significant difference of density between its medial and lateral parts (Bowery *et al.*, 1999). Additionally, low binding was observed in the Rt (Bowery *et al.*, 1999), as it had also been described in the monkey thalamus, in another binding study that used a $GABA_B$ receptor antagonist (Ambardekar *et al.*, 1999). Furthermore, this study is also in agreement with the previous (Bowery *et al.*, 1999), in what concerns the receptor binding density observed in most thalamic nuclei. Therefore, higher $GABA_B$ receptor binding was found in the AV, MD, Pulvinar (Pul), VPM, MG, and in the ventral anterior (VA) nuclei (Ambardekar *et al.*, 1999).

#### 2. *Immunohistochemistry and* In Situ *Hybridization Studies*

*a. $GABA_A$* In the rat thalamus, immunohistochemistry studies found intense immunoreactivity for the $GABA_A$ receptor/benzodiazepine receptor/chloride channel complex in the dorsal thalamic nuclei, such as the AV and the ventral nuclear complex, whereas labeling in the Rt was weaker (Bentivoglio *et al.*, 1991). The distribution of 13 different proteins of $GABA_A$ receptor subunits ($\alpha$1–6, $\beta$1–3, $\gamma$1–3, and $\delta$) was also studied by immunocytochemistry in the adult rat brain (Pirker *et al.*, 2000). In that study, labeling for subunits $\alpha1$, $\beta1$, $\beta2$, $\beta3$, and $\gamma2$ was found throughout the brain. In the thalamus, nuclei showed mostly high immunoreactivity for $\alpha1$, $\alpha4$, and $\beta2$ subunits with dense processes and/or diffuse staining, whereas labeling for the $\delta$ subunit was slightly weaker (Pirker *et al.*, 2000). In fact, expression of this subunit seems to be restricted to a few brain regions, including the thalamus (Benke *et al.*, 1991). Abundance of $\alpha4$ immunoreactivity (Khan *et al.*, 1996) as well as $\alpha3$ and $\alpha4$ mRNA labeling (Araki and Tohyama, 1992) was observed in the thalamus by other authors. In contrast, less immunoreactivity to $\alpha2$, $\alpha3$, $\alpha5$, $\alpha6$, $\gamma1$, $\gamma2$, and $\gamma3$ was observed in comparison to other brain areas (Pirker *et al.*, 2000). The Rt exhibited a different profile of immunoreactivity, with diffuse and/or processes staining for subunits $\alpha3$, $\beta1$, $\beta3$, and $\gamma2$, and cell bodies labeling for $\alpha1$ unit. Moreover, differences in the subunit content were found between individual thalamic nuclei, in addition to a differential expression of $GABA_A$ subunits in the dorsal and ventral portions of the LGN (Pirker *et al.*, 2000). Similarly, Miralles *et al.* (1999) have found high $\beta2$ diffuse labeling of the neuropil but little or no expression of $\beta3$ in all thalamic nuclei except the Rt. In this nucleus, however, a previous study has not found any immunolabeling for the $\beta3$ subunit (Spreafico *et al.*, 1993).

In the monkey, a detailed *in situ* hybridization study showed that in most dorsal thalamic nuclei, the mRNA for the $\alpha1$, $\beta2$, and $\gamma2$ subunits were the most expressed, followed by the $\alpha5$ transcript, and then by the $\alpha2$, $\alpha3$, $\alpha4$, $\beta1$, $\beta3$, and $\gamma1$ subunits mRNA (Huntsman *et al.*, 1996). Abundant mRNA expression for the $\alpha1$, $\alpha3$, $\alpha5$, $\beta2$, and $\gamma2$ subunits was found in the anterior nuclear complex (AM, AV, and anterodorsal, AD nuclei) of the thalamus, whereas in the ventral group of nuclei (VA, VL, VM, VPL, VPM, and ventroposteroinferior, VPI nuclei) and in the MD, moderate levels of expression were evident for the same subunits, with the exception of $\alpha3$ in the ventral group of nuclei, where its expression was low (Huntsman *et al.*, 1996). Additionally, high levels of most subunit transcripts, especially $\alpha1$, $\alpha5$, $\beta2$, and $\gamma2$, were observed in the lateral group of nuclei (LD, LP, and dLGN), with the highest levels of hybridization for every subunit transcript observed in the dLGN (Huntsman *et al.*, 1996). The Pul nuclei showed a heterogeneous distribution of receptor subunit transcripts, $\alpha1$ being the dominant subunit (Huntsman *et al.*, 1996), while the intralaminar nuclei and the MG showed moderate-to-high levels of almost all of the receptor subunit transcripts examined. Levels of $\alpha2$, $\alpha3$, $\beta1$, $\beta3$, and $\gamma1$ expression were surprisingly moderate in intralaminar nuclei as compared to the remaining thalamic nuclei, where low levels of these subunits were observed (Huntsman *et al.*, 1996). In contrast, the posterior group of nuclei showed overall low levels of expression of all receptor subunit transcripts, and in the Rt no expression of any of the subunit transcripts was detected, except for $\gamma2$ that was expressed at modest levels (Huntsman *et al.*, 1996).

In other animal species, such as chicken, immunoreactivity for $\alpha1$ and $\gamma2$ $GABA_A$ receptor subunits was observed in nuclei of the dorsal thalamus, the later being less abundant. Moreover, $\alpha1$ was present in diffusely stained neuropil in which no cell somata could be recognized individually, while $\gamma2$ was observed in cell somata (Aller *et al.*, 2003). In agreement, *in situ* hybridization histochemistry revealed that also the mRNAs for these two $GABA_A$ subunits are present in the dorsal thalamus of the chicken brain (Glencorse *et al.*, 1991). In fact, $GABA_A$ receptors seem to be most dense in the dorsal thalamus, with considerably lesser amounts in the ventral thalamus, across a wide range of vertebrate species, mammals and nonmammals, as evaluated by receptor binding studies (Glendenning, 2003; Veenman *et al.*, 1994) or by immunoreactivity to subunits $\beta 2$ and $\beta 3$ (Anzelius *et al.*, 1995).

*b. GABA$_B$* The distribution of GABA$_B$ receptor subunits was evaluated by immunohistochemistry in different brain areas. Labeling for the GABA$_B$ receptor revealed evident neuropil staining in different thalamic regions, such as the ventrobasal complex (VB, which is composed of the VPL and the VPM) and midline nuclei, but labeling of cell bodies was also observed in this region (Princivalle *et al.*, 2000). Immunoreactivity could also be found in cell bodies and neuropil of the Rt and in the dLGN. In contrast, the vLGN along with the MD nuclei showed low signal both in neuropil and somata (Princivalle *et al.*, 2000). In what concerns GABA$_B$ subunits, GABA$_{B1}$ and GABA$_{B2}$, immunoreactivity was evident throughout thalamic regions both in human and rat brain tissues. Thus, in the human thalamus GABA$_{B1}$ labeling was particularly intense in the Rt and ventral nuclei cell bodies, but the neuropil of the Rt and the MD nuclei was also darkly stained (Billinton *et al.*, 2000). In contrast, GABA$_{B2}$ staining prevailed in the neuropil and showed a much weaker cellular localization, with faintly labeled neurons visible in the Rt and ventral nuclei (Billinton *et al.*, 2000). Moreover, Calver *et al.* (2000) found that, in contrast to other human brain regions, the expression of GABA$_{B(1b)}$ mRNA in the thalamus was several times higher relatively to that of GABA$_{B(1a)}$. In fact, this overexpression of GABA$_{B(1b)}$ over GABA$_{B(1a)}$ was also observed in the thalamus of rat (Bischoff *et al.*, 1999; Fritschy *et al.*, 1999). In this species, GABA$_{B(1a)}$, GABA$_{B(1b)}$, and GABA$_{B2}$ immunoreactivity was high in cell bodies and the neuropil throughout the thalamus, with the GABA$_{B(1b)}$ distribution being homogenously dense in all nuclei, and GABA$_{B(1a)}$ and GABA$_{B2}$ being most dense in the ventral and medial thalamic nuclei as well as in the Rt (Charles *et al.*, 2001). However, there are contradictory reports in what respects GABA$_{B1}$ immunoreactivity in the Rt of rat, since Margeta-Mitrovic *et al.* (1999) observed relatively low staining of cell bodies and almost no staining of the neuropil. In the same study, glutamic acid decarboxylase (GAD) positive neurons were found in this nucleus, whereas immunofluorescent double labeling for GABA$_{B1}$ and GAD only revealed very few cells coexpressing both markers, therefore suggesting that the GABA$_{B1}$ subunit does not function as an autoreceptor in the Rt (Margeta-Mitrovic *et al.*, 1999). In the remaining thalamus, very intense staining of the neuropil as well as clear labeling of cell bodies was detected in the AM, LP, AD, VM, and LD nuclei (Margeta-Mitrovic *et al.*, 1999). Moreover, moderate to high immunoreactivity levels were also found in the centrolateral (CL), CM, VPL, VPM, and posterior (Po) nuclei of the thalamus (Margeta-Mitrovic *et al.*, 1999). In another study, Princivalle *et al.* (2001) have found that GABA$_{B(1a)}$ and GABA$_{B(1b)}$ were present in many thalamic nuclei including the LD, CL, MD, and Rt nuclei. However, the cellular structures labeled were different for the two subunits, especially in the VB and Rt. Immunoreactivity for $GABA_{B(1a)}$ was observed mainly in the cell bodies but also in dendrites in the Rt and within the neuropil in the VB, whereas the signal for $GABA_{B(1b)}$ was evident exclusively in the neuropil in the Rt and in processes and some scattered cells in the VB (Princivalle *et al.*, 2001). The $GABA_{B2}$ expression was associated to both neuropil and cell bodies in every thalamic nuclei, although it was more intense in the neuropil in the Rt, while in the VB it was more marked in the cell bodies (Princivalle *et al.*, 2001). Based on these findings, the same authors suggest that in the thalamocortical circuit the $GABA_{B(1b)}$ and $GABA_{B(1a)}$ are part of the pre- and postsynaptic receptor, respectively (Princivalle *et al.*, 2001). However, pre- and postembedding immunohistochemistry studies, combined with electron microscopy and three-dimensional reconstruction of labeled profiles, revealed that immunolabeling for $GABA_{B(1a)/(1b)}$ and $GABA_{B2}$ in the VB was very intense in the neuropil over the dendritic field of thalamocortical cells and was entirely localized extrasynaptically in postsynaptic elements, whereas no immunoreactivity was detectable in presynaptic elements or glial cells (Kulik *et al.*, 2002). The same study has shown an extensive colocalization (more than 95%) of $GABA_{B(1a)/(1b)}$ and $GABA_{B2}$ immunolabeling on thalamocortical cells dendrites of the VB (Kulik *et al.*, 2002).

As observed by immunohistochemistry, *in situ* hybridization studies also suggest that the $GABA_{B(1b)}$ subunit exhibits higher levels of expression than $GABA_{B(1a)}$ in the thalamus of rat (Bischoff *et al.*, 1999). In fact, with the exception of the MGN and vLGN nuclei, which had abundant $GABA_{B(1a)}$ transcript expression, in most of the dorsal and medial thalamic nuclei the $GABA_{B(1a)}$ transcript levels were generally low to moderate, whereas the $GABA_{B(1b)}$ subunit showed high to very high mRNA expression levels (Bischoff *et al.*, 1999). However, in the PVP, Re, Rt, and the ventral part of the LG, the expression level of the $GABA_{B(1b)}$ transcript was lower than that for $GABA_{B(1a)}$ (Bischoff *et al.*, 1999). A similar proportion was observed in two separate *in situ* hybridization studies performed in some somatosensitive nuclei of the rat thalamus. A moderate expression of the $GABA_{B(1b)}$ and $GABA_{B2}$ subunits mRNA was found in particular nuclei, such as the VB, Po, and CM/CL, whereas no expression was found in the Rt (Ferreira-Gomes *et al.*, 2004, 2005). In contrast, no significant mRNA expression of the $GABA_{B(1a)}$ was detected in any of these regions (Ferreira-Gomes *et al.*, 2005). Equally, Liang and coworkers (2000) have not found any significant hybridization signal for $GABA_{B(1b)}$ within the Rt, as well as in the vLGN. However, the mRNA levels were medium to high for both $GABA_{B(1a)}$ and $GABA_{B(1b)}$ subunits in the majority of the dorsal thalamus, while they were low to medium within the Rt in the case of the $GABA_{B(1a)}$ transcript. Moreover, the levels of expression for the $GABA_{B(1a)}$ and $GABA_{B(1b)}$ mRNAs were higher in neurons of AD, MD, LD, MGN, and dLGN nuclei, whereas cells in intralaminar nuclei displayed weaker hybridization signals

(Liang *et al.*, 2000). Additionally, the VPM and VPL exhibited moderate signal intensities for the $GABA_{B(1a)}$ and $GABA_{B(1b)}$ mRNAs (Liang *et al.*, 2000). In another *in situ* hybridization study, $GABA_{B1}$ and $GABA_{B2}$ mRNAs were moderately expressed in the VPM and VPL, while the Po showed a weak signal for both transcripts (Li *et al.*, 2003). In addition, the lateral and medial geniculate bodies had higher levels of both mRNAs, particularly $GABA_{B2}$ (Li *et al.*, 2003). $GABA_{B2}$ mRNA signal was also observed in relatively high amounts over the cell bodies in the AD and MD nuclei, the LD as well as the VA, VL, and VP nuclei (Durkin *et al.*, 1999). Heavy labeling of the $GABA_{B2}$ mRNA was equally detected in the Re and Rh nuclei, and slightly less in the PV, CM, and paracentral (PC) nuclei. As in other *in situ* hybridization studies, low levels of $GABA_{B2}$ mRNA were detected in the Rt (Durkin *et al.*, 1999). In what respects the variant $GABA_{B(1c)}$, Pfaff *et al.* (1999) reported a wide distribution of its transcripts in the CNS of rat that overlapped that of the $GABA_{B(1a)}$ and $GABA_{B(1b)}$, showing high mRNA levels in the thalamus.

In rhesus monkey, *in situ* hybridization with cRNA probes revealed that the density of the $GABA_B$ transcript is much higher in the dorsal thalamus than in the ventral thalamus or the Rt (Münoz *et al.*, 1998), in similarity to the $GABA_A$ receptor. In the dorsal thalamus, the highest $GABA_B$ mRNA levels were found both in relay cells and interneurons of the AV and parafascicular nucleus (Pf). The ventral group of nuclei showed moderate $GABA_B$ expression, the VA showing the highest, and the VL and VP nuclei the lowest $GABA_B$ expression levels in the dorsal thalamus. Within these nuclei, the VPM displayed higher levels of expression than the VPL and the VPI nuclei. Additionally, moderately dense levels of hybridization were also observed in the MD, Pul, and CM nuclei, as well as in the medial and lateral geniculate nuclei (Münoz *et al.*, 1998). This distribution of the $GABA_B$ transcript in the rhesus monkey thalamus was corroborated by different binding studies (Ambardekar *et al.*, 1999; Bowery *et al.*, 1999) (Section III.A.1).

*c. $GABA_C$* Contrary to the ubiquitous distribution of $GABA_A$ and $GABA_B$ receptors, $GABA_C$ receptors are only found in the retina and in a restricted number of structures mainly related with the visual system, as well as in the hippocampus, spinal cord, and cerebellum (Alakuijala *et al.*, 2005; Boué-Grabot *et al.*, 1998; Enz *et al.*, 1995, 1996; Fletcher *et al.*, 1998; Lukasiewicz, 1996; Rozzo *et al.*, 2002; Schlicker *et al.*, 2004; Wegelius *et al.*, 1998; Zhang *et al.*, 1995). In fact, within the thalamus *in situ* hybridization studies revealed expression of the $\rho 2$ subunit only in the LGN (Alakuijala *et al.*, 2005; Wegelius *et al.*, 1998), known to be involved in the perception of visual stimuli, while $\rho 1$ mRNA was not found in any brain regions studied (Wegelius *et al.*, 1998). However, by using the reverse transcriptase–polymerase chain reaction the same authors found some expression of $\rho 1$ in the thalamus (Wegelius *et al.*, 1998).

## B. Distribution during Development in the Thalamus

Expression of receptor subunits varies during differentiation, in registry with the formation of neuronal circuits that serve specific functions, which may differ from those of the adult brain. In spite of this, research on the expression of GABA receptors in the developing brain has not attracted a great deal of attention.

### 1. $GABA_A$

Bentivoglio *et al.* (1991) observed that during the first postnatal weeks there was a progressive reduction of $GABA_A$ receptor complex immunoreactivity in the Rt and a parallel increase in the dorsal thalamus. In agreement, Xia and Haddad (1992), using quantitative receptor binding autoradiography to examine postnatal expression of $GABA_A$ receptors in different brain areas at five postnatal ages of the rat (postnatal day 1, 5, 10, 21, and 120), reported that $GABA_A$ receptor densities increased with age in some brain regions, including the thalamus, especially between postnatal days 10 and 21. An *in situ* hybridization detailed study found abundant expression of $\alpha 2$, $\alpha 3$, $\alpha 5$, and $\beta 3$ mRNA in both embryonic and early postnatal thalamus (Laurie *et al.*, 1992). This expression was decreased in the adult thalamocortical cells and was replaced by the $\alpha 1$, $\alpha 4$, $\beta 2$, and $\delta$ subunit mRNAs, suggesting that the composition and associated properties of $GABA_A$ receptors in the embryonic/early postnatal rat brain differ remarkably from those of the adult (Laurie *et al.*, 1992). In another *in situ* hybridization study, however, expression of $\beta 2$, $\beta 3$, and $\gamma 2$ subunits mRNAs was equally detected in the thalamus of the embryonic rat brain (Poulter *et al.*, 1993). The differential expression of some $GABA_A$ receptor subunits, particularly $\alpha 1$ and $\alpha 2$, seems to have a similar developmental profile in rodents and primates, suggesting that the regulation of receptor subtypes might be conserved across species (Hornung and Fritschy, 1996; Laurie *et al.*, 1992; Paysan and Fritschy, 1998). In fact, immunohistochemistry studies performed in the marmoset monkey between embryonic day 100 (6 weeks before birth) and adulthood revealed that the $\alpha 2$ subunit was detected in the fetal thalamus and until the first postnatal weeks, in contrast to what happened in other brain regions (Hornung and Fritschy, 1996). The levels of this subunit were transient, gradually decreasing shortly after birth in the sensory relay nuclei, up to postnatal day 60 in the medial thalamus and up to 1 year after birth in the intralaminar nuclei. On the contrary, staining for $\alpha 1$ subunit in the thalamus during embryonic life was detected only after embryonic day 130 in the VP nuclei and LGN (Hornung and Fritschy, 1996). However, the levels increased throughout the thalamus during the first postnatal weeks, before the $\alpha 2$ subunit disappeared, indicating a change in the subunit composition of $GABA_A$ receptors during development. In the same study, the $\beta 2/3$ subunits staining was observed at every age examined, suggesting their association with either the $\alpha 1$ or the $\alpha 2$ subunits (Hornung and Fritschy, 1996).

Overall, data suggest that anatomical and cellular expression of $GABA_A$ subunits during development is a complex and dynamic process leading to a distribution pattern that differs from that observed in the adult brain.

### 2. *GABA*$_B$

Densitometric analysis of Western blots revealed a distinct expression pattern of $GABA_{B(1a)}$ and $GABA_{B(1b)}$ isoforms in the brain during postnatal development (Fritschy *et al.*, 1999). In that study, $GABA_{B(1a)}$ staining was five times higher than that of $GABA_{B(1b)}$ at postnatal day (P) 0 and remained the highest within the first postnatal days (P0–P5), then decreasing abruptly within 2 weeks, to almost adult levels. On the contrary, the signal for $GABA_{B(1b)}$ increased after P5, reaching a maximum around P10, a time point when both $GABA_{B(1a)}$ and $GABA_{B(1b)}$ subunits were expressed at equal levels and exceeded adult values (Fritschy *et al.*, 1999). After P10, $GABA_{B(1b)}$ gradually decreased in juvenile rats, reaching in the adult cerebral cortex, thalamus and cerebellum, twice the levels of $GABA_{B(1a)}$ isoform (Fritschy *et al.*, 1999).

In the thalamus, immunoreactivity for $GABA_B$ receptors was higher than in the adulthood during the first postnatal days and until the second postnatal week, especially in the neuropil of the Rt and medial nuclei (Princivalle *et al.*, 2000). Additionally, during the first postnatal days immunoreactivity in the rat VB was predominant in cell bodies, whereas after the second postnatal week the immunolabeling increased in the neuropil, hiding the stained cells (Princivalle *et al.*, 2000). On the contrary, the signal in the MD was higher in the neuropil during the first postnatal days, decreasing from P7 to adulthood in the neuropil and increasing in cell bodies. The remaining midline and intralaminar nuclei showed a very high immunolabeling in the neuropil whereas in the LGN the signal was higher in cell bodies (Princivalle *et al.*, 2000). From P22, the differences in $GABA_B$ receptor expression between young and adult rats decreased gradually (Princivalle *et al.*, 2000).

*In situ* hybridization studies observed $GABA_{B1}$ receptor mRNA in the thalamus of fetal rats at gestational day (GD) 11.5 and 12.5 (Kim *et al.*, 2003b). At those time points, RNAse protection assays corroborated that $GABA_{B1}$ receptor mRNA was abundant in the thalamus as well as in most of the brain, while at GD 10.5 the signal was lower. In contrast, $GABA_{B2}$ receptor mRNA was not detected on GD 10.5, 11.5, and 12.5, neither by *in situ* hybridization nor by RNAse protection assays (Kim *et al.*, 2003b). These observations were confirmed in a similar study, and additionally,

$GABA_{B1}$ and $GABA_{B2}$ mRNA levels were analyzed at other gestational days (Li *et al.*, 2004). Thus, on GD 13.5 and 15.5 $GABA_{B1}$ subunit mRNA showed higher expression than on GD 11.5 and 12.5 in all brain regions, and on GD 17.5 distinct hybridization signals were found in some brain regions including the thalamus. On GD 19.5 and 21.5, the labeling for $GABA_{B1}$ mRNA increased in the thalamus to levels similar to the adult brain both by *in situ* hybridization and by RNAse protection assays (Li *et al.*, 2004). Regarding $GABA_{B2}$ subunit mRNA, it was first weakly detected on GD 13.5 in discrete brain regions, including the thalamus, then increasing from GD 17.5 to GD 21.5 and reaching adult levels (Li *et al.*, 2004). Therefore, at this stage $GABA_{B1}$ and $GABA_{B2}$ subunit had a similar expression pattern, with a higher expression level of $GABA_{B1}$ (Li *et al.*, 2004).

In summary, $GABA_{B1}$ and $GABA_{B2}$ subunit mRNAs have different expression patterns, during brain maturation, with the $GABA_{B1}$ subunit expressed earlier and in higher amounts, possibly indicating that this subunit might have a more important role than $GABA_{B2}$ in the early development of rat CNS (Kim *et al.*, 2003b). Furthermore, an opposite regulation in the expression of the $GABA_{B(1a)}$ and $GABA_{B(1b)}$ seems to occur, leading to a prevalence of $GABA_{B(1a)}$ at birth and of $GABA_{B(1b)}$ in the adult (Fritschy *et al.*, 1999), suggesting that the two isoforms might serve distinct roles during development and adulthood (Möhler *et al.*, 2001).

### 3. $GABA_C$

Distribution of $GABA_C$ during development is poorly studied and thus incomplete. However, an *in situ* hybridization study by Alakuijala *et al.* (2005) described the expression of the $\rho 2$ subunit mRNA, revealing that, in the thalamus, it was only detected in the dLGN at P60. Thus, as it happens in adulthood (Section III.A.2.c), $GABA_C$ subunits in the thalamus during development appear to be selectively expressed in the dLGN, a visual related region.

## IV. Role of GABA Receptors in Nociception Within the Thalamus

GABAergic mechanisms appear to be involved in antinociceptive processes in some regions of the CNS (Jasmin *et al.*, 2004). The effects in the nociceptive behavior of administering GABAergic agents, either agonists or antagonists, in the spinal cord have been thoroughly studied (Enna and McCarson, this volume; Hammond and Washington, 1993; Jasmin *et al.*, 2004; Malan *et al.*, 2002; Malcangio *et al.*, 1992; Sluka *et al.*, 1993, 1994; Smith *et al.*, 1994). Moreover, at the spinal level, GABAergic mechanisms seem to interact with the supraspinal opioidergic system in order to produce antinociception (Holmes and Fujimoto, 1994; Suh *et al.*, 1996). At supraspinal levels, GABAergic mechanisms seem to modulate nociceptive transmission in the brainstem through $GABA_B$ receptors (Thomas *et al.*, 1995, 1996), while in the thalamus comparatively little is known about the role of GABA receptors in nociceptive mechanisms.

## A. $GABA_A$ Receptors

Studies suggest that in some thalamic nuclei, opioid-induced antinociception might be mediated by the GABAergic system. Thus, on the microinjection of bicuculline, an antagonist of $GABA_A$ receptors, into the Sm, Jia *et al.* (2004) observed a significant enhancement of the morphine (injected into the Sm)-evoked inhibition of the tail-flick reflexes, while the same effect was attenuated when muscimol (a selective $GABA_A$ receptor agonist) was injected. These studies suggest that $GABA_A$ receptors in the Sm are involved in the modulation of Sm morphine-induced antinociception. In another nucleus of the medial thalamus, the Pf, most neurons were excited by noxious stimuli and this neuronal excitation was reduced by GABA and by THIP (4,5,6,7-tetrahydroisothiazolo-[5,4-c]pyridine-3-ol), a $GABA_A$ agonist (Reyes-Vazquez *et al.*, 1986). Moreover, behavioral tests using the rat tail-immersion assay showed that the injection of GABA or THIP in this nucleus induced an antinociceptive effect, suggesting that $GABA_A$ receptors located in the Pf might be responsible for this antinociceptive response (Reyes-Vazquez *et al.*, 1986). Changes in the spontaneous activities of VPM neurons induced by formalin injection in the hind paw, another nociceptive test, were altered by injection of muscimol in the somatosensory cortex, implying that pain reactivity of the VPM cells, during the generation of inflammatory pain, may be modulated via corticothalamic pathways through $GABA_A$ receptors (Jung *et al.*, 2004). Furthermore, microinjection of picrotoxin in the VB produced "wet-dog" shakes, whereas a "pain-like" behavior was observed in rats when this ligand was applied in the Rt (Oliveras and Montagne-Clavel, 1994). In cat, the spontaneous resting activity of single thalamic neurons was decreased upon GABA application and nociceptive thalamic cells were inhibited by electrical stimulation of the dorsal column nucleus. These mechanisms seemed to involve not only the $GABA_A$ but also the $GABA_B$ receptor subtypes (Olausson *et al.*, 1994).

In the somatosensory thalamus, the temporal characteristics of phasic neuronal responses seem to be mediated, at least in part, by $GABA_A$ receptors (Hicks *et al.*, 1986; Salt, 1989; Vahle-Hinz and Hicks, 2003). In the rat VB, there is a widely distributed inhibitory system operating in both the medial (VPM) and lateral (VPL) nuclei of this complex that is partly mediated by $GABA_A$ receptors, suggesting that these receptors might play a role in the plasticity of the sensory thalamus associated with deafferentation pain (Roberts *et al.*, 1992). In fact, long-term dorsal rhizotomies in monkeys lead to a downregulation of $GABA_A$ receptors, even in the absence of major loss of GABA neurons, in principal somatosensory thalamic nuclei deprived from sensory stimulation, such as the VP, possibly representing a reduction in pre- and/or postsynaptic receptors and resulting in disinhibition and increased activity of the somatosensory neurons (Rausell *et al.*, 1992). This disinhibition could then unmask previously hidden inputs to these thalamic neurons, which would then be relayed to the cortex, as the authors suggest. Therefore, these receptors might play a role in the mechanisms underlying the perturbations of sensory perception, such as severe "central" pain that arise with chronic deafferentation, by causing an imbalance of the normal inputs to the somatosensory cortex. In fact, Hicks *et al.* (1986) have shown that, in cat, somatosensory thalamic neurons from the VPL often show small increases of their peripheral receptive fields into adjacent areas of skin upon blockade of $GABA_A$ receptors by iontophoresis of bicuculline. Moreover, upon unilateral spinal cord dorsal root section, some neurons of the contralateral VP nuclei and zona incerta exhibit high frequency discharges (hyperactive neurons), which are significantly suppressed by iontophoretic application of GABA (Yamashiro *et al.*, 1994). These studies strongly implicate GABA receptors, especially $GABA_A$, in the thalamic processing of neuropathic pain, although the mechanisms are far from being completely elucidated.

## B. $GABA_B$ Receptors

The role of $GABA_B$ receptors in the thalamus in response to a noxious input is also poorly studied. Systemic administration of tiagabine, an antiepileptic drug, caused an increase of endogenous GABA levels in the medial thalamus and induced an antinociceptive behavior that was evaluated on mechanical, chemical, and thermal noxious stimulation (Ipponi *et al.*, 1999). This antinociception was reverted by a selective $GABA_B$ receptor antagonist, suggesting that the antinociceptive effect of tiagabine in the thalamus was mediated through $GABA_B$ receptors (Ipponi *et al.*, 1999). In other thalamic nuclei, such as the relay VB region and the Po, *in situ* hybridization studies have shown that the expression levels of $GABA_{B(1b)}$ mRNA were altered in response to a prolonged noxious input arising from a monoarthritic ankle in the rat (Ferreira-Gomes *et al.*, 2004). Actually, decreases of mRNA levels were observed in the VB contralateral to the inflamed ankle at different time points of inflammation, whereas in the Po a bilateral increase was detected in the early phases of the disease (Ferreira-Gomes *et al.*, 2004). Moreover, yet unpublished studies from our group show that also $GABA_{B2}$ mRNA expression decreased in the contralateral VB at different stages of the monoarthritis and in the ipsilateral Po in the early phase of the disease (Ferreira-Gomes *et al.*, 2006). These data suggest that $GABA_B$ receptors take part in the plastic changes occurring in thalamic relay nuclei in response to chronic peripheral inflammatory pain and might possibly contribute to the processing of noxious stimuli at this level. In fact, in another study in which monoarthritic rats were stereotaxically injected with baclofen in the VB contralateral to the inflamed joint, a significant decrease of nociceptive behavior was observed whereas saline injection had no effect (Potes *et al.*, 2006a). In addition, the animal response to baclofen injection was dependent on the time course of the disease, suggesting the occurrence of different excitatory states of thalamic VB neurons during the evolution of the monoarthritis. In a different model of peripheral inflammatory pain, the formalin test, stereotaxic injection of baclofen in the VB also caused a specific inhibition of pain-related behaviors, in both the acute and tonic phases of the test (Potes *et al.*, 2006b), suggesting a role for $GABA_B$ receptors not only in chronic but also in acute inflammatory pain processing in the thalamus. In a study using mice lacking $\alpha$1G T-type $Ca^{2+}$ channels, which in the thalamus are activated by $GABA_B$ inhibitory postsynaptic potentials (IPSPs), Kim *et al.* (2003a) observed hyperalgesia in response to visceral pain. Moreover, electrophysiology recordings showed that T-type $Ca^{2+}$ channels in the VPL neurons are activated after noxious stimulation of viscera. Results from this study suggested that T-type $Ca^{2+}$ channels underlie an antinociceptive mechanism in the thalamus and support the idea that burst firing plays a critical role in sensory gating in the thalamus (Kim *et al.*, 2003a). However, the authors also propose that this antinociceptive mechanism may not be effective in controlling acute pain responses, but it is active only after persistent influx of noxious signals to the thalamus (Kim *et al.*, 2003a).

In conclusion, both $GABA_A$ and $GABA_B$ receptors are extensively expressed in thalamic nuclei. However, only a few studies addressed the role of GABA receptors in the processing of noxious stimuli in this region. Although the sparse reports strongly implicate these receptors in nociceptive mechanisms in the thalamus, there are only a few hints on how exactly GABA receptors play this role.

## References


Alakuijala, A., Palgi, M., Wegelius, K., Schmidt, M., Enz, R., Paulin, L., Saarma, M., and Pasternack, M. (2005). GABA receptor rho subunit expression in the developing rat brain. *Brain Res. Dev. Brain Res.* **154**, 15–23.

Albrecht, B. E., and Darlison, M. G. (1995). Localization of the rho 1- and rho 2-subunit messenger RNAs in chick retina by in situ hybridization predicts the existence of gamma-aminobutyric acid type C receptor subtypes. *Neurosci. Lett.* **189**, 155–158.

Aller, M. I., Paniagua, M. A., Pollard, S., Stephenson, F. A., and Fernandez-Lopez, A. (2003). The GABA(A) receptor complex in the chicken brain: Immunocytochemical distribution of alpha 1- and gamma 2-subunits and autoradiographic distribution of BZ1 and BZ2 binding sites. *J. Chem. Neuroanat.* **25**, 1–18.

Ambardekar, A. V., Ilinsky, I. A., Forestl, W., Bowery, N. G., and Kultas-Ilinsky, K. (1999). Distribution and properties of GABA(B) antagonist [3H]CGP 62349 binding in the rhesus monkey thalamus and basal ganglia and the influence of lesions in the reticular thalamic nucleus. *Neuroscience* **93**, 1339–1347.

Ambardekar, A. V., Surin, A., Parts, K., Ilinsky, I. A., and Kultas-Ilinsky, K. (2003). Distribution and binding parameters of $GABA_A$ receptors in the thalamic nuclei of *Macaca mulatta* and changes caused by lesioning in the globus pallidus and reticular thalamic nucleus. *Neuroscience* **118**, 1033–1043.

Anzelius, M., Ekstrom, P., Mohler, H., and Richards, J. G. (1995). Immunocytochemical localization of $GABA_A$ receptor beta 2/beta 3-subunits in the brain of Atlantic salmon (*Salmo salar* L). *J. Chem. Neuroanat.* **8**, 207–221.

Araki, T., and Tohyama, M. (1992). Region-specific expression of $GABA_A$ receptor alpha 3 and alpha 4 subunits mRNAs in the rat brain. *Brain Res. Mol. Brain Res.* **12**, 293–314.

Benke, D., Mertens, S., Trzeciak, A., Gillessen, D., and Mohler, H. (1991). Identification and immunohistochemical mapping of $GABA_A$ receptor subtypes containing the delta-subunit in rat brain. *FEBS Lett.* **283**, 145–149.

Bentivoglio, M., Spreafico, R., Alvarez-Bolado, G., Sanchez, M. P., and Fairen, A. (1991). Differential expression of the $GABA_A$ receptor complex in the dorsal thalamus and reticular nucleus: An immunohistochemical study in the adult and developing rat. *Eur. J. Neurosci.* **3**, 118–125.

Billinton, A., Ige, A. O., Wise, A., White, J. H., Disney, G. H., Marshall, F. H., Waldvogel, H. J., Faull, R. L., and Emson, P. C. (2000). GABA(B) receptor heterodimer-component localisation in human brain. *Brain Res. Mol. Brain Res.* **77**, 111–124.

Bischoff, S., Leonhard, S., Reymann, N., Schuler, V., Shigemoto, R., Kaupmann, K., and Bettler, B. (1999). Spatial distribution of $GABA_BR1$ receptor mRNA and binding sites in the rat brain. *J. Comp. Neurol.* **412**, 1–16.

Bloom, F. E., and Iversen, L. L. (1971). Localizing $^3$H-GABA in nerve terminals of rat cerebral cortex by electron microscopic autoradiography. *Nature* **229**, 628–630.

Bonnert, T. P., McKernan, R. M., Farrar, S., le Bourdelles, B., Heavens, R. P., Smith, D. W., Hewson, L., Rigby, M. R., Sirinathsinghji, D. J., Brown, N., Wafford, K. A., and Whiting, P. J. (1999). Theta, a novel gamma-aminobutyric acid type A receptor subunit. *Proc. Natl. Acad. Sci. USA* **96**, 9891–9896.

Bormann, J. (2000). The "ABC" of GABA receptors. *Trends Pharmacol. Sci.* **21**, 16–19.

Boué-Grabot, E., Roudbaraki, M., Bascles, L., Tramu, G., Bloch, B., and Garret, M. (1998). Expression of GABA receptor $\rho$ subunits in rat brain. *J. Neurochem.* **70**, 899–907.

Bowery, N. G., Doble, A., Hill, D. R., Hudson, A. L., Shaw, J. S., Turnbull, M. J., and Warrington, R. (1981). Bicuculline-insensitive GABA receptors on peripheral autonomic nerve terminals. *Eur. J. Pharmacol.* **71**, 53–70.

Bowery, N. G., Hudson, A. L., and Price, G. W. (1987). $GABA_A$ and $GABA_B$ receptor site distribution in the rat central nervous system. *Neuroscience* **20**, 365–383.

Bowery, N. G., Parry, K., Goodrich, G., Ilinsky, I., and Kultas-Ilinsky, K. (1999). Distribution of GABA(B) binding sites in the thalamus and basal ganglia of the rhesus monkey (*Macaca mulatta*). *Neuropharmacology* **38**, 1675–1682.

Bowery, N. G., Bettler, B., Froestl, W., Gallagher, J. P., Marshall, F., Raiteri, M., Bonner, T. I., and Enna, S. J. (2002). International Union of Pharmacology. XXXIII. Mammalian gamma-aminobutyric acid(B) receptors: Structure and function. *Pharmacol. Rev.* **54**, 247–264.

Calver, A. R., Medhurst, A. D., Robbins, M. J., Charles, K. J., Evans, M. L., Harrison, D. C., Stammers, M., Hughes, S. A., Hervieu, G., Couve, A., Moss, S. J., Middlemiss, D. N., *et al.* (2000). The expression of GABA(B1) and GABA(B2) receptor subunits in the CNS differs from that in peripheral tissues. *Neuroscience* **100**, 155–170.

Calver, A. R., Davies, C. H., and Pangalos, M. N. (2002). $GABA_B$ receptors: From monogamy to promiscuity. *Neurosignals* **11**, 299–314.

Calver, A. R., Michalovich, D., Testa, T., Robbins, M. J., Jaillard, C., Hill, J., Szekeres, P. G., Charles, K. J., Jourdain, S., Holbrook, J. D., Boyfield, I., Patel, N., *et al.* (2003). Molecular cloning and characterisation of a novel $GABA_B$-related G-protein coupled receptor. *Brain Res. Mol. Brain Res.* **110**, 305–317.

Charles, K. J., Evans, M. L., Robbins, M. J., Calver, A. R., Leslie, R. A., and Pangalos, M. N. (2001). Comparative immunohistochemical localisation of $GABA_{B1a}$, $GABA_{B1b}$ and $GABA_{B2}$ subunits in rat brain, spinal cord and dorsal root ganglion. *Neuroscience* **106**, 447–467.

Chebib, M. (2004). $GABA_C$ receptor ion channels. *Clin. Exp. Pharmacol. Physiol.* **31**, 800–804.

Chebib, M., and Johnston, G. A. R. (2000). GABA activated ion channel: Medicinal chemistry and molecular biology. *J. Med. Chem.* **43**, 1427–1447.

Chu, D. C., Albin, R. L., Young, A. B., and Penney, J. B. (1990). Distribution and kinetics of $GABA_B$ binding sites in rat central nervous system: A quantitative autoradiographic study. *Neuroscience* **34**, 341–357.

Coyle, J. T. (2004). The GABA-glutamate connection in schizophrenia: Which is the proximate cause? *Biochem. Pharmacol.* **68**, 1507–1514.

Cutting, G. R., Lu, L., O'Hara, B. F., Kasch, L. M., Montrose-Rafizadeh, C., Donovan, D. M., Shimada, S., Antonarakis, S. E., Guggino, W. B., Uhl, G. R., and Kazazian, H. H., Jr. (1991). Cloning of the g-aminobutyric acid (GABA) r1 cDNA: A GABA receptor subunit highly expressed in the retina. *Proc. Natl. Acad. Sci. USA* **88**, 2673–2677.

Cutting, G. R., Curristin, S., Zoghbi, H., O'Hara, B. F., Seldin, M. F., and Uhl, G. R. (1992). Identification of a putative g-aminobutyric acid (GABA) receptor subunit r2 cDNA and colocalization of the genes encoding rho 2 (GABRR2) and rho 1 (GABRR1) to human chromosome 6q14-q21 and mouse chromosome 4. *Genomics* **12**, 801–806.

Duggan, A. W., and McLennan, H. (1971). Bicuculline and inhibition in the thalamus. *Brain Res.* **25**, 188–191.

Durkin, M. M., Gunwaldsen, C. A., Borowsky, B., Jones, K. A., and Branchek, T. A. (1999). An *in situ* hybridization study of the distribution of the $GABA_{B2}$ protein mRNA in the rat CNS. *Brain Res. Mol. Brain Res.* **71**, 185–200.

Enz, R. (2001). $GABA_C$ receptors: A molecular view. *Biol. Chem.* **382**, 1111–1122.

Enz, R., and Cutting, G. R. (1998). Molecular composition of $GABA_C$ receptors. *Vision Res.* **38**, 1431–1441.

Enz, R., Brandstätter, J. H., Hartveit, E., Wässle, H., and Bormann, J. (1995). Expression of GABA receptor rho 1 and rho 2 subunits in the retina and brain of the rat. *Eur. J. Neurosci.* **38**, 1431–1441.

Enz, R., Brandstätter, J. H., Wässle, H., and Bormann, J. (1996). Immunocytochemical localization of the $GABA_C$ receptor $\rho$ subunits in the mammalian retina. *J. Neurosci.* **16**, 4479–4490.

Ferreira-Gomes, J., Neto, F. L., and Castro-Lopes, J. M. (2004). Differential expression of $GABA_{B(1b)}$ receptor mRNA in the thalamus of normal and monoarthritic animals. *Biochem. Pharmacol.* **68**, 1603–1611.

Ferreira-Gomes, J., Neto, F. L., and Castro-Lopes, J. M. (2006). $GABA_{B2}$ receptor subunit mRNA decreases in the thalamus of monoarthritic animals. (submitted).

Fletcher, E. L., Koulen, P., and Wässle, H. (1998). $GABA_A$ and $GABA_C$ receptors on mammalian rod bipolar cells. *J. Comp. Neurol.* **396**, 351–365.

Fritschy, J. M., Meskenaite, V., Weinmann, O., Honer, M., Benke, D., and Mohler, H. (1999). GABAB-receptor splice variants GB1a and GB1b in rat brain: Developmental regulation, cellular distribution and extrasynaptic localization. *Eur. J. Neurosci.* **11**, 761–768.

Frolund, B., Ebert, B., Kristiansen, U., Liljefors, T., and Krogsgaard-Larsen, P. (2002). $GABA_A$ receptor ligands and their therapeutic potentials. *Curr. Top. Med. Chem.* **2**, 817–832.

Futatsugi, Y., and Riviello, J. J., Jr. (1998). Mechanisms of generalized absence epilepsy. *Brain Dev.* **20**, 75–79.

Gage, P. W. (1992). Activation and modulation of neuronal $K^+$ channels by GABA. *Trends Neurosci.* **15**, 46–51.

Gardner, C. R., Tully, W. R., and Hedgecock, J. R. (1993). The rapidly expanding range of neuronal benzodiazepine ligands. *Prog. Neurobiol.* **40**, 1–61.

Glencorse, T. A., Bateson, A. N., Hunt, S. P., and Darlison, M. G. (1991). Distribution of the $GABA_A$ receptor alpha 1- and gamma 2-subunit mRNAs in chick brain. *Neurosci. Lett.* **133**, 45–48.

Glendenning, K. K. (2003). Distribution of muscimol, QNB, and 5HT binding in the vertebrate diencephalon: A comparative study of eight mammals and three non-mammals. *Microsc. Res. Tech.* **62**, 247–261.

Hammond, D. L., and Washington, J. D. (1993). Antagonism of L-baclofen-induced antinociception by CGP 35348 in the spinal cord of the rat. *Eur. J. Pharmacol.* **234**, 255–262.

Harris, R. M., and Hendrickson, A. E. (1987). Local circuit neurons in the rat ventrobasal thalamus: A GABA immunocytochemical study. *Neuroscience* **21**, 229–236.

Heaulme, M., Chambon, J. P., Leyris, R., Wermuth, C. G., and Biziere, K. (1987). Characterization of the binding of [3H]SR 95531, a $GABA_A$ antagonist, to rat brain membranes. *J. Neurochem.* **48**, 1677–1686.

Hechler, V., Gobaille, S., and Maitre, M. (1992). Selective distribution pattern of gamma-hydroxybutyrate receptors in the rat forebrain and midbrain as revealed by quantitative autoradiography. *Brain Res.* **572**, 345–348.

Hendry, S. H., Schwark, H. D., Jones, E. G., and Yan, J. (1987). Numbers and proportions of GABA-immunoreactive neurons in different areas of monkey cerebral cortex. *J. Neurosci.* **7**, 1503–1519.

Hicks, T. P., Metherate, R., Landry, P., and Dykes, R. W. (1986). Bicuculline induced alterations of response properties in functionally identified ventroposterior thalamic neurones. *Exp. Brain Res.* **63**, 248–264.

Hill, D. R., and Bowery, N. G. (1981). 3H-Baclofen and 3H-GABA bind to bicuculline-insensitive GABA B sites in rat brain. *Nature* **290**, 149–152.

Holmes, B. B., and Fujimoto, J. M. (1994). [D-Pen2-D-Pen5]enkephalin, a delta opioid agonist, given intracerebroventricularly in the mouse produces antinociception through medication of spinal GABA receptors. *Pharmacol. Biochem. Behav.* **49**, 675–682.

Hornung, J. P., and Fritschy, J. M. (1996). Developmental profile of $GABA_A$-receptors in the marmoset monkey: Expression of distinct subtypes in pre- and postnatal brain. *J. Comp. Neurol.* **367**, 413–430.

Huguenard, J. R. (1999). Neuronal circuitry of thalamocortical epilepsy and mechanisms of antiabsence drug action. *Adv. Neurol.* **79**, 991–999.

Huntsman, M. M., Leggio, M. G., and Jones, E. G. (1996). Nucleus-specific expression of GABA(A) receptor subunit mRNAs in monkey thalamus. *J. Neurosci.* **16**, 3571–3589.

Ipponi, A., Lamberti, C., Medica, A., Bartolini, A., and Malmberg-Aiello, P. (1999). Tiagabine antinociception in rodents depends on GABA(B) receptor activation: Parallel antinociception testing and medial thalamus GABA microdialysis. *Eur. J. Pharmacol.* **368**, 205–211.

Iversen, L. L., and Bloom, F. E. (1972). Studies of the uptake of $^3$H-GABA and $^3$H-glycine in slices and homogenates of rat brain and spinal cord by electron microscopic autoradiography. *Brain Res.* **41**, 131–143.

Jasmin, L., Wu, M. V., and Ohara, P. T. (2004). GABA puts a stop to pain. *Curr. Drug Targets CNS Neurol. Disord.* **3**, 487–505.

Jia, H., Xie, Y. F., Xiao, D. Q., and Tang, J. S. (2004). Involvement of GABAergic modulation of the nucleus submedius (Sm) morphine-induced antinociception. *Pain* **108**, 28–35.

Jung, S. C., Kim, J. H., Choi, I. S., Cho, J. H., Bae, Y. C., Lee, M. G., Shin, H. C., and Choi, B. J. (2004). Corticothalamic modulation on formalin-induced change of VPM thalamic activities. *Neuroreport* **15**, 1405–1408.

Kaupmann, K., Huggel, K., Heid, J., Flor, P. J., Bischoff, S., Mickel, S. J., McMaster, G., Angst, C., Bittiger, H., Froestl, W., and Bettler, B. (1997). Expression cloning of GABA(B) receptors uncovers similarity to metabotropic glutamate receptors. *Nature* **386**, 239–246.

Kaupmann, K., Malitschek, B., Schuler, V., Heid, J., Froestl, W., Beck, P., Mosbacher, J., Bischoff, S., Kulik, A., Shigemoto, R., Karschin, A., and Bettler, B. (1998a). GABA(B)-receptor subtypes assemble into functional heteromeric complexes. *Nature* **396**, 683–687.

Kaupmann, K., Schuler, V., Mosbacher, J., Bischoff, S., Bittiger, H., Heid, J., Froestl, W., Leonhard, S., Pfaff, T., Karschin, A., and Bettler, B. (1998b). Human $\gamma$-aminobutyric acid type B receptors are differentially expressed and regulated inwardly rectifying $K^+$ channels. *Proc. Natl. Acad. Sci. USA* **95**, 14991–14996.

Khan, Z. U., Gutierrez, A., Mehta, A. K., Miralles, C. P., and De Blas, A. L. (1996). The alpha 4 subunit of the $GABA_A$ receptors from rat brain and retina. *Neuropharmacology* **35**, 1315–1322.

Kim, D., Park, D., Choi, S., Lee, S., Sun, M., Kim, C., and Shin, H. S. (2003a). Thalamic control of visceral nociception mediated by T-type $Ca^{2+}$ channels. *Science* **302**, 117–119.

Kim, M. O., Li, S., Park, M. S., and Hornung, J. P. (2003b). Early fetal expression of $GABA_{B1}$ and $GABA_{B2}$ receptor mRNAs on the development of the rat central nervous system. *Brain Res. Dev. Brain Res.* **143**, 47–55.

Kulik, A., Nakadate, K., Nyíri, G., Notomi, T., Malitschek, B., Bettler, B., and Shigemoto, R. (2002). Distinct localization of $GABA_B$ receptors relative to synaptic sites in the rat cerebellum and ventrobasal thalamus. *Eur. J. Neurosci.* **15**, 291–307.

Kultas-Ilinsky, K., Fogarty, J. D., Hughes, B., and Ilinsky, I. A. (1988). Distribution and binding parameters of GABA and benzodiazepine receptors in the cat motor thalamus and adjacent nuclear groups. *Brain Res.* **459**, 1–16.

Kuner, R., Kohr, G., Grunewald, S., Eisenhardt, G., Bach, A., and Kornau, H. C. (1999). Role of heterodimer formation in $GABA_B$ receptor function. *Science* **283**, 74–77.

Laurie, D. J., Wisden, W., and Seeburg, P. H. (1992). The distribution of thirteen $GABA_A$ receptor subunit mRNAs in the rat brain. III. Embryonic and postnatal development. *J. Neurosci.* **12**, 4151–4172.

Li, S. P., Park, M. S., Yoon, H., Rhee, K. H., Bahk, J. Y., Lee, J. H., Park, J. S., and Kim, M. O. (2003). Differential distribution of $GABA_{B1}$ and $GABA_{B2}$ receptor mRNAs in the rat brain. *Mol. Cells* **16**, 40–47.

Li, S., Park, M. S., and Kim, M. O. (2004). Prenatal alteration and distribution of the $GABA_{B1}$ and $GABA_{B2}$ receptor subunit mRNAs during rat central nervous system development. *Brain Res. Dev. Brain Res.* **150**, 141–150.

Liang, F., Hatanaka, Y., Saito, H., Yamamori, T., and Hashikawa, T. (2000). Differential expression of gamma-aminobutyric acid type B receptor-1a and -1b mRNA variants in GABA and non-GABAergic neurons of the rat brain. *J. Comp. Neurol.* **416**, 475–495.

Lloyd, K. G., Morselli, P. L., and Bartholini, G. (1987). GABA and affective disorders. *Med. Biol.* **65**, 159–165.

Lukasiewicz, P. D. (1996). $GABA_C$ receptors in the vertebrate retina. *Mol. Neurobiol.* **12**, 181–194.

Malan, T. P., Mata, H. P., and Porreca, F. (2002). Spinal GABA(A) and GABA(B) receptor pharmacology in a rat model of neurophatic pain. *Anesthesiology* **96**, 1161–1167.

Malcangio, M., Malmberg-Aiello, P., Giotti, A., Ghelardini, C., and Bartolini, A. (1992). Desensitization of $GABA_B$ receptors and antagonism by CGP 35348, prevent bicuculline- and picrotoxin-induced antinociception. *Neuropharmacology* **31**, 783–791.

Margeta-Mitrovic, M., Mitrovic, I., Riley, R. C., Jan, L. Y., and Basbaum, A. I. (1999). Immunohistochemical localization of GABA(B) receptors in the rat central nervous system. *J. Comp. Neurol.* **405**, 299–321.

Marshall, F. H., Jones, K. A., Kaupmann, K., and Bettler, B. (1999). $GABA_B$ receptors—the first 7TM heterodimers. *Trends Pharmacol. Sci.* **20**, 396–399.

Medina, J. H. M., Violoa, H., Wolfman, C., Marder, M., Wasowskj, C., Calvo, D., and Paladini, A. C. (1998). Neuroactive flavonoids; new ligands for the benzodiazepine receptors. *Phytomedicine* **5**, 235–243.

Miralles, C. P., Li, M., Mehta, A. K., Khan, Z. U., and De Blas, A. L. (1999). Immunocytochemical localization of the beta(3) subunit of the gamma-aminobutyric acid(A) receptor in the rat brain. *J. Comp. Neurol.* **413**, 535–548.

Misgeld, U., Bijak, M., and Jarolimek, W. (1995). A physiological role for $GABA_B$ receptors and the effects of baclofen in the mammalian central nervous system. *Prog. Neurobiol.* **46**, 423–462.

Möhler, H., Benke, D., and Fritschy, J. M. (2001). GABA(B)-receptor isoforms molecular architecture and distribution. *Life Sci.* **68**, 2297–2300.

Montpied, P., Martin, B. M., Cottingham, S. L., Stubblefield, B. K., Ginns, E. I., and Paul, S. M. (1988). Regional distribution of the GABAA/benzodiazepine receptor (alpha subunit) mRNA in rat brain. *J. Neurochem.* **51**, 1651–1654.

Münoz, A, Huntsman, M. M., and Jones, E. G. (1998). GABA(B) receptor gene expression in monkey thalamus. *J. Comp. Neurol.* **394**, 118–126.

Oertel, W. H., Graybiel, A. M., Magnaini, E., Elde, R. P., Schmechel, D. E., and Kopin, I. J. (1983). Co-existence of glutamic acid decarboxylase and somatostatin-like immunoreactivity in neurons of the feline nucleus reticularis thalami. *J. Neurosci.* **3**, 1322–1332.

Ogurusu, T., and Shingai, R. (1996). Cloning of a putative $\gamma$-aminobutyric acid (GABA) receptor subunit r3 cDNA. *Biochim. Biophys. Acta* **1305**, 15–18.

Ogurusu, T., Taira, H., and Shingai, R. (1995). Identification of $GABA_A$ receptor subunits in the rat retina: Cloning of the rat $GABA_A$ receptor r2 subunit cDNA. *J. Neurochem.* **65**, 964–968.

Olausson, B., Xu, Z. Q., and Shyu, B. C. (1994). Dorsal column inhibition of nociceptive thalamic cells mediated by gamma-aminobutyric acid mechanisms in the cat. *Acta Physiol. Scand.* **152**, 239–247.

Oliveras, J. L., and Montagne-Clavel, J. (1994). The $GABA_A$ receptor antagonist picrotoxin induces a "pain-like" behavior when administered into the thalamic reticular nucleus of the behaving rat: A possible model for "central" pain? *Neurosci. Lett.* **179**, 21–24.

Olsen, R. W., and DeLorey, T. M. (1999). GABA and glycine. *In* "Basic Neurochemistry: Molecular, Cellular and Medical Aspects" (G. J. Siegel, Ed.), pp. 335–346. Lippincott Williams & Willkins, Philadelphia.

Olsen, R. W., McCabe, R. T., and Wamsley, J. K. (1990). $GABA_A$ receptor subtypes: Autoradiographic comparison of GABA, benzodiazepine, and convulsant binding sites in the rat central nervous system. *J. Chem. Neuroanat.* **3**, 59–76.

Ottersen, O. P., and Storm-Mathisen, J. (1984). GABA-containing neurons in the thalamus and pretectum of the rodent: And immunocytochemical study. *Anat. Embryol.* **170**, 197–207.

Palacios, J. M., Wamsley, J. K., and Kuhar, M. J. (1981). High affinity GABA receptors-autoradiographic localization. *Brain Res.* **222**, 285–307.

Paysan, J., and Fritschy, J. M. (1998). $GABA_A$-receptor subtypes in developing brain. Actors or spectators? *Perspect. Dev. Neurobiol.* **5**, 179–192.

Pfaff, T., Malitschek, B., Kaupmann, K., Prezeau, L., Pin, J. P., Bettler, B., and Karschin, A. (1999). Alternative splicing generates a novel isoform of the rat metabotropic GABA(B) R1 receptor. *Eur. J. Neurosci.* **11**, 2874–2882.

Pirker, S., Schwarzer, C., Wieselthaler, A., Sieghart, W., and Sperk, G. (2000). GABA(A) receptors: Immunocytochemical distribution of 13 subunits in the adult rat brain. *Neuroscience* **101**, 815–850.

Potes, C. S., Neto, F. L., and Castro-Lopes, J. M. (2006a). Administration of baclofen, a $GABA_B$ agonist, in the thalamic ventrobasal complex attenuates allodynia in monoarthritic rats subjected to the ankle-bend test. *J. Neurosci. Res.* **83**, 515–523.

Potes, C. S., Neto, F. L., and Castro-Lopes, J. M. (2006b). Inhibition of pain behaviour by $GABA_B$ receptor activation in the thalamic ventrobasal complex: Effect on normal rats subjected to the formalin test of nociception. (submitted).

Poulter, M. O., Barker, J. L., O'Carroll, A. M., Lolait, S. J., and Mahan, L. C. (1993). Coexistent expression of $GABA_A$ receptor beta 2, beta 3 and gamma 2 subunit messenger RNAs during embryogenesis and early postnatal development of the rat central nervous system. *Neuroscience* **53**, 1019–1033.

Price, J. L. (1995). Thalamus. *In* "The Rat Nervous System" (G. Paxinos, Ed.), 2nd edn., pp. 629–648. Academic Press, San Diego.

Princivalle, A., Regondi, M. C., Frassoni, C., Bowery, N. G., and Spreafico, R. (2000). Distribution of GABA(B) receptor protein in somatosensory cortex and thalamus of adult rats and during postnatal development. *Brain Res. Bull.* **52**, 397–405.

Princivalle, A. P., Pangalos, M. N., Bowery, N. G., and Spreafico, R. (2001). Distribution of $GABA_{B(1a)}$, $GABA_{B(1b)}$ and $GABA_{B2}$ receptor protein in cerebral cortex and thalamus of adult rats. *Neuroreport* **12**, 591–595.

Rabow, L. E., Russek, S. J., and Farb, D. H. (1995). From ion currents to genomic analysis: Recent advances in $GABA_A$ receptor research. *Synapse* **21**, 189–274.

Ralston, H. J., and Ralston, D. D. (1994). Medial lemniscal and spinal projections to the macaque thalamus: An electron microscopic study of differing GABAergic circuit serving thalamic somatosensory mechanisms. *J. Neurosci.* **14**, 2485–2502.

Rausell, E., Cusick, C. G., Taub, E., and Jones, E. G. (1992). Chronic deafferentation in monkeys differentially affects nociceptive and non-nociceptive pathways distinguished by specific calcium-binding proteins and down-regulates gamma-aminobutyric acid type A receptors at thalamic levels. *Proc. Natl. Acad. Sci. USA* **89**, 2571–2575.

Reyes-Vazquez, C., Enna, S. J., and Dafny, N. (1986). The parafasciculus thalami as a site for mediating the antinociceptive response to GABAergic drugs. *Brain Res.* **383**, 177–184.

Roberts, E. (1986). GABA: The road to neurotransmitter status. *In* "Benzodiazepine/GABA Receptors and Chloride Channels: Structural and Functional Properties" (R. W. Olsen and C. J. Venter, Eds.), pp. 1–39. Wiley, New York.

Roberts, W. A., Eaton, S. A., and Salt, T. E. (1992). Widely distributed GABA-mediated afferent inhibition processes within the ventrobasal thalamus of rat and their possible relevance to pathological pain states and somatotopic plasticity. *Exp. Brain Res.* **89**, 363–372.

Rozzo, A., Armellin, M., Franzot, J., Chiaruttini, C., Nistri, A., and Tongiorgi, E. (2002). Expression and dendritic mRNA localization of $GABA_C$ receptor $\rho 1$ and $\rho 2$ subunits in the developing rat brain and spinal cord. *Eur. J. Neurosci.* **15**, 1747–1758.

Rustioni, A., Schmechel, D. E., Spreafico, R., Cheema, S., and Cuénod, M. (1983). Excitatory and inhibitory amino acid putative neurotransmitters in the ventralis posterior complex: An autoradiographic and immunocytochemical study in rats and cats. *In* "Somatosensory Integration in the Thalamus" (G. Macchi, A. Rustioni, and R. Spreafico, Eds.), pp. 365–383. Elsevier, Amsterdam.

Salt, T. E. (1989). Gamma-aminobutyric acid and afferent inhibition in the cat and rat ventrobasal thalamus. *Neuroscience* **28**, 17–26.

Sanacora, G., Gueorguieva, R., Epperson, C. N., Wu, Y. T., Appel, M., Rothman, D. L., Krystal, J. H., and Mason, G. F. (2004). Subtype-specific alterations of gamma-aminobutyric acid and glutamate in patients with major depression. *Arch. Gen. Psychiatry* **61**, 705–713.

Saporta, S., and Kruger, L. (1977). The organization of thalamocortical realy neurons in the rat ventrobasal complex studied by the retrograde transport of horseradish peroxidase. *J. Comp. Neurol.* **174**, 187–208.

Schlicker, K., Boller, M., and Schmidt, M. (2004). $GABA_C$ receptor mediated inhibition in acutely isolated neurons of the rat dorsal lateral geniculate nucleus. *Brain Res. Bull.* **63**, 91–97.

Shinotoh, H., Yamasaki, T., Inoue, O., Itoh, T., Suzuki, K., Hashimoto, K., Tateno, Y., and Ikehira, H. (1986). Visualization of specific binding sites of benzodiazepine in human brain. *J. Nucl. Med.* **27**, 1593–1599.

Sieghart, W. (1995). Structure and pharmacology of $\gamma$-aminobutyric $acid_A$ receptor subtypes. *Pharmacol. Rev.* **47**, 181–234.

Sieghart, W., Fuchs, K., Tretter, V., Ebert, V., Jechlinger, M., Hoger, H., and Adamiker, D. (1999). Structure and subunit composition of $GABA_A$ receptors. *Neurochem. Int.* **34**, 379–385.

Sluka, K. A., Willis, W. D., and Westlund, N. K. (1993). Joint inflammation and hyperalgesia are reduced by spinal bicuculline. *Neuroreport* **5**, 109–112.

Sluka, K. A., Willis, W. D., and Westlund, N. K. (1994). Inflammation-induced release of excitatory amino acids is prevented by spinal administration of a $GABA_A$ but not by a $GABA_B$ receptor antagonist in rats. *J. Pharmacol. Exp. Ther.* **271**, 76–82.

Smith, G. D., Harrison, S. M., Birch, P. J., Elliot, P. J., Malcangio, M., and Bowery, N. G. (1994). Increased sensitivity to the antinociceptive activity of (+/−)-baclofen in an animal model of chronic neuropathic, but not inflammatory hyperalgesia. *Neuropharmacology* **33**, 1103–1108.

Spreafico, R., De Biasi, S., Amadeo, A., and De Blas, A. L. (1993). $GABA_A$-receptor immunoreactivity in the rat dorsal thalamus: An ultrastructural investigation. *Neurosci. Lett.* **158**, 232–236.

Steiger, J. L., and Russek, S. J. (2004). $GABA_A$ receptors: Building the bridge between subunit mRNAs, their promoters, and cognate transcription factors. *Pharmacol. Ther.* **101**, 259–281.

Suh, H. W., Kim, Y. H., Choi, Y. S., Choi, S. R., and Song, D. K. (1996). Effects of GABA antagonists injected spinally on antinociception induced by opioids administered supraspinally in mice. *Eur. J. Pharmacol.* **27**, 141–147.

Thomas, D. A., McGowan, M. K., and Hammond, D. L. (1995). Microinjection of baclofen in the ventromedial medulla of rats: Antinociception at low doses and hyperalgesia at high doses. *J. Pharmacol. Exp. Ther.* **275**, 274–284.

Thomas, D. A., Navarrete, I. M., Graham, B. A., McGowan, M. K., and Hammond, D. L. (1996). Antinociception produced by systemic R(+)-baclofen hydrochloride is attenuated by CGP 35348 administered to the spinal cord or ventromedial medulla of rats. *Brain Res.* **718**, 129–137.

Vahle-Hinz, C., and Hicks, T. P. (2003). Temporal shaping of phasic neuronal responses by GABA- and non-GABA-mediated mechanisms in the somatosensory thalamus of the rat. *Exp. Brain Res.* **153**, 310–321.

Veenman, C. L., Albin, R. L., Richfield, E. K., and Reiner, A. (1994). Distributions of $GABA_A$, $GABA_B$, and benzodiazepine receptors in the forebrain and midbrain of pigeons. *J. Comp. Neurol.* **344**, 161–189.

Vogt, L. J., Vogt, B. A., and Sikes, R. W. (1992). Limbic thalamus in rabbit: Architecture, projections to cingulate cortex and distribution of muscarinic acetylcholine, $GABA_A$, and opioid receptors. *J. Comp. Neurol.* **319**, 205–217.

Wafford, K. A. (2005). $GABA_A$ receptor subtypes: Any clues to the mechanism of benzodiazepine dependence? *Curr. Opin. Pharmacol.* **5**, 47–52.

Wang, J., Huo, F. Q., Li, Y. Q., Chen, T., Han, F., and Tang, J. S. (2005). Thalamic nucleus submedius receives GABAergic projection from thalamic reticular nucleus in the rat. *Neuroscience* **134**, 515–523.

Wegelius, K., Reeben, M., Rivera, C., Kaila, K., Saarma, M., and Pasternack, M. (1996). The r1 GABA receptor cloned from the rat retina is down-modulated by protons. *Neuroreport* 7, 2005–2009.

Wegelius, K., Pasternack, M., Hiltunen, J. O., Rivera, C., Kaila, K., Saarma, M., and Reeben, M. (1998). Distribution of GABA receptor rho subunit transcripts in the rat brain. *Eur. J. Neurosci.* **10**, 350–357.

White, J. H., Wise, A., Main, M. J., Green, A., Fraser, N. J., Disney, G. H., Barnes, A. A., Emson, P., Foord, S. M., and Marshall, F. H. (1998). Heterodimerization is required for the formation of a functional GABA(B) receptor. *Nature* **396**, 679–682.

Wilke, K., Gaul, R., Klauck, S. M., and Poustka, A. (1997). A gene in human chromosome band Xq28 (GABRE) defines a putative new subunit class of the $GABA_A$ neurotransmitter receptor. *Genomics* **45**, 1–10.

Wong, C. G., Bottiglieri, T., and Snead, O. C., III. (2003). GABA, gamma-hydroxybutyric acid and neurological disease. *Ann. Neurol.* **54**, 3–12.

Wu, L. G., and Saggau, P. (1997). Presynaptic inhibition of elicited neurotransmitter release. *Trends Neurosci.* **20**, 204–212.

Xia, Y., and Haddad, G. G. (1992). Ontogeny and distribution of $GABA_A$ receptors in rat brainstem and rostral brain regions. *Neuroscience* **49**, 973–989.

Yamashiro, K., Mukawa, J., Terada, Y., Tomiyama, N., Ishida, A., Mori, K., Tasker, R. R., and Albe-Fessard, D. (1994). Neurons with high-frequency discharge in the central nervous system in chronic pain. *Stereotact. Funct. Neurosurg.* **62**, 290–294.

Zhang, D., Pan, Z. H., Zhang, X., Brideau, A. D., and Lipton, S. A. (1995). Cloning of a gamma-aminobutyric acid type c receptor subunit in rat retina with a methionine residue is critical for picrotoxinin channel block. *Proc. Natl. Acad. Sci. USA* **92**, 11756–11760.

**Povl Krogsgaard-Larsen, Bente Frølund, and Tommy Liljefors**

Department of Medicinal Chemistry
The Danish University of Pharmaceutical Sciences
2 Universitetsparken, DK-2100 Copenhagen, Denmark

# $GABA_A$ Agonists and Partial Agonists: THIP (Gaboxadol) as a Non-Opioid Analgesic and a Novel Type of Hypnotic[1]

## I. Chapter Overview

The $GABA_A$ receptor system is implicated in a number of central nervous system (CNS) disorders, making $GABA_A$ receptor ligands interesting as potential therapeutic agents. Only a few different classes of structures are currently known as ligands for the GABA recognition site on the heteropentameric $GABA_A$ receptor complex, reflecting the very strict structural requirements for $GABA_A$ receptor recognition and activation. A majority of compounds showing agonist activity at the $GABA_A$ receptor site are structurally derived from the $GABA_A$ agonists muscimol, THIP (Gaboxadol), or isoguvacine, which we developed at the initial stage of the project. Using

[1] This is a revised and updated version of an article entitled "$GABA_A$ agonists and partial agonists: THIP (Gaboxadol) as a non-opioid analgesic and a novel type of hypnotic" that appeared in *Biochem. Pharmacol.* **68**, 1573–1580 (2004).

*Advances in Pharmacology, Volume 54* 1054-3589/06 $35.00

DOI: 10.1016/S1054-3589(06)54003-7

recombinant $GABA_A$ receptors, functional selectivity has been shown for a number of compounds, including THIP, showing subunit-dependent potency and maximal response. The pharmacological and clinical activities of THIP probably reflect its very potent effects at extrasynaptic $GABA_A$ receptors insensitive to benzodiazepines (BZDs) and containing $\alpha4\beta3\delta$ subunits. The results of ongoing phase III clinical studies on the effect of the partial $GABA_A$ agonist THIP on human sleep pattern show that the functional consequences of a directly acting agonist are distinctly different from those seen after administration of $GABA_A$ receptor modulators such as BZDs. In the light of the interest in partial $GABA_A$ receptor agonists as potential therapeutics, structure–activity studies of a number of analogs of 4-PIOL, a low-efficacy partial $GABA_A$ agonist derived from THIP have been performed. In this connection, a series of $GABA_A$ ligands has been developed showing pharmacological profiles ranging from moderately potent low-efficacy partial $GABA_A$ agonist activity to potent and selective antagonist effect.

## II. GABA Receptors: Multiplicity, Structure, and Function

The discovery of GABA in the early 1950s and the identification of the alkaloid bicuculline (Curtis *et al.*, 1970) and its quaternized analog bicuculline methochloride (BMC) (Johnston *et al.*, 1972) as competitive GABA antagonists in CNS tissues initiated the pharmacological characterization of GABA receptors. The subsequent design of isoguvacine, 4,5,6,7-tetrahydroisoxazolo[5,4-*c*]pyridin-3-ol (THIP, Gaboxadol) (Krogsgaard-Larsen *et al.*, 1977) (Fig. 1), and piperidine-4-sulphonic acid (P4S) (Krogsgaard-Larsen *et al.*, 1981) as a novel class of specific GABA agonists further stimulated studies of the pharmacology of the GABA receptors.

The GABA analog baclofen did, however, disturb the picture of a uniform class of GABA receptors. Baclofen, which was designed as a lipophilic analog of GABA capable of penetrating the blood–brain barrier (BBB), is an antispastic agent, but its GABA agonistic effect could not be antagonized by BMC. In the early 1980s, Bowery and coworkers demonstrated that baclofen, or rather (*R*)-(–)-baclofen, was selectively recognized

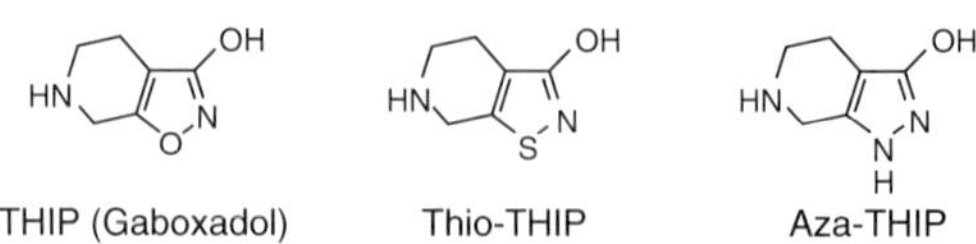


**FIGURE 1** Structures of the $GABA_A$ agonist/partial agonist THIP, the $GABA_A$ partial agonist/antagonist Thio-THIP, and the $GABA_C$ antagonist Aza-THIP.

as an agonist by a distinct subpopulation of GABA receptors, which was named $GABA_B$ receptors (Bowery *et al.*, 1980). Cloning of the $GABA_BR1$ and $GABA_BR2$ receptors and the identification of functional heterodimeric $GABA_B$ receptors have greatly stimulated $GABA_B$ receptor research (Martin *et al.*, 1999; Möhler and Fritschy, 1999). The "classical" BMC-sensitive GABA receptors were designated $GABA_A$ receptors. This receptor classification represents an important step in the development of the pharmacology of GABA.

During this period, the exploration of the GABA receptors was dramatically intensified by the observation that the binding site for the BZDs (Möhler and Okada, 1977; Squires and Braestrup, 1977) was associated with the $GABA_A$ receptors. After the cloning of a large number of $GABA_A$ receptor subunits, this area of the pharmacology of GABA continues to be in a state of very rapid development (Egebjerg *et al.*, 2002).

In connection with the design of conformationally restricted analogs of GABA, another "disturber of the peace" appeared on the GABA scene, namely *cis*-4-aminobut-2-enoic acid (CACA). This compound and the structurally related GABA analog, *cis*-2-aminomethylcyclopropanecarboxylic acid (CAMP) are GABA-like neuronal depressants, which are not sensitive to BMC, and they bind to a class of GABA receptor sites, which neither recognize isoguvacine nor (*R*)-(–)-baclofen. The phosphinic acid analog of isoguvacine, TPMPA (Murata *et al.*, 1996), and, more recently, 4,5,6,7-tetrahydropyrazolo[5,4-*c*]pyridin-3-ol (Aza-THIP) (Krehan *et al.*, 2003) (Fig. 1) have been shown to be selective antagonists at $GABA_C$ receptors (Johnston, 1996). These receptors have been named $GABA_C$ receptors or non-$GABA_A$, non-$GABA_B$ (NANB) receptors for GABA (Johnston, 1996; Murata *et al.*, 1996).

The $GABA_A$ receptor complex is a pentameric structure formed by coassembly of subunits from seven different classes ($\alpha$1–6, $\beta$1–3, $\gamma$1–3, $\delta$, ε, $\theta$, $\rho$1–3). The five subunits, which in native receptors usually are constituted by two α, two $\beta$, and a $\gamma$, $\delta$, or ε subunit, are situated in a circular array surrounding a central chloride-permeable pore (Sieghart and Sperk, 2002; Sieghart *et al.*, 1999).

Several studies have demonstrated the involvement of GABA and $GABA_A$ receptors in diseases like seizures, depression, anxiety, and sleep disorders (Sieghart *et al.*, 1999; Thomsen and Ebert, 2002). GABA and other directly acting $GABA_A$ receptor agonists (GABA-mimetics) bind specifically to a recognition site located at the interface between an $\alpha$ and a $\beta$ subunit (Amin and Weiss, 1993; Amin *et al.*, 1997; Ebert *et al.*, 1994) whereas the classical BZDs, such as diazepam, flunitrazepam, as well as the novel BZD ligands with a nonbenzodiazepine structure as for example zaleplon, zolpidem, zopiclone, and indiplon, bind to an allosteric site located at the interface between an $\alpha$ and a $\gamma$ subunit (Amin and Weiss, 1993; Amin *et al.*, 1997; Duncalfe *et al.*, 1996).

## III. GABA$_A$ Agonists

The basically inhibitory nature of the central GABA neurotransmission prompted the design and development of different structural types of GABA agonists. The conformational restriction of various parts of the molecule of GABA and bioisosteric replacements of the functional groups of this amino acid have led to a broad spectrum of specific GABA$_A$ agonists. Some of these molecules have played a key role in the development of the pharmacology of the GABA$_A$ receptor, or rather receptor family (Krogsgaard-Larsen *et al.*, 1994, 1997).

Muscimol, a constituent of the mushroom *Amanita muscaria*, has been extensively used as a lead for the design of different classes of GABA analogs (Fig. 2). The 3-isoxazolol carboxyl group bioisostere of muscimol can be replaced by a 3-isothiazolol or 3-hydroxyisoxazoline group to give thiomuscimol and dihydromuscimol, respectively, without significant loss of GABA$_A$ receptor agonism (Krogsgaard-Larsen *et al.*, 1979). (*S*)-Dihydromuscimol is the most potent GABA$_A$ agonist so far described (Krogsgaard-Larsen *et al.*, 1985). The structurally related muscimol analogs, isomuscimol and azamuscimol, on the other hand are virtually inactive, emphasizing the very strict

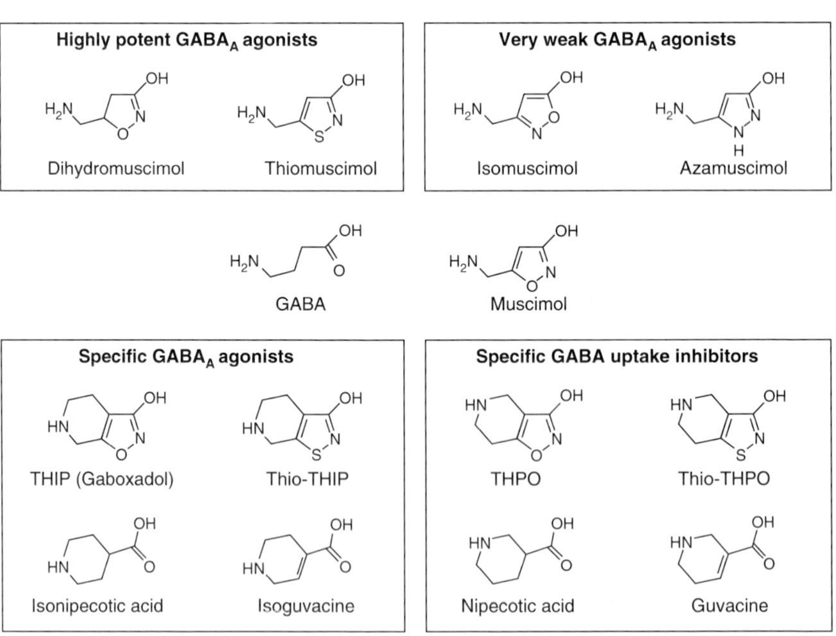


**FIGURE 2** Comparison of the structures of some GABA$_A$ agonists and GABA uptake inhibitors.

structural constraints imposed on agonist molecules by the $GABA_A$ receptors (Krogsgaard-Larsen *et al.*, 1979).

The conversion of muscimol into THIP (Gaboxadol) (Figs. 2 and 3) (Krogsgaard-Larsen *et al.*, 1977) and the isomeric compound 4,5,6,7-tetrahydroisoxazole[4,5-*c*]pyridin-3-ol (THPO) effectively separated $GABA_A$ receptor and GABA uptake affinity, THIP being a specific $GABA_A$ agonist and THPO a GABA uptake inhibitor (Fig. 2) (Krogsgaard-Larsen and Johnston, 1975).

Using THIP as a lead, a series of specific monoheterocyclic $GABA_A$ agonists, including isoguvacine and isonipecotic acid, was developed (Fig. 2) (Krogsgaard-Larsen *et al.*, 1977, 1979). Thio-THIP (Fig. 1) is weaker than THIP as a $GABA_A$ agonist, but studies have disclosed a unique pharmacological profile of this compound. Whereas Thio-THIP shows distinct $GABA_A$ agonist effects on cat spinal neurons (Krogsgaard-Larsen *et al.*, 1983), recent studies using human brain recombinant $GABA_A$ receptors have disclosed very low-efficacy partial agonism/antagonism of Thio-THIP (Brehm *et al.*, 1997).

In light of the structural similarity of THIP and Thio-THIP (Fig. 1) the markedly different pharmacology of these compounds is noteworthy and emphasizes the strict structural requirements of $GABA_A$ receptors. The p*K*a values of THIP (4.4; 8.5) and Thio-THIP (6.1; 8.5) (Krogsgaard-Larsen *et al.*, 1983) are different, and a significant fraction of the molecules of the latter compound must contain a nonionized 3-isothiazolol group at physiological pH. Furthermore, the different degree of charge delocalization of the zwitterionic forms of THIP and Thio-THIP and other structural parameters of these two compounds may have to be considered in order to explain their different potency and efficacy at $GABA_A$ receptors.

A series of cyclic amino acids derived from THPO, including nipecotic acid (Krogsgaard-Larsen and Johnston, 1975) and guvacine (Johnston *et al.*, 1975), was developed as GABA uptake inhibitors. Whereas nipecotic acid and guvacine potently inhibit neuronal as well as glial GABA uptake (Schousboe *et al.*, 1979), THPO interacts selectively with the latter uptake

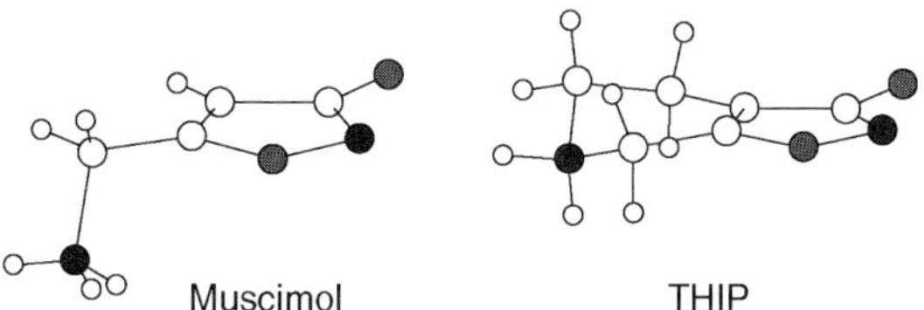


**FIGURE 3** The structures of muscimol and THIP as determined by x-ray crystallographic analyses (from Krogsgaard-Larsen *et al.*, 2002). (See Color Insert.)

system. Thio-THPO is slightly weaker than THPO as an inhibitor of GABA uptake (Krogsgaard-Larsen *et al.*, 1983).

## A. THIP (Gaboxadol), a Selective Agonist at $\delta$-Containing $GABA_A$ Receptors

The quantitatively most predominant $GABA_A$ receptor subunit combination throughout the brain is composed of $\alpha1\beta2/3\gamma2$ subunits, primarily synaptically located (Fritschy and Möhler, 1995; Nusser *et al.*, 1995; Pirker *et al.*, 2000; Wisden *et al.*, 1992). However, much attention has been focused on the less abundant but ostensibly functionally important receptor subtypes with a more restricted location and specialized function. Thus, the primarily extrasynaptically located $\alpha4\beta3\delta$ receptors, which are found in high concentrations not only in hippocampus and thalamus but also in neocortex (Pirker *et al.*, 2000; Sur *et al.*, 1999), seem to play a key role in sleep. Results from our ongoing research projects have suggested that these receptors are the main target for THIP (Gaboxadol), which at present is subjected to clinical phase III studies as a hypnotic.

Whereas Gaboxadol behaves as a partial agonist ($E_{max} = 70\%$) with a fairly low potency ($EC_{50} = 238$ μM) at $\alpha1\beta3\gamma2S$ receptors expressed in *Xenopus* oocytes (Ebert *et al.*, 1994, 1997), it acts as a highly potent ($EC_{50} = 1.3$ μM) full agonist in the rat cortical wedge preparation (Ebert *et al.*, 2002). Based on a series of *in vitro* and *in vivo* pharmacological studies (Stórustovu and Ebert, 2003; Voss *et al.*, 2003), it is hypothesized that Gaboxadol and the BZDs interact with two distinct receptor populations: the BZDs with synaptically located $\alpha1\beta3\gamma2S$ receptors and Gaboxadol with extrasynaptically located $\alpha4\beta3\delta$ receptors. Hence, the effects exerted at these separate populations will sum in an additive rather than a supraadditive manner (Stórustovu and Ebert, 2003). A functional selectivity for $\alpha4\beta3\delta$ receptors at which Gaboxadol acts as a highly potent agonist with an $E_{max}$ of 165% also explains that apparent potent and efficacious behavior of Gaboxadol in the rat cortical wedge preparation (Fig. 4).

$\alpha4\beta X\delta$ receptors have proven difficult to express in recombinant system and therefore only a few studies investigating the pharmacology of this receptor construct have been published. However, a novel murine L(tk) cell line stably expressing $\alpha4\beta3\delta$ receptors has been extensively used to study the basic pharmacology of this receptor subtype (Adkins *et al.*, 2001; Brown *et al.*, 2002). Other groups have published results from more specific studies in *Xenopus* oocytes expressing $\alpha4\beta2/3\delta$ receptors (Sundström-Poromaa *et al.*, 2002; Wallner *et al.*, 2003). A broad spectrum of agonists has been found to behave as full and partial agonists in $\alpha1$–$6\beta X\gamma2$ receptors expressed in *Xenopus* oocytes (Ebert *et al.*, 1994, 1997, 2001; Stórustovu and Ebert, 2005).

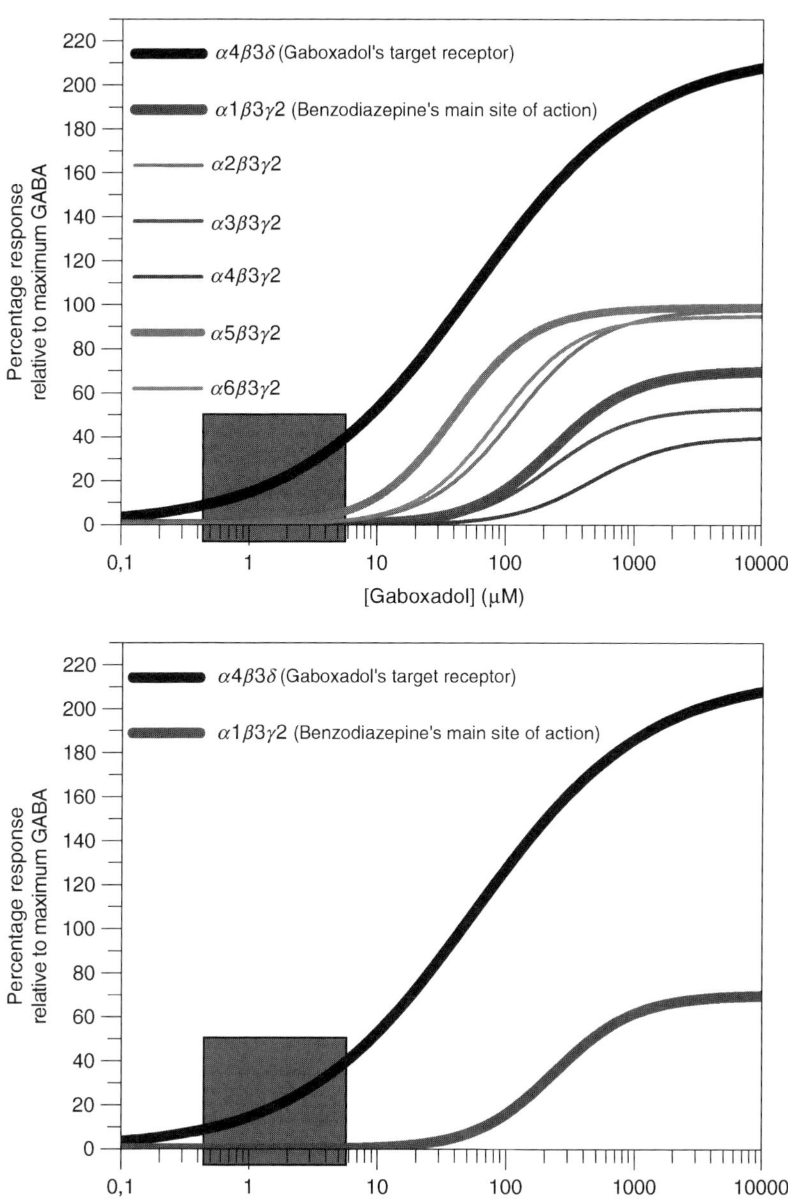


**FIGURE 4** Concentration–response curves for THIP (Gaboxadol) obtained from *Xenopus* oocytes expressing GABA$_A$ receptors of different subunit composition (Ebert *et al.*, 2001). In the lower figure, the effects on $\alpha4\beta3\delta$ and $\alpha1\beta3\gamma2$, the main GABA$_A$ receptor targets for Gaboxadol and the BZDs, respectively, are emphasized. The bar indicates the therapeutically relevant concentration area (Madsen *et al.*, 1983). (See Color Insert.)

## IV. Partial $GABA_A$ Agonists

Under clinical conditions where stimulation of the $GABA_A$ receptor system may be relevant, partial agonists displaying a relatively high efficacy may be particularly useful. The level of efficacy needed may be dependent on the disease in question. The potent analgesic effects of THIP (Gaboxadol) (see in a later section) seem to indicate that this relatively high level of efficacy (Krogsgaard-Larsen *et al.*, 1988; Maksay, 1994) is close to optimal with respect to treatment of pain. Analogously, very low-efficacy $GABA_A$ agonists showing predominant antagonists profiles may have clinical interest in conditions where a gentle reduction in $GABA_A$ receptor activity may be needed.

The nonfused THIP analog, 5-(4-piperidyl)isoxazol-3-ol (4-PIOL) (Fig. 5), is a low-affinity $GABA_A$ agonist (Mortensen *et al.*, 2004), which has been characterized as a partial $GABA_A$ agonist using functional patch-clamp techniques on cultured cerebral cortical and hippocampal neurons (Frølund *et al.*, 1995; Kristiansen *et al.*, 1991). In cortical neurons, the action of 4-PIOL was compared with those of the $GABA_A$ agonist isoguvacine and the $GABA_A$ antagonist BMC (Kristiansen *et al.*, 1991). Based on these studies, it is concluded that 4-PIOL is a low-efficacy partial agonist showing a predominant $GABA_A$ antagonist profile being about 30-fold weaker than BMC as an antagonist at the $GABA_A$ receptors. 4-PIOL has been proposed to possess some subtype-specific characteristics (Rabe *et al.*, 2000). On recombinant $GABA_A$ receptors of the $\alpha1\beta2\gamma2$ subtype expressed in HEK-293 cells, 4-PIOL acted as a weak agonist, whereas it was devoid of activity in the $\alpha6\beta2\gamma2$ receptor subtype.

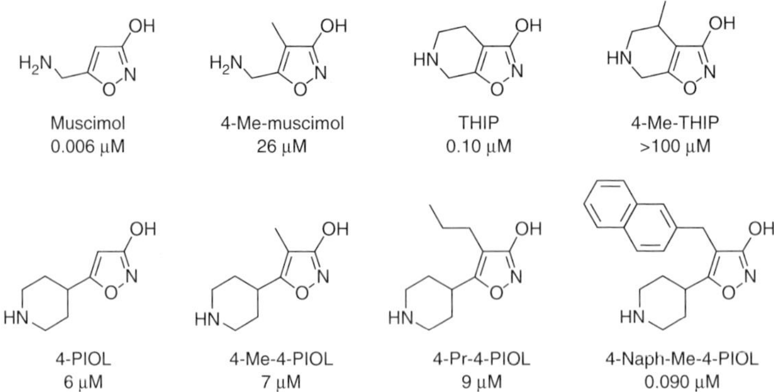


**FIGURE 5** $GABA_A$ agonist binding data ($IC_{50}$, μM) for muscimol, THIP, 4-PIOL, and some analogs of these $GABA_A$ agonist ligands.

## V. 4-PIOL Analogs as $GABA_A$ Antagonists

Introduction of alkyl groups into the 4-position of the 3-isoxazolol ring of muscimol and THIP severely inhibits interaction with the $GABA_A$ receptor recognition site as illustrated in Fig. 5. Thus, 4-Me-muscimol is three to four orders of magnitude weaker than muscimol as an inhibitor of $GABA_A$ receptor binding, whereas 4-Et-muscimol (Krogsgaard-Larsen and Johnston, 1978) and also 4-Me-THIP (Haefliger *et al.*, 1984) are inactive. In contrast, the $GABA_A$ recognition site tolerates introduction of alkyl groups into the 4-position of the 3-isoxazolol ring of 4-PIOL (Frølund *et al.*, 2000). These structure–activity relationships indicate that the binding modes of the $GABA_A$ agonists, muscimol, and THIP and in particular of the low-efficacy partial agonist 4-PIOL are different.

There is strong evidence that an arginine residue at the $GABA_A$ receptor recognition site is directly involved in the binding of the anionic part of the receptor ligand (Westh-Hansen *et al.*, 1999). Based on this observation, a hypothesis has been proposed concerning the binding modes of the bioactive conformations of muscimol and 4-PIOL (Frølund *et al.*, 2000) as illustrated in Fig. 6. In these binding modes, the two 3-isoxazolol rings do not overlap. This means that the 4-position of the 3-isoxazolol ring in muscimol does not correspond to the 4-position in the 3-isoxazolol ring of 4-PIOL during interaction of muscimol and 4-PIOL with the receptor recognition site.

A number of analogs of 4-PIOL have been synthesized with substituents in the 4-position of the 3-isoxazolol ring in order to further investigate

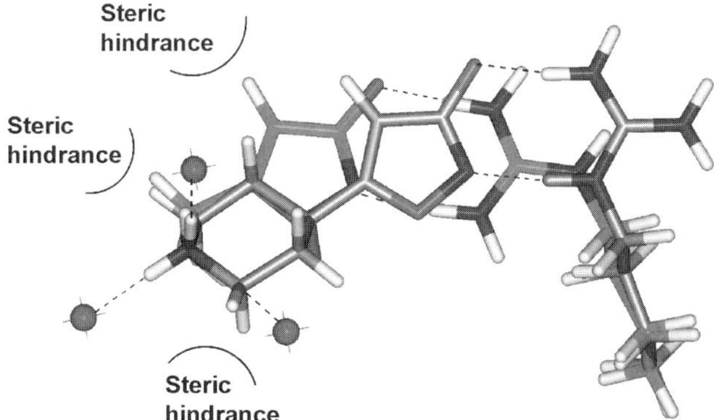


**FIGURE 6** A pharmacophore model for $GABA_A$ receptor agonists showing the proposed binding modes of muscimol (green bonds) and 4-PIOL (light grey bonds) and their interactions with two different conformations of an arginine residue. The red spheres indicate sites to which the ammonium group in muscimol interacts via hydrogen bonds (from Krogsgaard-Larsen *et al.*, 2002). (See Color Insert.)

the steric tolerance of this position (Frølund *et al.*, 2002; Krogsgaard-Larsen *et al.*, 2002). The results from these studies are exemplified in Fig. 5. Substitution of the 4-position with alkyl or benzyl groups resulted in affinity and potencies comparable with those of 4-PIOL. However, introduction of more bulky groups, such as diphenylalkyl and naphthylalkyl groups, as exemplified by the 2-naphthylmethyl analog, 4-Naph-Me-4-PIOL are not only tolerated but also resulted in a marked increase both in affinity and in potency.

Using whole-cell patch-clamp techniques on cultured cerebral cortical neurons in the electrophysiological testing, the pharmacology of the 4-PIOL analogs in the absence or presence of the specific $GABA_A$ receptor agonist isoguvacine was studied (Frølund *et al.*, 2002). The results demonstrated that the structural modifications led to a change in the pharmacological profile of the compounds from moderately potent low-efficacy partial $GABA_A$ receptor agonist activity to potent and selective antagonist effect. The 2-naphthylmethyl (Fig. 5) and the 4-biphenylmethyl analogs showed antagonist potency comparable with or markedly higher than that of the standard $GABA_A$ antagonist gabazine.

These structure–activity studies seem to support the proposed hypothesis concerning the distinct binding mode of 4-PIOL, implying that the 4-position in 4-PIOL does not correspond to the 4-position in muscimol (Figs. 5 and 6). Thus, a cavity of considerable binding capacity seems to exist at the 4-PIOL recognition site of the $GABA_A$ receptor.

Molecular modeling studies of the two high-affinity compounds containing a 2-naphthylmethyl and a 3,3-diphenylpropyl substituent, and the less active 1-naphthylmethyl and 4-biphenyl analogs, indicate that this proposed binding cavity may be exploited in two directions (Fig. 7). In both of these positions an aromatic ring seems to be highly favorable for the receptor affinity (Frølund *et al.*, 2002).

As mentioned earlier, the GABA-binding site in the $GABA_A$ receptor is assumed to be located at the interface between $\alpha$ and $\beta$ subunits (Smith and Olsen, 1995). It has been speculated that the $GABA_A$ antagonists bind to and stabilize a distinct inactive receptor conformation. In case of the 4-arylalkyl substituted 4-PIOL analogs it may be speculated that the large cavity accommodating the 4-substituent is located in the space between these subunits. $GABA_A$ receptors belong to the same superfamily as the nicotinic acetylcholine receptors. It has been proposed that the mechanism for ligand-induced channel opening in nicotinic acetylcholine receptors involves rotations of the subunits in the ligand-binding domain (Unwin, 1995). Assuming that the $GABA_A$ receptors utilize a similar mechanism for channel opening, large substituents may interfere with the channel opening resulting in antagonistic effects of the compounds (Frølund *et al.*, 2002).

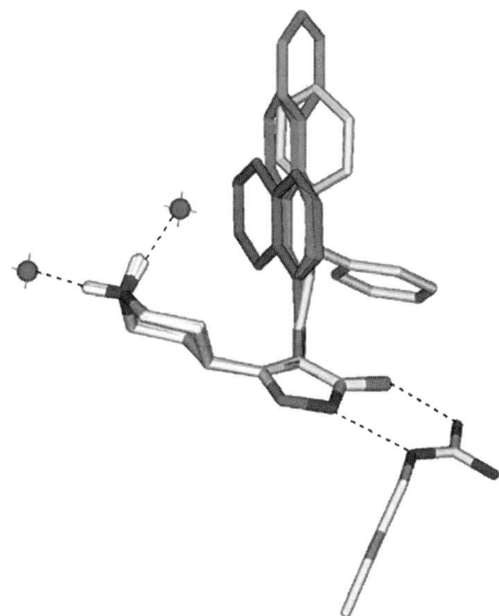

**FIGURE 7** Proposed bioactive conformations for the high-affinity 1-naphthylmethyl, 2-naphthylmethyl, 3,3-diphenylpropyl, and 4-biphenyl analogs of 4-PIOL (from Krogsgaard-Larsen *et al.*, 2002). (See Color Insert.)

## VI. Behavioral and Clinical Effects of the Partial $GABA_A$ Agonist THIP (Gaboxadol)

### A. Analgesia and Anxiety

The involvement of central $GABA_A$ receptors in pain mechanisms and analgesia has been thoroughly studied, and the results have been discussed and reviewed (DeFeudis, 1989; Krogsgaard-Larsen *et al.*, 1997; McCarson and Enna, this volume). The demonstration of potent antinociceptive effects of the specific and metabolically stable partial $GABA_A$ agonist THIP (Gaboxadol) in different animal models and the potent analgesic effects of Gaboxadol in man greatly stimulated studies in this area of pain research. Gaboxadol-induced analgesic effects were shown to be insensitive to the opiate antagonist naloxone indicating that these effects are not mediated by the opiate receptors (Zorn and Enna, 1987).

Gaboxadol and morphine are approximately equipotent as analgesics, although their relative potencies are dependent on the animal species and experimental models used. Acute injection of Gaboxadol potentiates morphine-induced analgesia, and chronic administration of Gaboxadol produces a certain degree of functional tolerance to its analgesic effects. In contrast to morphine, Gaboxadol does not cause respiratory depression. Clinical studies on postoperation patients, and patients with chronic pain of malignant origin have disclosed potent analgesic effects of Gaboxadol, in the latter group of patients at total doses of 5–30 mg (i.m.) of Gaboxadol.

In cancer patients and also in patients with chronic anxiety (Hoehn-Saric, 1983) the desired effects of Gaboxadol were accompanied by side effects, notably sedation, nausea, and in a few cases euphoria. The side effects of Gaboxadol have, however, been described as mild and similar in quality to those of other GABA-mimetics (Hoehn-Saric, 1983). This combination of analgesic and anxiolytic effects of THIP obviously has therapeutic prospects.

The neuronal and synaptic mechanisms underlying Gaboxadol- and, in general, GABA-induced analgesia are still only incompletely understood. The insensitivity of Gaboxadol-induced analgesia to naloxone has been consistently demonstrated. GABA-induced analgesia does not seem to be mediated primarily by spinal $GABA_A$ receptors but rather by GABA mechanisms in the forebrain, and it appears also to involve neurons in the midbrain. The naloxone insensitivity and apparent lack of dependence liability of $GABA_A$ agonist-mediated analgesia suggest that GABAergic drugs may play a role in future treatment of pain. Furthermore, it has been suggested that pharmacological manipulation of GABA mechanisms may have some relevance for future treatment of opiate drug addicts (DeFeudis, 1989).

Findings suggest that subtype-selective $GABA_A$ receptor agonists, such as Gaboxadol, may have some utility in alleviating neuropathic allodynia and hyperalgesia in human patients. Furthermore, the utility of Gaboxadol for improving sleep disorders may have additional benefits for neuropathic pain patients where disruption of sleep impacts negatively on quality of life measurements (Rode *et al.*, 2005).

## B. Sleep Disorders

GABAergic compounds acting at the barbiturate site, the neurosteroid site, or the BZD site of the $GABA_A$ receptor complex have been used as hypnotics for years. Most of these hypnotics interact with all subtypes of receptors. However, as $\alpha 4$ and $\delta$ containing receptors do not bind BZDs, effect of BZDs at these receptor subtypes is absent (Wafford *et al.*, 1996). It is generally agreed that the sedative effect of BZDs is mediated primarily via $\alpha 1$ containing receptors, whereas side effects related to amnesia may be mediated by $\alpha 5$, primarily located in the hippocampal region (Rudolph *et al.*, 1999). However, short-acting $\alpha 1$ selective BZD ligands like zaleplon, zopiclone, and zolpidem do produce memory impairment and hangover effects (Landolt and Gillin, 2000), suggesting that even an $\alpha 1$

selective compound with a very short half-life may produce side effects. The reason for this side effect profile may well be a consequence of the high degree of GABA receptor activation caused by the positive $GABA_A$ receptor modulator. The massive activation of GABA receptors will influence several other systems, ultimately resulting in a general acute modification of the overall function of the CNS. Electroencephalographic (EEG) measurements during sleep support this hypothesis. A normal sleep pattern involves a complex variation of different degrees of sleep, ranging from light sleep via deeper sleep stages to the dream-associated rapid eye movement (REM) stage of sleep. Present understanding of sleep quality and the relation to EEG patterns is still limited; however, not only the duration of REM sleep but also the transitions between the different sleep stages are important (Landolt and Gillin, 2000). The effect of BZDs at the sleep micro architecture is not limited to the onset of REM sleep, which is delayed.

In contrast to the observations with BZDs, barbiturates, and neurosteroids, a series of studies have shown that this perturbation of the sleep micro architecture may not arise with compounds acting directly at the $GABA_A$ recognition site (Lancel and Faulhaber, 1996; Lancel *et al.*, 1996). In this respect, Gaboxadol is an interesting compound. Gaboxadol appears to improve the quality of sleep, as measured using behavioral parameters. The compound shows no effect on the onset of REM sleep, as measured using EEG (Lancel and Faulhaber, 1996; Lancel *et al.*, 1996). Furthermore, studies in elderly patients suffering from significant reduction in non-REM sleep showed that Gaboxadol was able to normalize the sleep pattern (Lancel *et al.*, 2001). Following dosing with Gaboxadol, patients did not experience the hangovers or impaired attention as reported for BZDs. Similar results have been obtained with muscimol, with the GABA uptake inhibitor tiagabine (Lancel *et al.*, 1998), and with the glia-selective GABA uptake inhibitor, THPO (Fig. 2) (Juhász *et al.*, 1991), strongly suggesting that the functional consequences of a direct acting agonist or enhanced synaptic GABA concentration are different from those seen with $GABA_A$ receptor modulators.

Agonistic modulators of $GABA_A$ receptors, in particular short-acting compounds, typically induce rapid tolerance to their hypnotic effect (Huckle, 2004). The tolerance potential of Gaboxadol to its effects on sleep has been studied in rats (Lancel and Langebartels, 2000; Liang *et al.*, 2004). Results of this study suggest that there is no rapid induction of tolerance to Gaboxadol and that withdrawal of the drug does not affect future sleep.

The effects of combinations of Gaboxadol, ethanol, and structurally different BZD agonists (flunitrazepam, zolpidem, and indiplon) were studied in a rat rotarod model (Voss *et al.*, 2003). All compounds, including Gaboxadol, produced a dose-dependent impairment of motor function, and a supraadditive effect was observed when the BZD ligands and ethanol were administered together. Gaboxadol did not interact synergistically with any of the BZDs to potentiate motor coordination deficits, and ethanol did not significantly potentiate the effects of Gaboxadol. The results of this study led the researchers to suggest that Gaboxadol and zolpidem in the rotarod model interact with distinct receptor populations (Voss *et al.*, 2003).

## VII. Conclusions

Molecular biology studies have revealed a high degree of structural heterogeneity of the $GABA_A$ receptors. Development of subtype selective or specific compounds is of key importance for the understanding of the physiological and pathological roles of different GABA receptor subtypes and may lead to valuable therapeutic agents. Studies along these lines have, so far, been complicated by the lack of information about the topography of the recognition site(s) of the $GABA_A$ receptor complex. In the absence of a crystal structure of the $GABA_A$ receptor complex, 3D-pharmacophore models, based on the analysis of known receptor ligands, have been useful tools in the design of new ligands. Recombinant receptors play a key role in the pharmacological characterization of ligands for the $GABA_A$ receptor. However, problems regarding subunit composition of native receptors are far from being fully elucidated. Furthermore, the subtypes of receptors involved in different disorders are still largely unknown. Although the functional consequences of modifications of subunit compositions, so far, are unpredictable, it has been shown that functional selectivity is obtainable for a number of $GABA_A$ agonists. An important aspect is the selection of subunit combinations relevant for the prediction of *in vivo* activity.

The main $GABA_A$ receptor targets for Gaboxadol and the BZDs are distinctly different making Gaboxadol an interesting drug candidate, primarily in sleep disorders. In addition, the non-opioid analgesic effect of Gaboxadol has therapeutic prospects.

## Acknowledgments

This work was supported by grants from the Lundbeck Foundation, the Danish Medical Research Council, the Centre for Drug Design and Transport, the NeuroScience PharmaBiotec Centre, and the Danish State Biotechnology Programme. The secretarial assistance of Mrs. Maria McGrail is gratefully acknowledged.

## References

Adkins, C. E., Pillai, G. V., Kerby, J., Bonnert, T. P., Haldon, C., Mckernan, R. M., Gonzalez, J. E., Oades, K., Whiting, P. J., and Simpson, P. B. (2001). $\alpha_4\beta_3\delta$ $GABA_A$ receptors characterized by fluorescence resonance energy transfer-derived measurements of membrane potential. *J. Biol. Chem.* **276**, 38934–38939.

Amin, J., and Weiss, D. S. (1993). $GABA_A$ receptor needs two homologous domains of the $\beta$-subunit for activation by GABA but not by pentobarbital. *Nature* **366**, 565–569.

Amin, J., Brooks-Kayal, A., and Weiss, D. S. (1997). Two tyrosine residues on the $\alpha$ subunit are crucial for benzodiazepine binding and allosteric modulation of $\gamma$-aminobutyric $acid_A$ receptors. *Mol. Pharmacol.* **51**, 833–841.

Bowery, N. G., Hill, D. R., Hudson, A. L., Doble, A., Middlemiss, D. N., Shaw, J., and Turnbull, M. (1980). (–)Baclofen decreases neurotransmitter release in the mammalian CNS by an action at a novel GABA receptor. *Nature* **283**, 92–94.

Brehm, L., Ebert, B., Kristiansen, U., Wafford, K. A., Kemp, J. A., and Krogsgaard-Larsen, P. (1997). Structure and pharmacology of 4,5,6,7-tetrahydroisothiazolo[5,4-*c*]pyridin-3-ol (Thio-THIP), an agonist/antagonist at $GABA_A$ receptors. *Eur. J. Med. Chem.* **32**, 357–363.

Brown, N., Kerby, J., Bonnert, T. P., Whiting, P. J., and Wafford, K. A. (2002). Pharmacological characterization of a novel cell line expressing human $\alpha_4\beta_3\delta$ $GABA_A$ receptors. *Br. J. Pharmacol.* **136**, 965–974.

Curtis, D. R., Duggan, A. W., Felix, D., and Johnston, G. A. R. (1970). GABA, bicuculline and central inhibition. *Nature* **226**, 1222–1224.

DeFeudis, F. V. (1989). GABA agonists and analgesia. *Drug News Perspect* **2**, 172–173.

Duncalfe, L. L., Carpenter, M. R., Smillie, L. B., Martin, I. L., and Dunn, S. M. (1996). The major site of photoaffinity labeling of the $\gamma$-aminobutyric acid type A receptor by [$^3$H] flunitrazepam is histidine 102 of the $\alpha$ subunit. *J. Biol. Chem.* **271**, 9209–9214.

Ebert, B., Wafford, K. A., Whiting, P. J., Krogsgaard-Larsen, P., and Kemp, J. A. (1994). Molecular pharmacology of gamma-aminobutyric acid type A receptor agonists and partial agonists in oocytes injected with different alpha, beta, and gamma receptor subunit combinations. *Mol. Pharmacol.* **46**, 957–963.

Ebert, B., Thompson, S. A., Saounatsou, K., Mckernan, R., Krogsgaard-Larsen, P., and Wafford, K. A. (1997). Differences in agonist/antagonist binding affinity and receptor transduction using recombinant human $\gamma$-aminobutyric acid type A receptors. *Mol. Pharmacol.* **52**, 1150–1156.

Ebert, B., Mortensen, M., Thompson, S. A., Kehler, J., Wafford, K. A., and Krogsgaard-Larsen, P. (2001). Bioisosteric determinants for subtype selectivity of ligands for heteromeric $GABA_A$ receptors. *Bioorg. Med. Chem. Lett.* **11**, 1573–1577.

Ebert, B., Stórustovu, S., Mortensen, M., and Frølund, B. (2002). Characterization of $GABA_A$ receptor ligands in the rat cortical wedge preparation: Evidence for action at extrasynaptic receptors? *Br. J. Pharmacol.* **137**, 1–8.

Egebjerg, J., Schousboe, A., and Krogsgaard-Larsen, P. (2002). "Glutamate and GABA receptors and transporters: Structure, function and pharmacology." Taylor & Francis, London.

Fritschy, J.-M., and Möhler, H. (1995). $GABA_A$-receptor heterogeneity in the adult rat brain: Differential regional and cellular distribution of seven major subunits. *J. Comp. Neurol.* **359**, 154–194.

Frølund, B., Kristiansen, U., Brehm, L., Hansen, A. B., Krogsgaard-Larsen, P., and Falch, E. (1995). Partial $GABA_A$ receptor agonists. Synthesis and *in vitro* pharmacology of a series of nonannulated analogs of 4,5,6,7-tetrahydroisoxazolo[5,4-*c*]pyridin-3-ol. *J. Med. Chem.* **38**, 3287–3296.

Frølund, B., Tagmose, L., Liljefors, T., Stensbøl, T. B., Engblom, C., Kristiansen, U., and Krogsgaard-Larsen, P. (2000). A novel class of potent 3-isoxazolol $GABA_A$ antagonists: Design, synthesis and pharmacology. *J. Med. Chem.* **43**, 4930–4933.

Frølund, B., Jørgensen, A. T., Tagmose, L., Stensbøl, T. B., Vestergaard, H. T., Engblom, C., Kristiansen, U., Sanchez, C., Krogsgaard-Larsen, P., and Liljefors, T. (2002). Novel class of potent 4-arylalkyl substituted 3-isoxazolol $GABA_A$ antagonists: Synthesis, pharmacology, and molecular modeling. *J. Med. Chem.* **45**, 2454–2468.

Haefliger, W., Révész, L., Maurer, R., Römer, D., and Büscher, H.-H. (1984). Analgesic GABA agonists. Synthesis and structure-activity studies on analogues and derivatives of muscimol and THIP. *Eur. J. Med. Chem.* **19**, 149–156.

Hoehn-Saric, R. (1983). Effects of THIP on chronic anxiety. *Psychopharmacology (Berlin)* **80**, 338–341.

Huckle, R. (2004). Gaboxadol. *Curr. Opin. Investig. Drugs* **5**, 766–773.

Johnston, G. A. R. (1996). $GABA_A$ receptor pharmacology. *Pharmacol. Ther.* **69**, 173–198.

Johnston, G. A. R., Beart, P. M., Curtis, D. R., Game, C. J. A., McCulloch, R. M., and MacLachlan, R. M. (1972). Bicuculline methochloride as a GABA antagonist. *Nature New Biol.* **240**, 219–220.

Johnston, G. A. R., Krogsgaard-Larsen, P., and Stephanson, A. (1975). Betel nut constituents as inhibitors of $\gamma$-aminobutyric acid uptake. *Nature* **258**, 627–628.

Juhász, G., Kékesi, K. A., Emri, Z., Ujszászi, J., Krogsgaard-Larsen, P., and Schousboe, A. (1991). Sleep promoting effect of a putative glial $\gamma$-aminobutyric acid uptake blocker applied in the thalamus of cats. *Eur. J. Pharmacol.* **209**, 131–133.

Krehan, D., Frølund, B., Ebert, B., Nielsen, B., Krogsgaard-Larsen, P., Johnston, G. A. R., and Chebib, M. (2003). Aza-THIP and related analogues of THIP as $GABA_C$ antagonists. *Bioorg. Med. Chem.* **11**, 4891–4896.

Kristiansen, U., Lambert, J. D. C., Falch, E., and Krogsgaard-Larsen, P. (1991). Electrophysiological studies of the $GABA_A$ receptor ligand, 4-PIOL, on cultured hippocampal neurons. *Br. J. Pharmacol.* **104**, 85–90.

Krogsgaard-Larsen, P., and Johnston, G. A. R. (1975). Inhibition of GABA uptake in rat brain slices by nipecotic acid, various isoxazoles and related compounds. *J. Neurochem.* **25**, 797–802.

Krogsgaard-Larsen, P., and Johnston, G. A. R. (1978). Structure-activity studies on the inhibition of GABA binding to rat brain membranes by muscimol and related compounds. *J. Neurochem.* **30**, 1377–1382.

Krogsgaard-Larsen, P., Johnston, G. A. R., Lodge, D., and Curtis, D. R. (1977). A new class of GABA agonist. *Nature* **268**, 53–55.

Krogsgaard-Larsen, P., Hjeds, H., Curtis, D. R., Lodge, D., and Johnston, G. A. R. (1979). Dihydromuscimol, thiomuscimol and related heterocyclic compounds as GABA analogues. *J. Neurochem.* **32**, 1717–1724.

Krogsgaard-Larsen, P., Snowman, A., Lummis, S. C., and Olsen, R. W. (1981). Characterization of the binding of the GABA agonist [$^3$H]piperidine-4-sulfonic acid to bovine brain synaptic membranes. *J. Neurochem.* **37**, 401–409.

Krogsgaard-Larsen, P., Mikkelsen, H., Jacobsen, P., Falch, E., Curtis, D. R., Peet, M. J., and Leah, J. D. (1983). 4,5,6,7-Tetrahydroisothiazolo[5,4-*c*]pyridin-3-ol and related analogues of THIP. Synthesis and biological activity. *J. Med. Chem.* **26**, 895–900.

Krogsgaard-Larsen, P., Nielsen, L., Falch, E., and Curtis, D. R. (1985). GABA agonists. Resolution, absolute stereochemistry, and enantioselectivity of (S)-(+)- and (R)-(−)-dihydromuscimol. *J. Med. Chem.* **28**, 1612–1617.

Krogsgaard-Larsen, P., Hjeds, H., Falch, E., Jørgensen, F. S., and Nielsen, L. (1988). Recent advances in GABA agonists, antagonists and uptake inhibitors: Structure–activity relationships and therapeutic potential. *Adv. Drug Res.* **17**, 381–456.

Krogsgaard-Larsen, P., Frølund, B., Jørgensen, F. S., and Schousboe, A. (1994). $GABA_A$ receptor agonists, partial agonists, and antagonists. Design and therapeutic prospects. *J. Med. Chem.* **37**, 2489–2505.

Krogsgaard-Larsen, P., Frølund, B., Kristiansen, U., Frydenvang, K., and Ebert, B. (1997). $GABA_A$ and $GABA_B$ receptor agonists, partial agonists, antagonists and modulators: Design and therapeutic prospects. *Eur. J. Pharm. Sci.* **5**, 355–384.

Krogsgaard-Larsen, P., Frølund, B., and Liljefors, T. (2002). Specific $GABA_A$ agonists and partial agonists. *Chem. Rec.* **2**, 419–430.

Lancel, M., and Faulhaber, J. (1996). The $GABA_A$ agonist THIP (Gaboxadol) increases non-REM sleep and enhances delta activity in the rat. *Neuroreport* **7**, 2241–2245.

Lancel, M., and Langebartels, A. (2000). $\gamma$-Aminobutyric $acid_A$ ($GABA_A$) agonist 4,5,6,7-tetrahydroisoxazolol[5,4-*c*]pyridin-3-ol persistently increases sleep maintenance and intensify during chronic administration to rats. *J. Pharmacol. Exp. Ther.* **293**, 1084–1090.

Lancel, M., Cronlein, T. A., and Faulhaber, J. (1996). Role of $GABA_A$ receptors in sleep regulation. Differential effects of muscimol and midazolam on sleep in rats. *Neuropsychopharmacology* **15**, 63–74.

Lancel, M., Faulhaber, J., and Deisz, R. A. (1998). Effect of the GABA uptake inhibitor tiagabine on sleep and EEG power spectra in the rat. *Br. J. Pharmacol.* **123**, 1471–1477.

Lancel, M., Wetter, T. C., Steiger, A., and Mathias, S. (2001). Effect of the $GABA_A$ agonist gaboxadol on nocturnal sleep and hormone secretion in healthy elderly subjects. *Am. J. Physiol. Endocrinol. Metab.* **281**, E130–E137.

Landolt, H. P., and Gillin, J. C. (2000). $GABA_A$ $\alpha_1$ receptors: Involvement in sleep regulation and potential of selective agonists in the treatment of insomnia. *CNS Drugs* **13**, 185–199.

Liang, J., Cagetti, E., Olsen, R. W., and Spigelmann, I. (2004). Altered pharmacology of synaptic and extrasynaptic $GABA_A$ receptors on CA1 hippocampal neurons is consistent with subunit changes in a model of alcohol withdrawal and dependence. *J. Pharmacol. Exp. Ther.* **310**, 1234–1245.

Madsen, S. M., Lindeburg, T., Folsgard, S., Jacobsen, E., and Sillesen, H. (1983). Pharmacokinetics of the gamma-aminobutyric acid agonist THIP (Gaboxadol) following intramuscular administration to man, with observations in dog. *Acta Pharmacol. Toxicol. (Copenh.)* **53**, 353–357.

Maksay, G. (1994). Thermodynamics of gamma-aminobutyric acid type A receptor binding differentiate agonists from antagonists. *Mol. Pharmacol.* **46**, 386–390.

Martin, S. C., Russek, S. J., and Farb, D. H. (1999). Molecular identification of the human $GABA_BR2$: Cell surface expression and coupling to adenylyl cyclase in the absence of $GABA_BR1$. *Mol. Cell. Neurosci.* **13**, 180–191.

Mortensen, M., Kristiansen, U., Ebert, B., Frølund, B., Krogsgaard-Larsen, P., and Smart, T. G. (2004). Activation of single heteromeric $GABA_A$ receptor ion channels by full and partial agonists. *J. Physiol. (London)* **557**, 393–417.

Murata, Y., Woodward, R. M., Miledi, R., and Overman, L. E. (1996). The first selective antagonist for a $GABA_C$ receptor. *Bioorg. Med. Chem. Lett.* **6**, 2073–2076.

Möhler, H., and Fritschy, J.-M. (1999). $GABA_B$ receptors make it to the top—as dimers. *Trends Pharmacol. Sci.* **20**, 87–89.

Möhler, H., and Okada, T. (1977). Benzodiazepine receptors: Demonstration in the central nervous system. *Science* **198**, 849–851.

Nusser, Z., Roberts, J. D., Baude, A., Richards, J. G., and Somogyi, P. (1995). Relative densities of synaptic and extrasynaptic $GABA_A$ receptors on cerebellar granule cells as determined by a quantitative immunogold method. *J. Neurosci.* **15**, 2948–2960.

Pirker, S., Schwarzer, C., Wieselthaler, A., Sieghart, W., and Sperk, G. (2000). $GABA_A$ receptors: Immunocytochemical distribution of 13 subunits in the adult rat brain. *Neuroscience* **101**, 815–850.

Rabe, H., Picard, R., Uusi-Oukari, M., Hevers, W., Luddens, H., and Korpi, E. R. (2000). Coupling between agonist and chloride ionophore sites of the $GABA_A$ receptor: Agonist/antagonist efficacy of 4-PIOL. *Eur. J. Pharmacol.* **409**, 233–242.

Rode, F., Jensen, D. G., Blackburn-Munro, G., and Bjerrum, O. J. (2005). Centrally-mediated antinociceptive actions of $GABA_A$ receptor agonists in the rat spared nerve injury model of neuropathic pain. *Eur. J. Pharmacol.* **516**, 131–138.

Rudolph, U., Crestani, F., Benke, D., Brunig, I., Benson, J. A., Fritschy, J.-M., Martin, J. R., Bluethmann, H., and Möhler, H. (1999). Benzodiazepine actions mediated by specific $\gamma$-aminobutyric $acid_A$ receptor subtypes. *Nature* **401**, 796–800.

Schousboe, A., Thorbek, P., Hertz, L., and Krogsgaard-Larsen, P. (1979). Effects of GABA analogues of restricted conformation on GABA transport in astrocytes and brain cortex slices and on GABA receptor binding. *J. Neurochem.* **33**, 181–189.

Sieghart, W., and Sperk, G. (2002). Subunit composition, distribution and function of $GABA_A$ receptor subtypes. *Curr. Top. Med. Chem.* **2**, 795–816.

Sieghart, W., Fuchs, K., Tretter, V., Ebert, V., Jechlinger, M., Höger, H., and Adamiker, D. (1999). Structure and subunit composition of $GABA_A$ receptors. *Neurochem. Int.* **34**, 379–385.

Smith, G. B., and Olsen, R. W. (1995). Functional domains of $GABA_A$ receptors. *Trends Pharmacol. Sci.* **16**, 162–168.

Squires, R. F., and Braestrup, C. (1977). Benzodiazepine receptors in rat brain. *Nature* **266**, 732–734.

Stórustovu, S., and Ebert, B. (2003). Gaboxadol: *In vitro* interaction studies with benzodiazepines and ethanol suggest functional selectivity. *Eur. J. Pharmacol.* **467**, 49–56.

Stórustovu, S., and Ebert, B. (2006). Pharmacological characterisation of agonists at $\delta$-containing $GABA_A$ receptors: $\delta$ determines the potency in heterotrimeric receptor complexes. *J. Pharmacol. Exp. Ther.* **316**, 1351–1359.

Sundström-Poromaa, I., Smith, D. H., Gong, Q. H., Sabado, T. N., Li, X., Light, A., Wiedmann, M., Williams, K., and Smith, S. S. (2002). Hormonally regulated $\alpha_4\beta_2\delta$ $GABA_A$ receptors are a target for alcohol. *Nat. Neurosci.* **5**, 721–722.

Sur, C., Farrar, S. J., Kerby, J., Whiting, P. J., Atack, J. R., and Mckernan, R. M. (1999). Preferential coassembly of $\alpha$4 and $\delta$ subunits of the $\gamma$-aminobutyric $acid_A$ receptor in rat thalamus. *Mol. Pharmacol.* **56**, 110–115.

Thomsen, C., and Ebert, B. (2002). Modulators of the $GABA_A$ receptor complex: Novel therapeutic aspects. *In* "Glutamate and GABA Receptors and Transporters: Structure, Function and Pharmacology" (J. Egebjerg, A. Schousboe, and P. Krogsgaard-Larsen, Eds.), pp. 407–427. Taylor & Francis, London.

Unwin, N. (1995). Acetylcholine receptor channel imaged in the open state. *Nature* **373**, 37–43.

Voss, J., Sánchez, C., Michelsen, S., and Ebert, B. (2003). Rotarod studies in the rat of the $GABA_A$ receptor agonist gaboxadol: Lack of ethanol potentiation and benzodiazepine cross-tolerance. *Eur. J. Pharmacol.* **482**, 215–222.

Wafford, K. A., Thompson, S. A., Thomas, D., Sikela, J., Wilcox, A. S., and Whiting, P. J. (1996). Functional characterization of human gamma-aminobutyric acidA receptors containing the alpha 4 subunit. *Mol. Pharmacol.* **50**, 670–678.

Wallner, M., Hanchar, H. J., and Olsen, R. W. (2003). Ethanol enhances $\alpha_4\beta_3\delta$ and $\alpha_6\beta_3\delta$ $\gamma$-aminobutyric acid type A receptors at low concentrations known to affect humans. *Proc. Natl. Acad. Sci. USA* **100**, 15218–15223.

Westh-Hansen, S. E., Witt, M. R., Dekermendjian, K., Liljefors, T., Rasmussen, P. B., and Nielsen, M. (1999). Arginine residue 120 of the human $GABA_A$ receptor alpha1, subunit is essential for GABA binding and chloride ion current gating. *Neuroreport* **10**, 2417–2421.

Wisden, W., Laurie, D. J., Monyer, H., and Seeburg, P. H. (1992). The distribution of 13 $GABA_A$ receptor subunit mRNAs in the rat brain. I. Telencephalon, diencephalon, mesencephalon. *J. Neurosci.* **12**, 1040–1062.

Zorn, S. H., and Enna, S. J. (1987). The GABA agonist THIP, attenuates antinociception in the mouse by modifying central cholinergic transmission. *Neuropharmacology* **26**, 433–437.

**Francine M. Benes* and Barbara Gisabella†**

*Program in Structural and Molecular Neuroscience
McLean Hospital, Belmont, Massachusetts

†Program in Neuroscience and Department of Psychiatry
Harvard Medical School, Belmont, Massachusetts

# Rat Modeling for GABA Defects in Schizophrenia

## I. Chapter Overview

Postmortem studies of schizophrenia conducted over the past 15 years have demonstrated alterations in various markers for the $\gamma$-aminobutyric acid (GABA) system that are consistent with a reduction of inhibitory modulation in the limbic lobe. These changes show a preferential distribution in layer II of the anterior cingulate cortex (ACCx) and sectors CA3 and CA2 of the hippocampus. Both of these sites receive a rich projection from the basolateral amygdala (BLa), and this has suggested this latter region might play a pivotal role in the induction of abnormalities in the limbic lobe of schizophrenics. To explore this possibility, a "partial" rodent model for neural circuitry abnormalities in schizophrenia has been applied to the study of limbic lobe circuitry in this disorder. When the $GABA_A$ receptor antagonist, picrotoxin (PICRO), is stereotaxically infused into the BLa of awake, freely moving rats, reductions in the number of GABA cells have been

*Advances in Pharmacology, Volume 54*

1054-3589/06 $35.00
DOI: 10.1016/S1054-3589(06)54004-9

induced in sectors CA3/2 but not CA1, pattern that is remarkably similar to that seen in schizophrenia. To explore whether these changes reflect functional alterations in the inhibitory modulation of the trisynaptic pathway, whole cell recordings in individual pyramidal cells have demonstrated a pronounced reduction of GABA currents in sectors CA3/2 but not CA1. These results suggest that this "partial" rat model for abnormal GABAergic integration within the trisynaptic pathway will provide a potentially powerful tool for studying the pathophysiology of schizophrenia and other psychotic disorders.

## II. Introduction

Neurons that express the compound, GABA, are broadly present throughout the central nervous system, although telencephalic structures, such as the cerebral cortex, show the most abundant quantities of this neurotransmitter (Jones, 1987). The GABAergic system has been implicated in the pathophysiology of schizophrenia and, more recently, bipolar disorder. In the discussion that follows, the evidence from postmortem studies of these two disorders will be reviewed. In the limbic lobe, consisting of the ACCx, hippocampal formation, and amygdala (AMYG), the GABA system may play a particularly important role in psychotic disorders. The postmortem findings from studies of this and other systems have suggested that there may be discrete loci within the limbic lobe where GABA cells are particularly disturbed. These have generated a "partial" rodent model in which projections from the AMYG to the anterior cingulate region and hippocampus are thought to play a central role in the pathophysiology of schizophrenia and its treatment with neuroleptic drugs.

### A. Postmortem Studies of Schizophrenia

Many postmortem studies of schizophrenia brain have focused their attention on the limbic lobe, a key component that probably contributes to the cognitive and emotional disturbances commonly seen in this disorder (Benes, 2000). Several histopathologic studies have shown that there are significant structural alterations in the *ACCx* and *hippocampus*. For example, several studies have reported abnormalities in layer II of ACCx in schizophrenia, and these are thought to be related to a developmental disturbance (Benes, 1988, 1993; Weinberger, 1987). These latter changes in schizophrenias have included smaller neuronal clusters separated by wider distances (Benes and Bird, 1987) and an increased density of vertical axons visualized with antibodies against both NFP200K (Benes and Bird, 1987) and glutamate (Benes *et al.*, 1992a). Taken together, these two studies suggested that schizophrenia might involve in an increased flow of excitatory activity into layers I and II of ACCx (Benes *et al.*, 1992a). Other studies have demonstrated in layer II a preferential decrease in the density of nonpyramidal neurons (Benes *et al.*, 1991), a marked increase of specific $GABA_A$ receptor binding on pyramidal cell bodies (Benes *et al.*, 1992b), and a reduction of cells expressing GAD mRNA (Akbarian *et al.*, 1995), changes that could be related to a disturbance in cell migration (Rakic, 1974) and/or specific afferents (Benes and Berretta, 2000b). The various anomalies noted in schizophrenia ACCx generated a working model in which two separate abnormalities were thought to occur: a decrease of GABAergic inhibitory activity in layer II (Benes *et al.*, 1992b) and an excessive glutamatergic inputs to layer I (Benes *et al.*, 1992a). Together, these alterations would tend to increase the firing of pyramidal neurons in ACCx, which, in turn, could produce excitotoxic effects both within ACCx itself and downstream in regions like hippocampus to which it projects (Benes, 1999). The model also predicts that there is a "mis-wiring" of DA afferents on intrinsic neurons in ACCx (Benes *et al.*, 1997). Some studies from other laboratories have been unable to demonstrate a reduction of nonpyramidal neurons in the cortex of schizophrenias (Akbarian *et al.*, 1995; Arnold *et al.*, 1995; Selemon *et al.*, 1995). It is noteworthy that the decrease in the numerical density ($N_d$) of nonpyramidal neurons appears to covary with affective disorder, rather than schizophrenia (Benes, 2001), calling into question whether this change is a significant feature of schizophrenia. As shown in Fig. 1, our other studies have also demonstrated an increase of DA inputs to interneurons in ACCx-II of schizophrenias (Benes *et al.*, 1997). Since DA fibers exert an inhibitory effect on follower cells (Retaux *et al.*, 1991a,b), a decrease of GABAergic activity in schizophrenia could nevertheless arise from such a "mis-wiring," whether or not there is an over loss of inhibitory interneurons (Baldessarini *et al.*, 1997). This could account for the compensatory upregulation of the $GABA_A$ receptor noted in ACCx-II of schizophrenias.

In hippocampus, shrinkage (Bogerts *et al.*, 1985), PN loss (Bogerts *et al.*, 1986; Falkai and Bogerts, 1986; Jeste and Lohr, 1989), as well as other cytoarchitectural changes (Altschuler *et al.*, 1987; Kovelman and Scheibel, 1984), such as decreased neuronal size (Arnold *et al.*, 1995; Benes, 1991; Zaidel *et al.*, 1997), have been reported and could theoretically be related to either a degenerative process or a neurodevelopmental disturbance (Arnold, 2000; Benes, 2000; Kovelman and Scheibel, 1984). Although there have been some studies that have failed to replicate the findings of neuronal loss in the hippocampus of schizophrenics (Arnold *et al.*, 1995; Benes, 1991; Heckers *et al.*, 1991), a more recent report has suggested that a discrete reduction in the number of nonpyramidal neurons may be present preferentially in sector CA2 of schizophrenias (Benes and Coyle, 1998). Other more discrete alterations of specific transmitter systems have also been observed in the hippocampus of schizophrenias. For example, a reduction of non-*N*-methyl-D-aspartate (NMDA) glutamate receptors, particularly the kainate

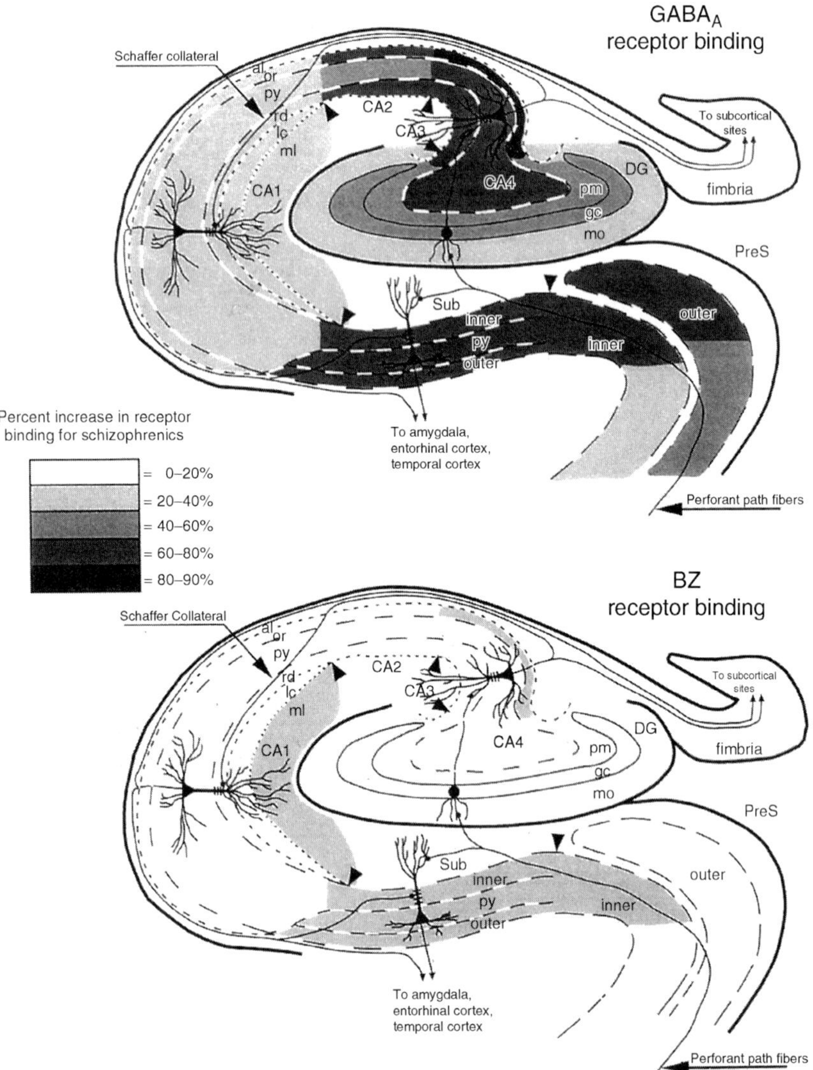


**FIGURE 1** Shadowgram showing percent increase of GABA$_A$ (upper) and BZ (lower) receptor binding activity in the hippocampus of schizophrenias vs cons. In schizophrenia subjects, there was a significant increase of GABA$_A$ receptor binding in sectors CA4, CA3, and CA2 but not in CA1. The BZ receptor did not show changes in regulation in schizophrenias, suggesting an uncoupling in the regulation of these two binding sites (Benes *et al.*, 1996).

subtype, has been observed in sectors CA4, 3, and 2 (Harrison *et al.*, 1991; Kerwin *et al.*, 1988, 1990; Porter *et al.*, 1997), as have a reduction of high affinity GABA reuptake (Reynolds *et al.*, 1990), increased GABA$_A$ receptor binding (Benes *et al.*, 1996) (Fig. 1) and a neuroleptic-dose–related increase of $GAD_{65}$-IR terminals (Todtenkopf and Benes, 1998). As with the non-NMDA receptors, the findings in these latter two studies were most significant in CA4, 3, and 2 but not in CA1; however, the most striking changes were in CA3/2. While typical inhibitory inputs to pyramidal neurons may be defective in CA1, a preferential increase of $GABA_A$ receptor binding has been found on nonpyramidal neurons in CA3, suggesting that *disinhibitory* activity may also be defective in this sector (Fig. 2). Other changes preferentially observed in sector CA2 of schizophrenias include a decrease of tyrosine hydroxylase- (TH-) immunoreactive (IR) varicosities (Todtenkopf and Benes, 1998) and a preferential decrease of IR for the $GluR_{5-7}$ subunits of the kainate receptor (Benes *et al.*, 2001b), both on pyramidal neurons. Most, if not all of these changes, have been associated directly or indirectly with GABAergic interneurons.

## B. Role of the Basolateral Amygdala in GABAergic Dysfunction

Why would preferential changes be observed in layer II of the anterior cingulate region and sectors CA3/CA2 of the hippocampus in schizophrenias? Several postmortem observations have pointed to the AMYG as a unifying factor that could account for this pattern (Benes *et al.*, 1992a; Longson *et al.*, 1996). The AMYG plays a pivotal role in the integration of emotional experience and the response to stress (Antoniadis and McDonald, 2000; Davis and Shi, 2000; LeDoux, 2000). It is differentiated into several nuclear subdivisions (Swanson and Petrovich, 1998) including the basolateral complex that provides a "massive" innervation to layer II in ACCx (Van Hoesen *et al.*, 1993), as well as CA3 and CA2 of the hippocampus (Pitkanen *et al.*, 2000). This latter projection passes through the stratum oriens of these sectors where we have noted the most pronounced changes in $GAD_{65}$-IR terminals (Todtenkopf and Benes, 1998) and $GABA_A$ receptor binding (Benes *et al.*, 1996) in schizophrenia and/or bipolar disorder. A rat model for neural circuitry changes in postmortem studies of schizophrenia and bipolar disorder has been developed (Benes and Berretta, 2000a). By injecting PICRO, an antagonist of the $GABA_A$ receptor into the basolateral nucleus (BLn), it has been possible to induce a reduction of GABAergic terminals preferentially in CA3 and CA2 but not in CA1. Changes of GABA cells in ACCx-II have also been noted in PICRO-treated rats. Taken together, this latter finding suggests that changes in the GABA system in hippocampus and ACCx of schizophrenias and bipolar disorder could be related, at least in part, to excessive discharges of excitatory activity from the AMYG.

The challenge now being faced by investigators who study schizophrenia is to define which cellular mechanism(s) may be contributing to the histopathologic changes reported to date in ACCx-II and hippocampus.

The trisynaptic pathway in normals vs schizophrenics

Normal control

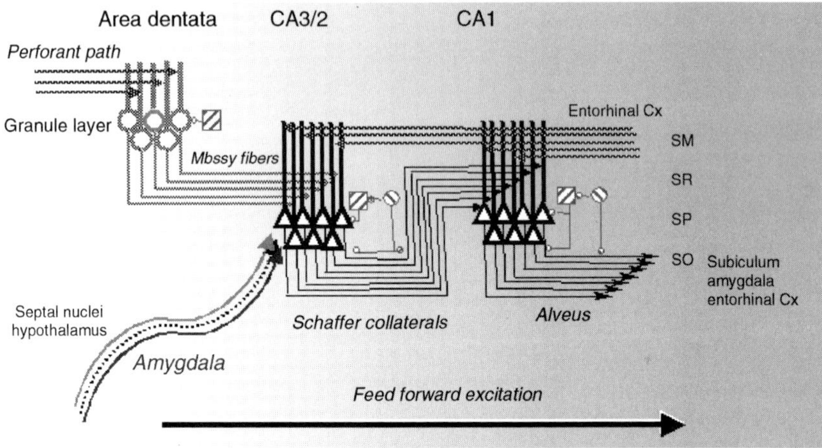


Schizophrenic

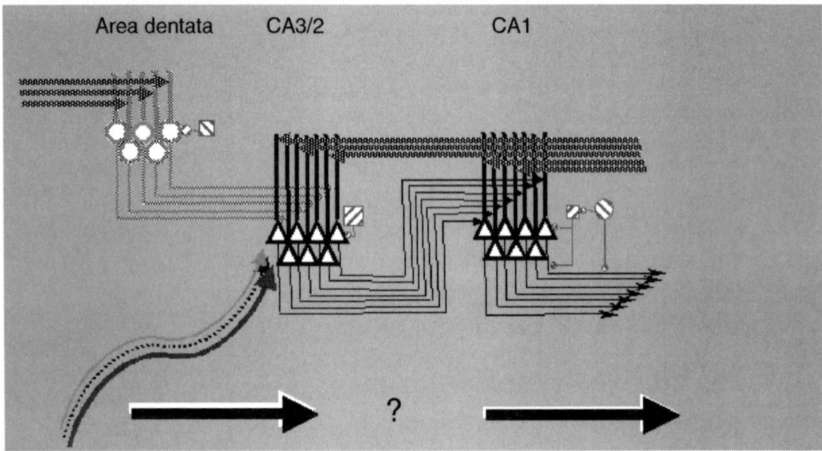


**FIGURE 2** Schematic diagram of the trisynaptic pathway in the hippocampusocampus of a normal control (upper) and schizophrenic (lower) subject. Perforant path fibers provide an excitatory input to dentate gyrus granule cells and the latter, in turn, send an excitatory input to the stratum radiatum-lacunosum of sector CA3. The pyramidal cells in this sector are modulated by both inhibitory and disinhibitory GABAergic interneurons, as excitatory activity is conveyed along Schaffer collater fibers that course toward rad of sector CA1, where they provide an excitatory input to pyramidal neurons of this sector. There is a progressive feed forward increase of excitation as the activity progresses toward CA1, and this is represented by the gradient of background shading. In the schizophrenic circuit, GABA cell dysfunction is present in CA3, and this causes an increase of excitatory activity flowing toward CA1 and a general increase in baseline levels of metabolic activity indicated by the loss of the feed forward

## C. Discrete Loci for Abnormalities in Postmortem Studies of Schizophrenia

Many lines of evidence indicate that emotionally stimulated learning and memory processing in the hippocampus is modulated by the AMYG (LeDoux, 1992; Nakao *et al.*, 2004). Projections from the amygdaloid complex reach several hippocampal regions, providing various routes by which it may potentially influence hippocampal function (Aggleton, 1986; Krettek and Price, 1977). Reports suggest that inputs from the AMYG to the hippocampus via two separate pathways, the indirect perforant path and the direct pathway to CA2/CA3, are responsible for alteration of the circuitry in CA4, CA3, CA2, and to a lesser extent in CA1 (Benes and Berretta, 2001; Berretta *et al.*, 2001). Electrical stimulation of the BLa in anesthetized rats generates synaptic potentials in the dentate gyrus of the hippocampus, indicating that they are connected through neuronal projections (Abe, 2001). In addition, emotional experiences are shown to activate the BLa, which in turn either enhances or impairs hippocampal long-term potentiation (LTP) (Akirav and Richter-Levin, 1999; Frey *et al.*, 2001; Mesches *et al.*, 1999). Direct evidence demonstrating that neuronal inputs from the AMYG modulate hippocampal synaptic plasticity has come from lesions in the basolateral nucleus of the amygdala (BLa) that result in decrease of LTP in rat hippocampus (Abe, 2001).

In the past 10 years, several studies have suggested that the relationship between the BLa and hippocampus may also contribute to the pathophysiology of schizophrenia (Dolan, 2002; Kim *et al.*, 2001; Richardson *et al.*, 2004). For example, brain imaging studies have demonstrated volume reductions in both regions of schizophrenics (Lawrie and Abukmeil, 1998). Moreover, several postmortem studies have pointed to a deficit of GABAergic activity in schizophrenia in cortical areas (Benes *et al.*, 2000, 2001a; Costa *et al.*, 2003, 2004) as well as subcortical areas, particularly hippocampal sectors, CA3 and CA2, which receive abundant projections from the BLa (Benes, 2000; Benes and Berretta, 2000a). There is also a report showing direct evidence of a decrease of high-affinity GABA uptake in the AMYG of the postmortem schizophrenic brain (Reynolds *et al.*, 1990). It has been postulated that these changes might induce an increased outflow of excitatory activity from the AMYG to the hippocampus and induce alterations of its intrinsic neural circuitry, particularly in GABAergic interneurons (Benes and Berretta, 2000a). Such changes could potentially influence LTP (Akirav and Richter-Levin, 2002; Ikegaya *et al.*, 1996), which may

---

gradient. The AMYG is shown sending excitatory afferents directly to CA3 and this is postulated to be increased in schizophrenics and possibly related to the GABA cell dysfunction. This model is consistent with PET scanning studies in which schizophrenics have been found to have an increase of baseline metabolic activity in the hippocampus. (See Color Insert.)

contribute to emotional learning during adolescence, the period when the schizophrenia phenotype is first manifest. To test this hypothesis, we have developed a "partial" rodent model in which a low, nonepileptogenic dose of PICRO, a noncompetitive antagonist of the $GABA_A$ receptor, is infused into the BLa to decrease GABAergic activity and increase the flow of excitatory activity to the hippocampus (Berretta *et al.*, 2001, 2004). With this "partial" model, it has been possible to generate changes in GABA cells similar to those reported in postmortem microscopic analyses of the hippocampus in schizophrenia (Berretta *et al.*, 2004).

As a general rule, it is not possible to study connectivity of corticolimbic networks in human brain since traditional tract tracing techniques cannot be employed. It is useful to consider how the postmortem findings concerning the circuitry within the hippocampus (Benes, 1999) might be related to the entorhinal cortex and BLa. As shown in Fig. 2, the trisynaptic pathway consists of: (1) perforant fibers from the entorhinal cortex that project to the area dentata; (2) mossy fibers from the granule cells of the area dentata that project to the stratum radiatum (rad) of CA3; and (3) Schaffer collaterals of pyramidal cells in CA3 that project to the rad of CA1. There are intrinsic GABAergic interneurons throughout the hippocampal formation (Fig. 2) that provide inhibitory modulation of the pyramidal cells. Many of these GABA neurons also send collateral branches that form disinhibitory connections with other GABA cells. The neuropathological and clinical observations described in the previous section are consistent with a model that predicts that an impairment of GABAergic function would be associated with an overall increase of excitation in the hippocampus (Fig. 2, lower panel). This model is noteworthy because it suggests that schizophrenics might show a deficit of not only inhibitory but also disinhibitory integration in CA3 (Benes, 1999). If this assumption were correct, an overall increase in the level of hippocampal activation, like that observed in schizophrenic subjects by Heckers *et al.* (1998), would be predicted to occur. As suggested in Fig. 2, these changes would likely bear some relationship to increased excitatory activity generated in the AMYG and entering the hippocampus either directly via the CA3 or indirectly from the AMYG via the entorhinal cortex. It might be expected from the previous discussion that the increased activation from the AMYG and, by inference, the entorhinal cortex could increase further the overall level of activation detected in the hippocampus using PET scanning and perhaps even be the primary cause of it.

As discussed previously, postmortem evidence from the study of schizophrenia has suggested that there may be a decreased number of interneurons in sector CA2 (Benes *et al.*, 1998) and those present in CA3 may be receiving a diminished GABA-to-GABA input (Benes *et al.*, 1996). The net effect of such a change would be a set of GABA cells in stratum pyramidale of CA3 with an unfettered ability to inhibit the pyramidal cells of CA3. Such an effect could hypothetically result in a decreased flow of activity along the

Schaffer collaterals projecting to CA1. It is noteworthy, although, that this proposed defect could potentially be compensated for in the stratum oriens, where the basal dendrites of pyramidal neurons receive a significant decrease of inhibitory modulation by GABAergic neurons in schizophrenics. Although the effect of GABA inputs directly to the neuronal cell bodies in the stratum pyramidale would tend to be more potent than that received via the basal dendrites in the stratum oriens, it is difficult to predict with certainty what pattern (i.e., disinhibitory vs inhibitory) might prevail in this sector. More precise information regarding the relative distribution of these changes in schizophrenia is needed. In CA1, on the other hand, there is no decrease of interneurons, and a modest upregulation of the $GABA_A$ receptor was observed only on pyramidal cells. This latter arrangement suggests that there may be small decrease of inhibitory modulation flowing from interneurons to projection cells in CA1.

An important component of the model shown in Fig. 2 is the implication that there might be an increase of activity flowing into the hippocampus from the AMYG and entorhinal region. As discussed previously, there is a direct projection from the caudal portion of the parvocellular subdivision of the basolateral nuclear complex of the AMYG to sector CA3 via the stratum oriens (Pitkanen *et al.*, 2000). A series of studies has demonstrated that infusion of a specific $GABA_A$ antagonist, PICRO, into this locus results in a rapid decrease in the density of $GAD_{65}$ and $GAD_{67}$-IR terminals in sectors CA3 and CA2 but not in CA1 (Berretta *et al.*, 2001). Since this same subdivision of the basolateral complex also sends an abundant projection to layer II of the ACCx (personal observation), it seems plausible that this hippocampal input could potential play a pivotal role in the pathophysiology of schizophrenia.

The results described previously demonstrate that disinhibition of neurons in the AMYG results in acute and selective changes in the density of GABAergic terminals in sectors $CA_{3/2}$ of the hippocampus. While changes in GAD-IR terminals were confined to $CA_3$ and $CA_2$, increases in the density of $GAD_{67}$-IR neuronal somata were observed in the $CA_4$ and the dentate gyrus. Overall, these results are consistent with the hypothesis that amygdalar activation can selectively affect specific subcircuits within the GABAergic system of the hippocampus.

## III. Rodent Model for Postmortem Findings in Schizophrenia

### A. Modeling for Reductions of GABAergic Interneurons

We have developed a rodent model for exploring whether an increased flow of excitatory activity from the AMYG could potentially account for the changes in the hippocampal GABA system seen in schizophrenia.

Our strategy has been to dissect out, from a complex network of corticolimbic circuitry, one potential source of abnormal afferent activity to the hippocampus and to use selective pharmacological manipulation as a way of inducing changes similar to those reported from the postmortem studies described previously. Toward this end, activation of the BLa has been induced using local intraparenchymal infusion of the $GABA_A$ receptor antagonist PICRO in awake, freely moving rats. Changes in the density of $GAD_{65}$- and $GAD_{67}$-(IR) somata and terminals have been used as an index of the response of the hippocampal GABA system to amygdalar activation. To our knowledge, this is the first study in the field of schizophrenia research in which a rodent model, other than those addressing neuroleptic effects (Eastwood and Harrison, 1999; Harrison, 1999), has been used to induce microscopic changes similar to those described in our postmortem investigations of schizophrenia.

As predicted, changes in both $GAD_{67}$- and $GAD_{65}$-IR terminals were detected on pyramidal neurons in both $CA_3$ and $CA_2$. This observation suggests that GABAergic interneurons affected by the AMYG might be those that make axo-somatic contacts with the neurons giving origin to the Schaffer collaterals. Ultimately those changes would impact on the flow of activity to sector $CA_1$ and on the resulting hippocampal output. A strikingly common feature among many hippocampal findings in postmortem schizophrenic brain is their prevalence for sectors $CA_3$ and $CA_2$ but not in $CA_1$ (Benes, 1999). This preferential localization is compelling when changes in hippocampal interneurons, and/or markers for the GABAergic system, are considered. For example, a reduction in nonpyramidal neurons was detected exclusively in $CA_2$ (Benes *et al.*, 1998) and increases in GABA receptor binding were found to be most intense in stratum oriens of $CA_3$ (Benes *et al.*, 1996). In a study in which $GAD_{65}$-IR terminals were measured, a lower density was found in stratum pyramidale in $CA_4$ and $CA_3$ and in stratum oriens of $CA_3$ and $CA_2$ of neuroleptic-free schizophrenics (Todtenkopf and Benes, 1998). Although there were only two subjects who had not received antipsychotic medication, a strong positive correlation between dose of neuroleptic and density of $GAD_{65}$-terminals was found on neuronal somata of $CA_3$ and $CA_4$, and in the stratum oriens of $CA_3$ and $CA_2$. Consistent with the general trend of this and other studies (see earlier), $CA_1$ showed no changes. Although the mechanism underlying these alterations in GABA terminals is not known, chronic haloperidol administration has been associated with a marked increase of GABA terminals in rat medial prefrontal cortex (Vincent *et al.*, 1994). It seems likely, however, that differences in connectivity might be responsible, at least in part, for the selectivity of these changes across the hippocampal sectors.

A key question that the findings obtained with the rat model for neural circuitry changes in postmortem studies of schizophrenia is whether they are accompanied by significant reductions in GABAergic activity. To explore this question, we have used single cell recording techniques (patch clamping) to measure the response of hippocampal pyramidal cells to amygdalar activation with PICRO infusion. These results are described in the next section.

## B. Using the "Partial" Model to Determine Functional Correlates of GABA Cell Anomalies

Using gene expression profiling, we have demonstrated that acute administration of PICRO in the BLa results in an upregulation of the M1, M2, and M3 cholinergic receptor subtypes (Benes *et al.*, 2004). The septo-hippocampal cholinergic fiber system ramifies extensively throughout the hippocampus formation and probably releases acetylcholine on these and other muscarinic receptor subtypes (Birdsall *et al.*, 1988; Dean *et al.*, 2003; Levey *et al.*, 1991; Smith *et al.*, 1988). This cholinergic system is believed to exert a strong influence on synaptic transmission and cellular excitability within hippocampal circuitry (de Sevilla *et al.*, 2002; Vogt and Regehr, 2001; Yun *et al.*, 2000) and may even modulate information processing via GABA inhibitory networks (Alreja *et al.*, 2000; Liu *et al.*, 1998; Wu *et al.*, 2000), like the ones that are postulated to be dysfunctional in schizophrenia (Bymaster *et al.*, 1999, 2003). The M1 subtype is the most abundant muscarinic receptor on pyramidal neurons in the hippocampus (Fornari *et al.*, 2000; Levey *et al.*, 1995; Marino *et al.*, 1998) and may potentially represent an important target for developing new strategies to treat this disorder. Studies in which M1 muscarinic receptor knockout mice have been employed have demonstrated a fundamental role of this receptor in cognition and, by inference, in schizophrenia (Liao *et al.*, 2003).

### 1. Activation of M3/M3 Receptors Increases LTP in CA1 and CA3 Area in the Rodent Model of Schizophrenia

As previously described (Gisabella *et al.*, 2005), we stereotaxically infused PICRO or saline (SAL) in rat BLa through over a period of 45 min and sacrificed the rats 96 h later. LTP was recorded following high-frequency stimulation (HFS) in rad of sectors CA1 and CA3 in a hippocampal slice preparation. Based on our earlier gene expression profiling study showing an upregulation of the M1 and M3 muscarinic receptors in PICRO-treated rats (Benes *et al.*, 2004), we investigated the possible modulatory role of the M1 agonist (McN-A-343) and the M1/M3 agonist (carbachol) on LTP (Cheong *et al.*, 2001; Yun *et al.*, 2000) in the hippocampus of rats receiving PICRO infusion in the BLa. After perfusing the hippocampal slices with the N6 M1/M3 receptor agonists (Anagnostaras *et al.*, 2003; Leung *et al.*, 2003) and applying tetanic stimulation, PICRO-treated rats showed an increased amplitude of LTP in sectors CA3 and CA1.

Hippocampal slices were infused with the M1 agonist, McN-A-343. LTP recorded from sector CA1 showed no significant effect of M1 receptor stimulation in either PICRO- or SAL-treated rats. In contrast, sector CA3 showed a marked decrease of LTP amplitude in control rats, but this inhibition was removed in the PICRO-treated animals ($P = 0.0005$) (Fig. 3D, C, and E, respectively). These last results also show how LTP is differentially regulated by the muscarinic system in these two hippocampal areas by amygdalar activation. Taken all together these data indicate that cholinergic input coming from M3 and M1 receptors facilitates synaptic plasticity in a model representing a GABA dysfunction in schizophrenia.

## 2. Quantification of Inhibitory GABA Currents

Using whole-cell recording techniques (Fig. 4) in the schizophrenia "partial" model, GABA currents have been measured in rat hippocampal slices. With a stimulating electrode placed in the rad, inhibitory postsynaptic currents (IPSCs) have been recorded in pyramidal cells in the CA3 and CA1 areas in hippocampal slices from both PICRO- and SAL-treated rats. Pyramidal neurons were distinguished from interneurons based on their morphological appearance and their ability to show spike frequency adaptation to a prolonged depolarizing current injection (Fig. 4). To isolate GABA currents, glutamatergic synaptic transmission was blocked by the NMDA receptor antagonist D-AP-5 (50 μM) and the α-amino-3-hydroxy-5-methyl-4-isoxazolepropionic acid (AMPA) receptor antagonist CNQX (20 μM) at a holding potential of −70 mV (Tsvetkov *et al.*, 2004). The input/output curves of the GABA IPSCs were obtained by recording 10–15 responses and averaging the recordings for each stimulation intensity tested. When the intensity of stimulation is gradually increased from a threshold stimulus (determined for each individual experiment), IPSCs of increasing amplitude can be induced. Statistical analyses of the input–output curves revealed that a significant decrease of GABA IPSCs occurred in sectors CA1 ($P = 0.037$) and CA3 ($P = 0.029$) of PICRO-treated rats when compared to SAL-treated rats (Fig. 5A and B). The observed decreases in the level of feed-forward GABAergic inhibition of principal neurons were more pronounced in sector CA3 than in CA1.

Spontaneous inhibitory postsynaptic currents (sIPSCs) were also used to test whether infusion of PICRO in the BLa can result in changes in the level of tonic inhibition in hippocampal neurons. The sIPSCs were recorded in hippocampal pyramidal neurons at a holding potential of −70 mV in the presence of D-APV and CNQX to abolish the contribution of glutamatergic inputs. The sIPSCs recorded under these conditions were completely blocked by PICRO (50 μM) in the bath, confirming that they are mediated by $GABA_A$ receptors. No change in the frequency of events (sIPSCs) was observed in PICRO-treated rats when compared to the SAL-treated group. The mean amplitude of sIPSCs was significantly decreased in CA3

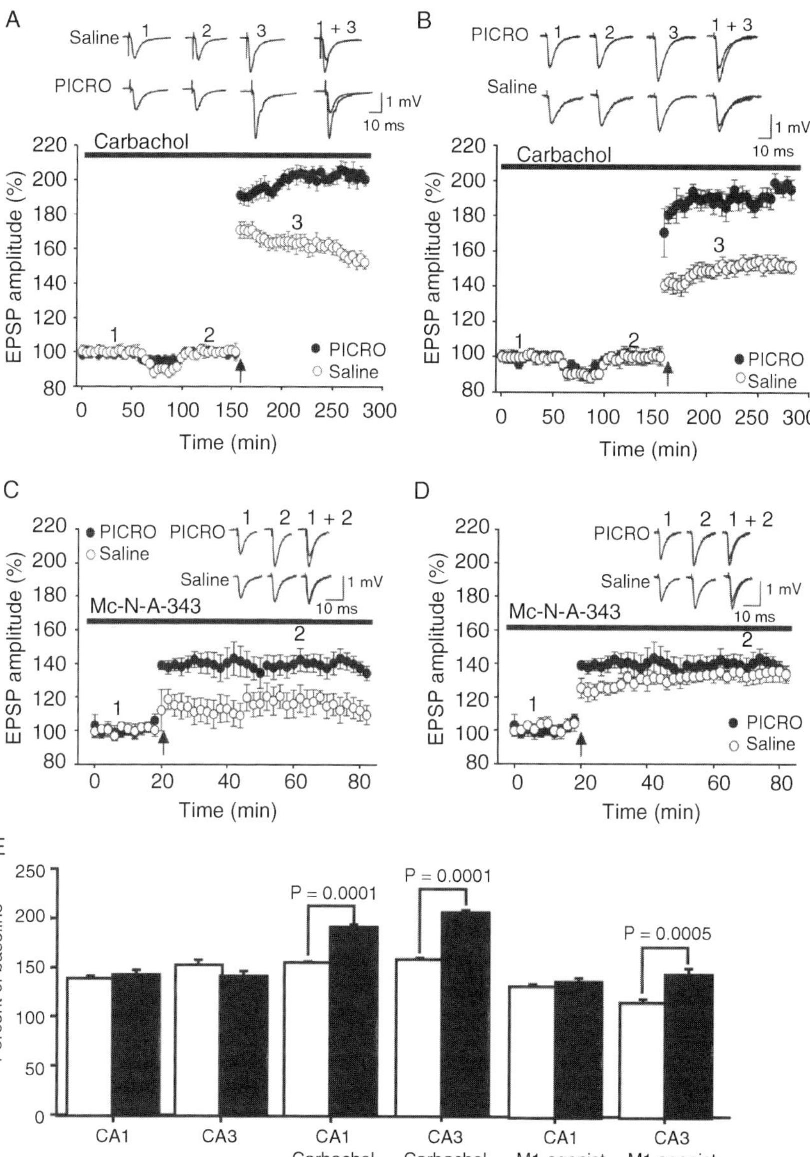


**FIGURE 3** Induction of LTP in the presence of carbachol binding in rats with a blockade of GABA activity in the BLa shifts synaptic plasticity toward higher amplitude in sectors CA3 and CA1, while application of Mc-N-A-343 resulted in a higher level of LTP amplitude only in sector CA3. Representative recordings of EPSP slopes before and after tetanus delivery are shown in the top graphs. (A and B) Continuous bath application of carbachol binding in CA3 and CA1 area increased LTP amplitude in PICRO-treated rats compared to control ($P = 0.0001$). (C) Continuous bath perfusion of Mc-N-A-343 in CA3 area induced potentiation of synaptic plasticity in PICRO-treated rats.

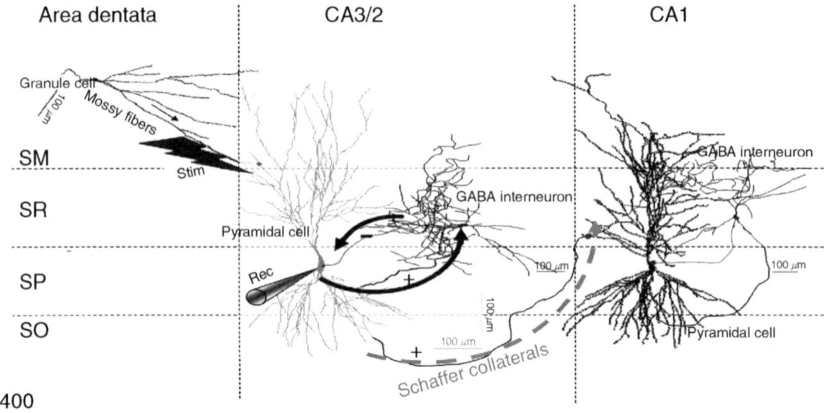


**FIGURE 4** Schematic diagram representing the position of the stimulator (Stim) and recording (Rec) electrodes on a pyramidal neuron stimulated by mossy fibers and inhibited by GABA interneurons. Pyramidal cells, in turn, activate other cells through Schaffer collaterals and their dendrites (Camera lucida drawing of pyramidal neuron and interneurons courtesy of Duke-Southampton archive; see http://www.cns.soton.ac.uk/~iachad/cellArchive). (See Color Insert.)

($P = 0.0009$) as evidenced by a significant shift of amplitude toward smaller events, while CA1 did not show any changes.

## IV. Commentary

Based on postmortem studies over the past 15 years, a decrease of GABAergic cells and/or activity has been postulated to occur in the limbic lobe of patients with schizophrenia. The latter studies have specifically pointed to two principal sites where changes in this and other neurotransmitter systems are present in this disorder. These sites include layer II of the ACCx and sectors CA3/2 of the hippocampus. Using a rodent model for altered neural circuitry in postmortem studies of schizophrenia, PICRO has been infused in the BLa. This has resulted in a decrease of GABA-mediated inhibition of principal neurons, particularly in sector CA3 and, to a much lesser degree in CA1 (Benes, 2000). Based on more experiments, reductions in the number of GABAergic neurons in CA3 appears to be accompanied by a marked reduction of GABA currents in pyramidal neurons of this sector but not in CA1. Taken together, these electrophysiological studies suggest that the "partial" rodent model has construct validity. Specifically, these results suggest that changes in the GABA system in postmortem studies and in those reproduced using the rodent model probably reflect a reduction in the amount of inhibitory modulation that is generated in the hippocampus of patients with schizophrenia. These results are consistent with a PET scanning study that demonstrated an increase in the basal metabolic activity

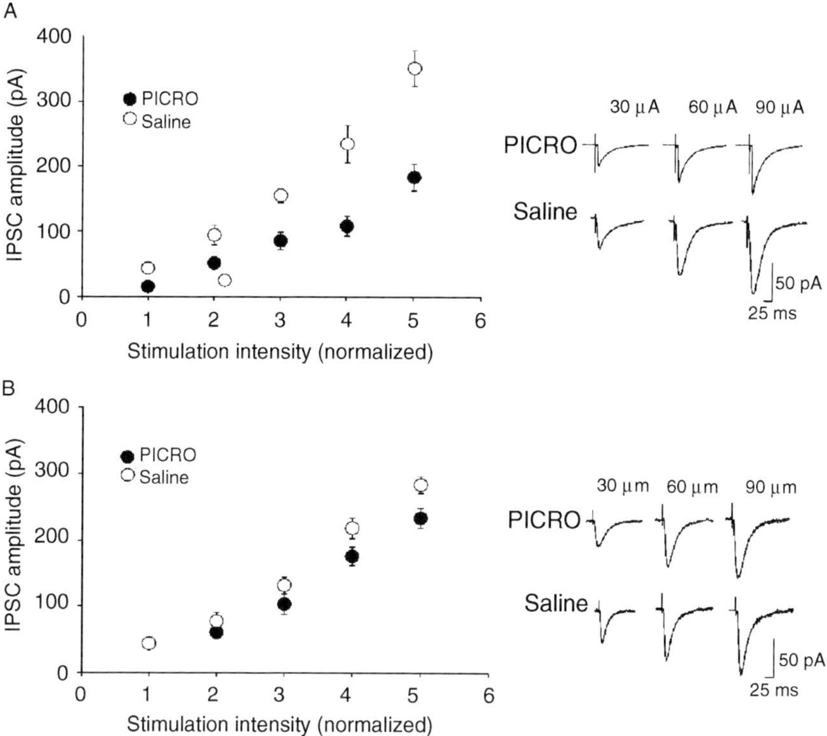


**FIGURE 5** GABA IPSCs evoked by different stimulus intensities showed decreased levels of IPSCs amplitude in both CA3 and CA1 in PICRO-treated rats compared to control. Input/output curves of the GABA IPSCs obtained by recording 10–15 responses averaged for each stimulation intensity tested. The intensity of stimulation was gradually increased from the threshold stimulus determined in each individual experiment, with an increment of 25 μA, to produce IPSCs of increasing amplitude. IPSCs evoked current exhibited a decreased ($P = 0.029$) (A) amplitude level in PICRO-treated rats, which was higher in CA3 compared to CA1 ($P = 0.037$) (B). Sample traces of IPSCs (right panel) showing unitary responses elicited at 30-, 60-, and 90-μA stimulus intensity.

in the hippocampus of patients with schizophrenia. Additionally, it will be useful to characterize prepulse inhibition (PPI) with acoustic startle. As noted previously, it has been postulated that the abnormalities seen in schizophrenia may be due to reduction of inhibitory modulation in a central filtering mechanism. If changes in PPI similar to those observed in schizophrenia can be induced with the "partial" rodent model, it would suggest that this model may also have predictive validity.

The electrophysiological changes observed in the hippocampal slice preparations obtained from SAL- and PICRO-treated rats could involve both presynaptic and postsynaptic elements, an idea that is in accordance with the demonstration that the BLa is capable of inducing changes in GABAergic axon terminals as well as second messengers and receptors

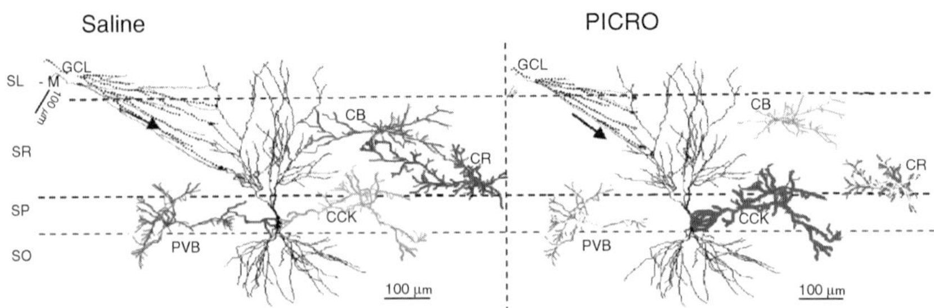


**FIGURE 6** Schematic diagram representing changes in various subtypes of GABAergic interneuron in the hippocampus of rats exposed to amygdalar activation in the rat model. Normally, the hippocampus contains at least four different subtypes of GABA cell defined by the presence of various peptides in the cytoplasm, including parvalbumin (PVB), calbinding (CB), calretinin (CR), and cholecystokinin (CCK). These cells provide inhibitory modulation of pyramidal cells at the level of the cell somata (PVB and CCK) and the dendritic tree (CB and CR). Rats receiving PICRO infusions in the BLa show a significant reduction of PVB-, CB-, and CR-containing interneurons. Those containing CCK show an increase of inhibitory terminals on the somata of pyramidal neurons. (See Color Insert.)

(Benes, 2000). The current finding confirms postmortem studies, which suggest a deficit of GABAergic activity associated with a decrease in high-affinity GABA uptake sites in schizophrenia subjects (Benes *et al.*, 1996) and the expression of mRNA for the 65-kDa isoform of glutamate decarboxylase (Heckers *et al.*, 2002), although the latter showed more pronounced reductions in bipolar subjects than in schizophrenics. The observed decrease in sIPSC amplitude, in the present work, complements previous human studies showing a compensatory upregulation of the $GABA_A$ receptor in the hippocampus of schizophrenics (Todtenkopf and Benes, 1998) and may therefore derive from a variety of pre- and/or postsynaptic factors, such as the GABA content of synaptic vesicles, that appears to be decreased in PICRO-treated rats. This decrease of GABA current in the rodent model of schizophrenia represents the first electrophysiological evidence of a deficit in hippocampal GABA activity in this disorder. Additionally, these findings are also consistent with a PET imaging study showing increased levels of metabolic activity in the hippocampus of schizophrenic subjects at baseline conditions and during auditory hallucinations (Heckers *et al.*, 1998). Understanding the influence of the BLa on the synaptic plasticity of GABAergic elements in the hippocampus may be beneficial in helping to develop novel pharmacological strategies for the treatment of schizophrenia and other psychotic disorders (Costa *et al.*, 2005; Guidotti *et al.*, 2005; Hyman and Fenton, 2003).

## Acknowledgments

This work was supported by grants from the National Institutes of Health (MH62822) and the generosity of Menachem and Carmella Abraham, John and Virginia Taplin.

## References


Abe, K. (2001). Modulation of hippocampal long-term potentiation by the amygdala: A synaptic mechanism linking emotion and memory. *Jpn. J. Pharmacol.* **86**, 18–22.

Aggleton, J. P. (1986). A description of the amygdalo-hippocampal interconnections in the macaque monkey. *Exp. Brain Res.* **64**, 515–526.

Akbarian, S., Kim, J. J., Potkin, S. G., Hagman, J. O., Tafazzoli, A., Bunney, W. E., and Jones, E. G. (1995). Gene expression for glutamic acid decarboxylase is reduced without loss of neurons in prefrontal cortex of schizophrenics. *Arch. Gen. Psychiatry* **52**, 258–278.

Akirav, I., and Richter-Levin, G. (1999). Biphasic modulation of hippocampal plasticity by behavioral stress and basolateral amygdala stimulation in the rat. *J. Neurosci.* **19**, 10530–10535.

Akirav, I., and Richter-Levin, G. (2002). Mechanisms of amygdala modulation of hippocampal plasticity. *J. Neurosci.* **22**, 9912–9921.

Alreja, M., Wu, M., Liu, W., Atkins, J. B., Leranth, C., and Shanabrough, M. (2000). Muscarinic tone sustains impulse flow in the septohippocampal GABA but not cholinergic pathway: Implications for learning and memory. *J. Neurosci.* **20**, 8103–8110.

Altschuler, L. L., Conrad, A., Kovelman, J., and Scheibel, A. (1987). Hippocampal pyramidal cell orientation in schizophrenia. A controlled neurohistology study of the Yakovlev collection. *Arch. Gen. Psychiat.* **44**, 1689–1701.

Anagnostaras, S. G., Murphy, G. G., Hamilton, S. E., Mitchell, S. L., Rahnama, N. P., Nathanson, N. M., and Silva, A. J. (2003). Selective cognitive dysfunction in acetylcholine M1 muscarinic receptor mutant mice. *Nat. Neurosci.* **6**, 51–58.

Antoniadis, E. A., and McDonald, R. J. (2000). Amygdala, hippocampus and discriminative fear conditioning to context. *Behav. Brain Res.* **108**, 1–19.

Arnold, S. E. (2000). "Hippocampal Pathology," pp. 57–80. Oxford University Press, Oxford, UK.

Arnold, S. E., Franz, B. R., Gur, R. C., Gur, R. E., Shapiro, R. M., Moberg, P. J., and Trojanowski, J. Q. (1995). Smaller neuron size in schizophrenia in hippocampal subfields that mediate cortical-hippocampal interactions. *Am. J. Psychiatry* **152**, 738–748.

Baldessarini, R. J., Hegarty, J. D., Bird, E. D., and Benes, F. M. (1997). Meta-analysis of postmortem studies of Alzheimer's disease-like neuropathology in schizophrenia. *Am. J. Psychiatry* **154**, 861–863.

Benes, F., and Coyle, J. T. (1998). Deja vu all over again. *Biol. Psychiatry* **43**, 781–782.

Benes, F. M. (1988). Post-mortem structural analyses of schizophrenic brain: Study designs and the interpretation of data. *Psychiatr. Dev.* **6**, 213–226.

Benes, F. M. (1991). Evidence for neurodevelopment disturbances in anterior cingulate cortex of post-mortem schizophrenic brain. *Schizophr. Res.* **5**, 187–188.

Benes, F. M. (1993). Neurobiological investigations in cingulate cortex of schizophrenic brain. *Schizophr. Bull.* **19**, 537–549.

Benes, F. M. (1999). Alterations of neural circuitry within layer II of anterior cingulate cortex in schizophrenia. *J. Psychiatr. Res.* **33**, 511–512.

Benes, F. M. (2000). Emerging principles of altered neural circuitry in schizophrenia. *Brain Res. Brain Res. Rev.* **31**, 251–269.

Benes, F. M. (2001). Carlsson and the discovery of dopamine. *Trends Pharmacol. Sci.* **22**, 46–47.

Benes, F. M., and Bird, E. D. (1987). An analysis of the arrangement of neurons in the cingulate cortex of schizophrenic patients. *Arch. Gen. Psychiatry* **44**, 608–616.

Benes, F. M., and Berretta, S. (2000a). Amygdalo-entorhinal inputs to the hippocampal formation in relation to schizophrenia. *Ann. NY Acad. Sci.* **911**, 293–304.

Benes, F. M., and Berretta, S. (2000b). Amygdalo-entorhinal inputs to the hippocampal formation in relation to schizophrenia. *Ann. NY Acad. Sci.* **911**, 293–304.

Benes, F. M., and Berretta, S. (2001). GABAergic interneurons: Implications for understanding schizophrenia and bipolar disorder. *Neuropsychopharmacology* **25**, 1–27.

Benes, F. M., McSparren, J., Bird, E. D., SanGiovanni, J. P., and Vincent, S. L. (1991). Deficits in small interneurons in prefrontal and cingulate cortices of schizophrenic and schizoaffective patients. *Arch. Gen. Psychiatry* **48**, 996–1001.

Benes, F. M., Sorensen, I., Vincent, S. L., Bird, E. D., and Sathi, M. (1992a). Increased density of glutamate-immunoreactive vertical processes in superficial laminae in cingulate cortex of schizophrenic brain. *Cereb. Cortex* **2**, 503–512.

Benes, F. M., Vincent, S. L., Alsterberg, G., Bird, E. D., and SanGiovanni, J. P. (1992b). Increased $GABA_A$ receptor binding in superficial layers of cingulate cortex in schizophrenics. *J. Neurosci.* **12**, 924–929.

Benes, F. M., Khan, Y., Vincent, S. L., and Wickramasinghe, R. (1996). Differences in the subregional and cellular distribution of $GABA_A$ receptor binding in the hippocampal formation of schizophrenic brain. *Synapse* **22**, 338–349.

Benes, F. M., Todtenkopf, M. S., and Taylor, J. B. (1997). Differential distribution of tyrosine hydroxylase fibers on small and large neurons in layer II of anterior cingulate cortex of schizophrenic brain. *Synapse* **25**, 80–92.

Benes, F. M., Kwok, E. W., Vincent, S. L., and Todtenkopf, M. S. (1998). A reduction of nonpyramidal cells in sector CA2 of schizophrenics and manic depressives (see comments). *Biol. Psychiatry* **44**, 88–97.

Benes, F. M., Todtenkopf, M. S., Logiotatos, P., and Williams, M. (2000). Glutamate decarboxylase(65)-immunoreactive terminals in cingulate and prefrontal cortices of schizophrenic and bipolar brain. *J. Chem. Neuroanat.* **20**, 259–269.

Benes, F. M., Vincent, S. L., and Todtenkopf, M. (2001a). The density of pyramidal and nonpyramidal neurons in anterior cingulate cortex of schizophrenic and bipolar subjects. *Biol. Psychiatry* **50**, 395.

Benes, F. M., Todtenkopf, M. S., and Kostoulakos, P. (2001b). GluR5,6,7 subunit immunoreactivity on apical pyramidal cell dendrites in hippocampus of schizophrenics and manic depressives. *Hippocampus* **11**, 482–491.

Benes, F. M., Burke, R. E., Walsh, J., Berretta, S., Matzilevich, D., Minns, M., and Konradi, C. (2004). Acute amygdalar activation induces an upregulation of multiple monoamine G protein coupled pathways in rat hippocampus. *Mol. Psychiatry* **9**, 895, 932–945.

Berretta, S., Munno, D. W., and Benes, F. M. (2001). Amygdalar activation alters the hippocampal GABA system: "Partial" modelling for postmortem changes in schizophrenia. *J. Comp. Neurol.* **431**, 129–138.

Berretta, S., Lange, N., Bhattacharyya, S., Sebro, R., Garces, J., and Benes, F. M. (2004). Long-term effects of amygdala GABA receptor blockade on specific subpopulations of hippocampal interneurons. *Hippocampus* **14**, 876–894.

Birdsall, N. J., Curtis, C. A., Eveleigh, P., Hulme, E. C., Pedder, E. K., Poyner, D., and Wheatley, M. (1988). Muscarinic receptor subtypes and the selectivity of agonists and antagonists. *Pharmacology* **37**(Suppl. 1), 22–31.

Bogerts, B., Meertz, E., and Schonfeldt-Bausch, R. (1985). Basal ganglia and limbic system pathology in schizophrenia. A morphometric study of brain volume and shrinkage. *Arch. Gen. Psychiatry* **42**, 784–791.

Bogerts, B., Falkai, P., and Tutsch, J. (1986). Cell numbers in the pallidum and hippocampus of schizophrenics. *In* "Biol. Psychiatry" (S. Cea, Ed.), pp. 1178–1180. Elsevier Press, Amsterdam.

Bymaster, F. P., Shannon, H. E., Rasmussen, K., DeLapp, N. W., Ward, J. S., Calligaro, D. O., Mitch, C. H., Whitesitt, C., Ludvigsen, T. S., Sheardown, M., Swedberg, M., Rasmussen, T., *et al.* (1999). Potential role of muscarinic receptors in schizophrenia. *Life Sci.* **64**, 527–534.

Bymaster, F. P., Felder, C. C., Tzavara, E., Nomikos, G. G., Calligaro, D. O., and McKinzie, D. L. (2003). Muscarinic mechanisms of antipsychotic atypicality. *Prog. Neuropsychopharmacol. Biol. Psychiatry* **27**, 1125–1143.

Cheong, M. Y., Yun, S. H., Mook-Jung, I., Joo, I., Huh, K., and Jung, M. W. (2001). Cholinergic modulation of synaptic physiology in deep layer entorhinal cortex of the rat. *J. Neurosci. Res.* **66**, 117–121.

Costa, E., Grayson, D. R., and Guidotti, A. (2003). Epigenetic downregulation of GABAergic function in schizophrenia: Potential for pharmacological intervention? *Mol. Interv.* **3**, 220–229.

Costa, E., Davis, J. M., Dong, E., Grayson, D. R., Guidotti, A., Tremolizzo, L., and Veldic, M. (2004). A GABAergic cortical deficit dominates schizophrenia pathophysiology. *Crit. Rev. Neurobiol.* **16**, 1–23.

Costa, E., Guidotti, A., and Veldic, M. (2005). Should allosteric positive modulators of GABA (A) receptors be tested in the treatment of schizophrenia? *Schizophr. Res.* **73**, 367–368.

Davis, M., and Shi, C. (2000). The amygdala. *Curr. Biol.* **10**, R131.

de Sevilla, D. F., Cabezas, C., de Prada, A. N., Sanchez-Jimenez, A., and Buno, W. (2002). Selective muscarinic regulation of functional glutamatergic Schaffer collateral synapses in rat CA1 pyramidal neurons. *J. Physiol.* **545**, 51–63.

Dean, B., Bymaster, F. P., and Scarr, E. (2003). Muscarinic receptors in schizophrenia. *Curr. Mol. Med.* **3**, 419–426.

Dolan, R. J. (2002). Emotion, cognition, and behavior. *Science* **298**, 1191–1194.

Eastwood, S. L., and Harrison, P. J. (1999). Detection and quantification of hippocampal synaptophysin messenger RNA in schizophrenia using autoclaved, formalin-fixed, paraffin wax-embedded sections. *Neuroscience* **93**, 99–106.

Falkai, P., and Bogerts, B. (1986). Cell loss in the hippocampus of schizophrenics. *Eur. Arch. Psychiat. Neurol. Sci.* **236**, 154–161.

Fornari, R. V., Moreira, K. M., and Oliveira, M. G. (2000). Effects of the selective M1 muscarinic receptor antagonist dicyclomine on emotional memory. *Learn Mem.* **7**, 287–292.

Frey, S., Bergado-Rosado, J., Seidenbecher, T., Pape, H. C., and Frey, J. U. (2001). Reinforcement of early long-term potentiation (early-LTP) in dentate gyrus by stimulation of the basolateral amygdala: Heterosynaptic induction mechanisms of late-LTP. *J. Neurosci.* **21**, 3697–3703.

Gisabella, B., Bolshakov, V. Y., and Benes, F. M. (2005). Regulation of synaptic plasticity in a schizophrenia model. *Proc. Natl. Acad. Sci. USA* **102**, 13301–13306.

Guidotti, A., Auta, J., Davis, J. M., Dong, E., Grayson, D. R., Veldic, M., Zhang, X., and Costa, E. (2005). GABAergic dysfunction in schizophrenia: New treatment strategies on the horizon. *Psychopharmacology (Berlin)* **180**, 191–205.

Harrison, P. J. (1999). The neuropathological effects of antipsychotic drugs. *Schizophr. Res.* **40**, 87–99.

Harrison, P. J., McLaughlin, D., and Kerwin, R. W. (1991). Decreased hippocampal expression of a glutamate receptor gene in schizophrenia. *The Lancet* **337**, 450–452.

Heckers, S., Heinsen, H., Heinsen, Y., and Beckmann, H. (1991). Cortex, white matter, and basal ganglia in schizophrenia: A volumetric postmortem study. *Biol. Psychiatry* **29**, 556–566.

Heckers, S., Rauch, S. L., Goff, D., Savage, C. R., Schacter, D. L., Fischman, A. J., and Alpert, N. M. (1998). Impaired recruitment of the hippocampus during conscious recollection in schizophrenia. *Nat. Neurosci.* **1**, 318–323.

Heckers, S., Stone, D., Walsh, J., Shick, J., Koul, P., and Benes, F. M. (2002). Differential hippocampal expression of glutamic acid decarboxylase 65 and 67 messenger RNA in bipolar disorder and schizophrenia. *Arch. Gen. Psychiatry* **59**, 521–529.

Hyman, S. E., and Fenton, W. S. (2003). Medicine. What are the right targets for psychopharmacology? *Science* **299**, 350–351.

Ikegaya, Y., Saito, H., and Abe, K. (1996). The basomedial and basolateral amygdaloid nuclei contribute to the induction of long-term potentiation in the dentate gyrus *in vivo*. *Eur. J. Neurosci.* **8**, 1833–1839.

Jeste, D., and Lohr, J. B. (1989). Hippocampal pathologic findings in schizophrenia. *Arch. Gen. Psychiatry* **46**, 1019–1024.

Jones, E. G. (1987). GABA-peptide neurons in primate cerebral cortex. *J. Mind Behav.* **8**, 519–536.

Kerwin, R., Patel, S., and Meldrum, B. (1990). Quantitative autoradiographic analysis of glutamate binding sites in the hippocampal formation in normal and schizophrenic brain post mortem. *Neuroscience* **39**, 25–32.

Kerwin, R. W., Patel, S., Meldrum, B. S., Czudek, C., and Reynolds, G. P. (1988). Asymmetrical loss of glutamate receptor subtype in left hippocampus in schizophrenia. *The Lancet* **1**, 583–584.

Kim, J. J., Lee, H. J., Han, J. S., and Packard, M. G. (2001). Amygdala is critical for stress-induced modulation of hippocampal long-term potentiation and learning. *J. Neurosci.* **21**, 5222–5228.

Kovelman, J. A., and Scheibel, A. B. (1984). A neurohistological correlate of schizophrenia. *Biol. Psychiat.* **19**, 1601–1621.

Krettek, J. E., and Price, J. L. (1977). Projections from the amygdaloid complex and adjacent olfactory structures to the entorhinal cortex and to the subiculum in the rat and cat. *J. Comp. Neurol.* **172**, 723–752.

Lawrie, S. M., and Abukmeil, S. S. (1998). Brain abnormality in schizophrenia. A systematic and quantitative review of volumetric magnetic resonance imaging studies. *Br. J. Psychiatry.* **172**, 110–120.

LeDoux, J. E. (1992). Brain mechanisms of emotion and emotional learning. *Curr. Opin. Neurobiol.* **2**, 191–197.

LeDoux, J. E. (2000). Emotion circuits in the brain (In process citation). *Annu. Rev. Neurosci.* **23**, 155–184.

Leung, L. S., Shen, B., Rajakumar, N., and Ma, J. (2003). Cholinergic activity enhances hippocampal long-term potentiation in CA1 during walking in rats. *J. Neurosci.* **23**, 9297–9304.

Levey, A. I., Kitt, C. A., Simonds, W. F., Price, D. L., and Brann, M. R. (1991). Identification and localization of muscarinic acetylcholine receptor proteins in brain with subtype-specific antibodies. *J. Neurosci.* **11**, 3218–3226.

Levey, A. I., Edmunds, S. M., Koliatsos, V., Wiley, R. G., and Heilman, C. J. (1995). Expression of m1-m4 muscarinic acetylcholine receptor proteins in rat hippocampus and regulation by cholinergic innervation. *J. Neurosci.* **15**, 4077–4092.

Liao, D. L., Hong, C. J., Chen, H. M., Chen, Y. E., Lee, S. M., Chang, C. Y., Chen, H., and Tsai, S. J. (2003). Association of muscarinic m1 receptor genetic polymorphisms with psychiatric symptoms and cognitive function in schizophrenic patients. *Neuropsychobiology* **48**, 72–76.

Liu, W., Kumar, A., and Alreja, M. (1998). Excitatory effects of muscarine on septohippocampal neurons: Involvement of M3 receptors. *Brain Res.* **805**, 220–233.

Longson, D., Deakin, J. F., and Benes, F. M. (1996). Increased density of entorhinal glutamate-immunoreactive vertical fibers in schizophrenia. *J. Neural. Transm.* **103**, 503–507.

Marino, M. J., Rouse, S. T., Levey, A. I., Potter, L. T., and Conn, P. J. (1998). Activation of the genetically defined m1 muscarinic receptor potentiates N-methyl-D-aspartate (NMDA) receptor currents in hippocampal pyramidal cells. *Proc. Natl. Acad. Sci. USA* **95**, 11465–11470.

Mesches, M. H., Fleshner, M., Heman, K. L., Rose, G. M., and Diamond, D. M. (1999). Exposing rats to a predator blocks primed burst potentiation in the hippocampus *in vitro*. *J. Neurosci.* **19**, RC18.

Nakao, K., Matsuyama, K., Matsuki, N., and Ikegaya, Y. (2004). Amygdala stimulation modulates hippocampal synaptic plasticity. *Proc. Natl. Acad. Sci. USA* **101**, 14270–14275.

Pitkanen, A., Pikkarainen, M., Nurminen, N., and Ylinen, A. (2000). Reciprocal connections between the amygdala and the hippocampal formation, perirhinal cortex, and postrhinal cortex in rat: A review (In process citation). *Ann. NY Acad. Sci.* **911**, 369–391.

Porter, R. H., Eastwood, S. L., and Harrison, P. J. (1997). Distribution of kainate receptor subunit mRNAs in human hippocampus, neocortex and cerebellum, and bilateral reduction of hippocampal GluR6 and KA2 transcripts in schizophrenia. *Brain Res.* **751**, 217–231.

Rakic, P. (1974). Neurons in rhesus monkey visual cortex. Systematic relation between time of origin and eventual disposition. *Science* **183**, 425–427.

Retaux, S., Besson, M. J., and Penit-Soria, J. (1991a). Opposing effects of dopamine D2 receptor stimulation on the spontaneous and the electrically evoked release of [3H]GABA on rat prefrontal cortex slices. *Neuroscience* **42**, 61–71.

Retaux, S., Besson, M. J., and Penit-Soria, J. (1991b). Synergism between D1 and D2 dopamine receptors in the inhibition of the evoked release of [3H]GABA in the rat prefrontal cortex. *Neuroscience* **43**, 323–329.

Reynolds, G. P., Czudek, C., and Andrews, H. B. (1990). Deficit and hemispheric asymmetry of GABA uptake sites in the hippocampus in schizophrenia. *Biol. Psychiatry* **27**, 1038–1044.

Richardson, M. P., Strange, B. A., and Dolan, R. J. (2004). Encoding of emotional memories depends on amygdala and hippocampus and their interactions. *Nat. Neurosci.* **7**, 278–285.

Selemon, L. D., Rajkowska, G., and Goldman-Rakic, P. S. (1995). Abnormally high neuronal density in the schizophrenic cortex. A morphometric analysis of prefrontal area 9 and occipital area 17. *Arch. Gen. Psychiatry* **52**, 805–818; discussion 819–820.

Smith, C. J., Perry, E. K., Perry, R. H., Candy, J. M., Johnson, M., Bonham, J. R., Dick, D. J., Fairbairn, A., Blessed, G., and Birdsall, N. J. (1988). Muscarinic cholinergic receptor subtypes in hippocampus in human cognitive disorders. *J. Neurochem.* **50**, 847–856.

Swanson, L. W., and Petrovich, G. D. (1998). What is the amygdala? (see comments). *Trends Neurosci.* **21**, 323–331.

Todtenkopf, M. S., and Benes, F. M. (1998). Distribution of glutamate decarboxylase65 immunoreactive puncta on pyramidal and nonpyramidal neurons in hippocampus of schizophrenic brain. *Synapse* **29**, 323–332.

Tsvetkov, E., Shin, R. M., and Bolshakov, V. Y. (2004). Glutamate uptake determines pathway specificity of long-term potentiation in the neural circuitry of fear conditioning. *Neuron* **41**, 139–151.

Van Hoesen, G. W., Morecraft, R. J., and Vogt, B. A. (1993). Connections of the monkey cingulate cortex. *Neurobiol. Cingulate Cortex Limbic Thalamus* 249–284.

Vincent, S. L., Adamec, E., Sorensen, I., and Benes, F. M. (1994). The effects of chronic haloperidol administration on GABA-immunoreactive axon terminals in rat medial prefrontal cortex. *Synapse* **17**, 26–35.

Vogt, K. E., and Regehr, W. G. (2001). Cholinergic modulation of excitatory synaptic transmission in the CA3 area of the hippocampus. *J. Neurosci.* **21**, 75–83.

Weinberger, D. R. (1987). Implications of normal brain development for the pathogenesis of schizophrenia. *Arch. Gen. Psychiatry* **44**, 660–669.

Wu, M., Shanabrough, M., Leranth, C., and Alreja, M. (2000). Cholinergic excitation of septohippocampal GABA but not cholinergic neurons: Implications for learning and memory. *J. Neurosci.* **20**, 3900–3908.

Yun, S. H., Cheong, M. Y., Mook-Jung, I., Huh, K., Lee, C., and Jung, M. W. (2000). Cholinergic modulation of synaptic transmission and plasticity in entorhinal cortex and hippocampus of the rat. *Neuroscience* **97**, 671–676.

Zaidel, D. W., Esiri, M. M., and Harrison, P. J. (1997). Size, shape, and orientation of neurons in the left and right hippocampus: Investigation of normal asymmetries and alterations in schizophrenia. *Am. J. Psychiatry* **154**, 812–818.

**E. Costa, E. Dong, D. R. Grayson, W. B. Ruzicka, M. V. Simonini, M. Veldic, and A. Guidotti**

Department of Psychiatry, Psychiatric Institute
University of Illinois at Chicago, Chicago, Illinois 60612

# Epigenetic Targets in GABAergic Neurons to Treat Schizophrenia

## I. Chapter Overview

In the cortical GABAergic neurons of schizophrenia (SZ) patients, transcriptional downregulation of genes encoding several proteins critical for neuronal plasticity, such as reelin and $GAD_{67}$, is related to an epigenetic hypermethylation of their corresponding promoters by DNA methyltransferase 1 (DNMT1), which is selectively overexpressed in these neurons. Epigenetic changes in the regulation of reelin and $GAD_{67}$ are believed to contribute to the sculpting of specific neuroanatomical, neurochemical, and behavioral endophenotypes in SZ. It is very likely that these changes can be treated by targeting the aberrations in epigenetic function detected in the cortical GABAergic neurons of SZ patients.

A multicenter double-blind study shows that atypical antipsychotics (risperidone and olanzapine) have a faster onset of response when combined with valproic acid (VPA) (Stahl and Grady, 2004). VPA is a histone deacetylase

*Advances in Pharmacology, Volume 54*

1054-3589/06 $35.00
DOI: 10.1016/S1054-3589(06)54005-0

(HDAC) inhibitor, which suggests that supplementation of atypical antipsychotics with HDAC inhibitors elicits a faster onset of specific epigenetic transcriptional changes underlying antipsychotic efficacy.

Mice treated for a prolonged period with large doses (1 g/kg, twice a day in 15 days) of methionine (MET) mimic many of the neurochemical and behavioral features characteristic of SZ (Tremolizzo *et al.*, 2002), including the reduced expression of reelin and $GAD_{67}$. When VPA is coadministered with MET, VPA dramatically enhances reelin and $GAD_{67}$ expression and prevents the MET-induced reelin and $GAD_{67}$ promoter hypermethylation.

These findings offer new opportunities for "epigenetic treatments" aimed at decreasing the hypermethylation of promoters (reelin, $GAD_{67}$, and possibly others) that are associated with GABAergic dysfunction in SZ.

## II. Introduction

In the nucleus, DNA is tightly packaged into chromatin, which is a DNA-protein complex. In its heterochromatic state, chromatin is highly compact and refractory to transcription (Fig. 1). A major protein component of chromatin is an octamer of highly basic proteins known as histones (Varga-Weisz and Becker, 1998). The octamers include four histone (H) core proteins, H2A, H2B, H3, and H4. These histones coalesce along with DNA to form the nucleosome, a fundamental unit of nuclear chromatin, which represents the higher order structure that serves as the substrate for DNA replication and transcription (Schalch *et al.*, 2005). Each histone protein has a long N-terminal tail that comprises nearly a quarter of its length. These eight tails extend outward from the octameric nucleosome, reaching out to neighboring nucleosomes and helping them keep tightly bound together. The positively charged lysine residues affiliated with the histone tails (largely those in positions 4, 9, and 14 of the tails of histones H3, and 5, 8, 12, and 16 of H4) mediate most of the DNA–histone interactions. Unmodified native histones bind tightly to DNA and reduce DNA interactions with other proteins, including those with RNA polymerase II, which is required for transcriptional activity (Angus-Hill *et al.*, 1999, Cheung *et al.*, 2000; Freedman, 1999). The barrier against transcription created by native chromatin structures must be overcome for transcription to occur (Fig. 1). This is accomplished through H3/H4 acetylation by histone acetyl transferases (HAT) and other modifications of the histone tails, which open up the chromatin at the same time as promoter expression occurs. Acetylation of the $\epsilon$ amino group of lysine residues (i.e., lysine 4 and 14, in H3 tails) by HATs neutralizes the positive charge of histones, disrupting the histone–DNA interaction (Fig. 1) (Angus-Hill *et al.*, 1999; Varga-Weisz and Becker, 1998). Some HATs can selectively acetylate lysine 14 in H3, which is one of the histone residues

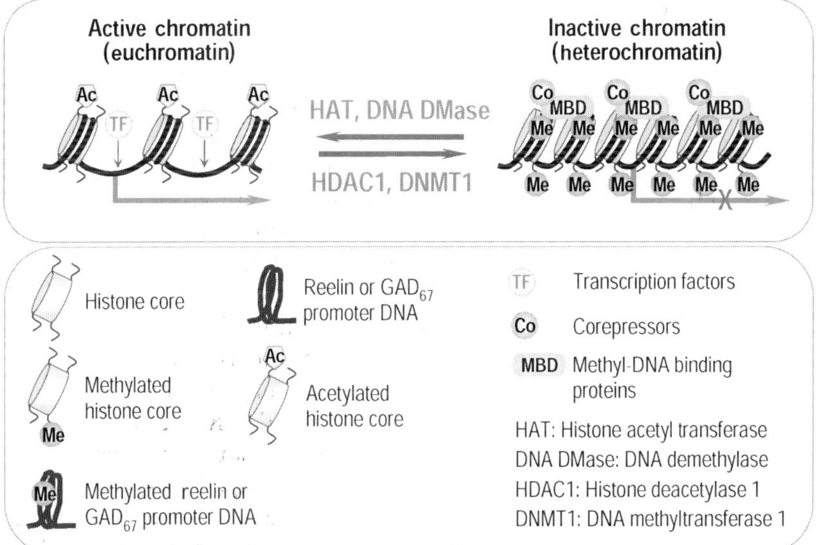


**FIGURE 1** Regulation of *RELN* and *GAD*$_{67}$ promoter CpG island methylation and transcription. Genes (*RELN*, *GAD*$_{67}$) expressing CpG islands in their promoters can be reversibly controlled (transcriptional repression or activation) by altered levels of histone acetylation, DNA promoter methylation and the presence or absence of transcription factors and repressors at their promoters. The chromatin structural changes that allow transition from an inactive to an active gene can be schematically represented by a two-conformational state model: (1) Inactive chromatin conformation (heterochromatin) associated with gene transcriptional repression achieved by CpG promoter island methylation, recruitment of MBD proteins, and recruitment of corepressors. This closed conformational state prevents DNA interaction with RNA polymerase II. (2) Active chromatin conformation (euchromatin) associated with gene transcriptional activation achieved by a combination of demethylation of CpG promoter islands, dissociation of MBD proteins from their promoters, covalent histone tail acetylation and recruitment of transcription factors, including recruitment of RNA polymerase II by DNA. (See Color Insert.)

implicated in transcription regulation (Cheung *et al.*, 2000; Freedman, 1999). Histone acetylation also appears to facilitate the association and binding of transcription factor complexes, ultimately bringing about the activity of RNA polymerase II on DNA and hence initiating transcription (Orphanides and Reinberg, 2000; Turner, 2002). In some instances, histone acetylation can be self-perpetuating—this characteristic favors the development of long-term cellular memory, creating a functional stable chromatin state that brings about long-lasting changes in the expression rates of specific genes (Battaglioli *et al.*, 2002; Crosio *et al.*, 2003; Lunyak *et al.*, 2000).

## III. Regulation of Histone Acetylation

Acetylation of nuclear histones is regulated by the balance between HAT and HDAC activities (De Ruijter *et al.*, 2003; Monneret, 2005). There are two main classes of HAT, Types A and B, which are expressed in the nucleus or the cytoplasm, respectively. All the members of these two enzyme families acetylate histones but their specificity is defined by their association with transcription factors. There are also two major classes of HDACs. Class I members (HDAC1, HDAC2, HDAC3, and HDAC8) are widely expressed and predominantly located in cell nuclei. Their structure includes a dominant catalytic domain. In contrast, Class II members (HDAC4, HDAC5, HDAC7, HDAC9a, HDAC9b, and HDAC10) include a proportionally smaller catalytic domain and can shuttle from the cytosol to the nucleus in response to specific extracellular signals. They express an N-terminal extension that mediates the enzyme's interactions with coactivators and corepressors and also confers signal responsiveness to $Ca^{2+}$-dependent kinases (De Ruijter *et al.*, 2003). The Class II HDACs are also widely expressed but have been preferentially found in striated muscles and the brain (De Ruijter *et al.*, 2003).

The identification of HDAC inhibitors, such as VPA (De Ruijter *et al.*, 2003), which is active in the treatment of mood disorders and SZ (Stahl and Grady, 2004; Wassef *et al.*, 2003), is of pharmacological importance because it permits the pharmacological manipulation of histone acetylation levels in the brain (Tremolizzo *et al.*, 2002, 2005). Further, the inhibition of brain HDACs may represent a new strategy for the treatment of psychiatric disorders. In fact, evidence is accumulating that HDAC activities play a fundamental role in regulating gene expression and chromatin remodeling in neurons (Dong *et al.*, 2005; Tremolizzo *et al.*, 2002, 2005).

## IV. Chromatin Remodeling at Neuromuscular Junction

How afferent neuronal inputs regulate changes in the expression of nuclear histone acetylation (histone code) and chromatin remodeling in postsynaptic cells is still poorly understood.

The signal transduction at postsynaptic nicotinic acetylcholine receptors expressed in skeletal muscle is one of the best-characterized models to investigate the regulation of gene expression in excitable tissues. In skeletal muscle, chemically induced electrical activity has long been known to control gene expression (Sanes and Lichtman, 2001). How electrical activity, through specific signal transduction cascades, is converted into a modification of transcriptional responses is only beginning to be understood. However, it seems likely that chromatin remodeling and histone tail acetylation participate in the regulation of skeletal muscle gene expression that is mediated by motor innervation (Méjat *et al.*, 2005).

Nicotinic receptor signal transduction comprises a heteropentameric cationic-gated channel defined by $\alpha_2$, $\beta$, $\delta$, and $\gamma/\epsilon$ receptor subunits. Before motor innervation, the expression of the skeletal muscle nicotinic receptor genes encoding the above-mentioned receptor subunits is regulated by the transcription of myogenin basic helix-loop-helix (bHLH) proteins (Méjat *et al.*, 2005; Sanes and Lichtman, 2001; Schaeffer *et al.*, 1998). The transcription of the $\epsilon$ subunit is not regulated by the myogenin factors operative in the expression of other nicotinic receptor subunits because these factors appear in subsynaptic nuclei only after birth. In these nuclei, the expression of nicotinic receptor subunits is upregulated by a number of neuronal signals, including the proteoglycan agrin. These signals stimulate acetylcholine postsynaptic receptor subunit redistribution, and this process is terminated by neuregulin (Fromm and Burden, 1998). The stimulation of skeletal muscle innervation triggers a $Ca^{2+}$-dependent signaling that lowers the expression of bHLH myogenin transcription factors and prevents the expression of extra-synaptic acetylcholine nicotinic receptor subunits (Fromm and Burden, 1998; Sanes and Lichtman, 2001; Schaeffer *et al.*, 1998, 2001). Muscle denervation activates the reexpression of myogenin and shortly thereafter, nicotinic receptor subunits begin returning to their previous positions along the muscle fiber lengths (Sanes and Lichtman, 2001; Schaeffer *et al.*, 2001).

One line of independent investigation conducted in both heart and skeletal muscles suggests that an HDAC, SHARP-1, is preferentially involved in the coordinated regulation of chromatin histone tail acetylation. This acetylation is operative in mediating striated muscle responses to physiological and stress stimuli via the expression of several muscle genes (Garriga-Canut *et al.*, 2001). These responses include the perinatal regulation of myogenin gene expression and the transcriptional regulation of genes encoding muscarinic acetylcholine receptor subunits (Garriga-Canut *et al.*, 2001). The role of bHLH proteins in the regulation of specific genes is not restricted to the neuromuscular junction. In fact in neurogenesis and neuronal differentiation, the bHLH proteins repress the transcription of specific genes in an HDAC-coordinated manner (Garriga-Canut *et al.*, 2001). It must be understood that under normal circumstances, histone proteins tend to downregulate transcription by protecting heterochromatin stability. Hence, the covalent acetylation of histone tails, which neutralizes their positively charged ends, is an attempt to reduce the chromatin-mediated inhibition of transcription (Fig. 1).

## V. Chromatin Remodeling During Memory Formation

Formation of long-term memory is associated with and depends on the regulation of gene expression. First, patterns of high frequency synaptic activity arising from NMDA receptor activation (Dingledine, 1983) facilitate $Ca^{2+}$ influx (Adams and Sweatt, 2002; Dingledine, 1983; Fanselow *et al.*, 1994; Harris *et al.*, 1984). This increase in intracellular $Ca^{2+}$ brings about the activation of a variety of signaling pathways that functionally converge in the activation of extracellular signal regulated kinase (ERK) (Adams and Sweatt, 2002; Davis *et al.*, 2000; Sananbenesi *et al.*, 2002). In turn, ERK directly or indirectly recruits and activates several transcription factors.

Evidence suggests that a high frequency pattern of synaptic activity is also associated with chromatin remodeling, for example:

1. Guan and coworkers (2003a,b) have shown that integration of long-term memory related to synaptic plasticity involves a bidirectional regulation of gene expression associated with chromatin remodeling. In *Aplysia californica*, stimuli generating long-term potentiation (LTP) induce H4 tail acetylation around the promoters of the *Aplysia* CCAAT-enhancer binding protein (Ap/EBP), whereas cues provoking long-term depression (LTD) recruit HDACs (Guan *et al.*, 2003a,b; Méjat *et al.*, 2005).
2. Histone acetylation is activated in rat hippocampal neurons in the contextual fear-conditioning paradigm during long-term memory formation (Levenson and Sweatt, 2005; Levenson *et al.*, 2004). Rats receiving HDAC inhibitors exhibit enhanced LTP and memory formation facilitation. These increases are associated with an increase of acetylated histone content in the hippocampus around the chromatin sites of pyramidal neurons, which are believed to be operative in increasing long-term memory (Levenson *et al.*, 2004). This effect is triggered by the NMDA receptor ligand occupancy and ERK activation, and this process is impaired by NMDA receptor antagonists (Davis *et al.*, 2000; English and Sweatt, 1997; Levenson *et al.*, 2004; Morris *et al.*, 1986).
3. In the heterozygous cyclic AMP response-element (CREB)-binding protein mouse ($CBP^{+/-}$), which also expresses a HAT haploinsufficiency, H2B acetylation, LTP expression, and learning and memory formation are impaired (Alarcon *et al.*, 2004; Korzus *et al.*, 2004). Treatment of $CBP^{+/-}$ mouse hippocampal slices with HDAC inhibitors significantly improves late-phase LTP induction, suggesting that inhibition of HDACs may have a compensatory action on HAT haploinsufficiency (Korzus *et al.*, 2004).
4. Gross modifications in chromatin structure have been demonstrated in the suprachiasmatic nucleus (the molecular clock) when animals are exposed to phase resetting light pulses (Levenson and Sweatt, 2005). Pulses of light induce changes in the transcription of several genes that comprise the molecular clock. These changes are mediated by the regulation of the epigenetic state of the suprachiasmatic nucleus and are considered a core molecular mechanism of the circadian clock that establishes a close relationship between gene expression and animal behavior.

Hence, it is very likely that changes in chromatin remodeling are associated with synaptic plasticity and the formation of long-term memory and that these changes can have lasting effects on behavior (Levenson and Sweatt, 2005).

## VI. Role of Reelin and Apolipoprotein E Receptors in Hippocampal Plasticity and Learning

Apolipoprotein E (ApoE) receptors (ApoER) are components operative in the transport and receptor-mediated uptake of ApoE by tissues (Schmechel *et al.*, 1993). Several tissues express ApoE and in the brain ApoE function is transacted predominantly in astrocytes (Schmechel *et al.*, 1993). However in the brain, the physiological significance of ApoE secretion and its binding to cognate ApoER requires additional clarification (Herz and Beffert, 2000).

In the general human population, ApoE is expressed in three major isoforms—ApoE2, ApoE3, and ApoE4—with ApoE3 as the most common isoform. In 1993, Schmechel *et al.* showed that ApoE4 overexpression is genetically associated with a late onset form of Alzheimer's disease. This disease is characterized by a loss of synapses and neurons and by the accumulation of amyloid plaques and neurofibrillary tangles. The mechanism by which ApoE4 predisposes to Alzheimer's disease is currently under debate. A model that has been proposed by Herz and Beffert (2000) is that members of the ApoER family, which are abundantly expressed on the surface of neurons may be involved in the pathogenesis of Alzheimer's disease. Two members of the ApoE receptor family, the very low-density lipoprotein receptor (VLDLR) and ApoER2, very likely participate in the regulation of the migration and layering of cortical neurons during development (Schmechel *et al.*, 1993). This pathway involves the signaling molecule reelin, which is a large protein of ~400 kDa that is secreted during embryogenesis by Cajal–Retzius cells transiently located in the superficial cortical layers (Rice and Curran, 2001). The downregulation of reelin (D'Arcangelo *et al.*, 1995) expression and that of the cognate receptors VLDLR and ApoER2 combined with a decrease of the cytoplasmic adapter protein mouse disabled-1 (DAB1) (Howell *et al.*, 1997; Sheldon *et al.*, 1997; Trommsdorff *et al.*, 1999; Ware *et al.*, 1997), create a phenotype characterized by severe cerebellar hypoplasia and disorganization of pyramidal neuronal layering in the brain cortex. These abnormalities are epitomized in the reeler mutant mouse. VLDLR and ApoER2 are both components of the reelin signal transduction cascade of migrating neurons, yet only mild neuroanatomical abnormalities are present in the brains of mice that have a deficit of only one of these two receptors (Drakew *et al.*, 2002). In embryos that lack both ApoER2 and VLDL, the reelin-dependent positioning of olivo-coclear and facial visual motor nuclear neurons is normal (Rossel *et al.*, 2005), suggesting that the present understanding of receptors that mediate reelin's action in the midbrain is incomplete.

After the fetal phase, the expression of Cajal–Retzius neurons that synthesize reelin disappear from the subpial layer. Subsequently in the cortex, reelin synthesis becomes restricted to cortical GABAergic interneurons, which synthesize and secrete reelin into the extracellular matrix (Pesold *et al.*, 1998; Rodriguez *et al.*, 2000). In this context, reelin likely contributes to neuronal plasticity by modulating axon branching via a signal transduction modality, including ApoER2 and VLDLR and the adapter protein DAB1 (Niu *et al.*, 2004). That reelin may play a role in synaptic plasticity is suggested by the decrease in dendritic branching and spine expression in apical or basilar dendrites of cortical pyramidal or hippocampal neurons in haploinsufficient heterozygous reeler mice (Costa *et al.*, 2001; Liu *et al.*, 2001). It is also important to mention that the downregulation of reelin expression in the cortex and hippocampus of SZ and bipolar disorder patients (Guidotti *et al.*, 2000) is associated with a decrease in the number of dendritic spines and in neuropil hypoplasticity (Guidotti *et al.*, 2005). A contiguity of reelin with dendritic spine synapses has been detected in wild-type mice but this contiguity is decreased in heterozygous reeler mice and is absent in reeler null mutant mice (Costa *et al.*, 2001; Rodriguez *et al.*, 2000). Reeler mice exhibit important gait abnormalities (Rice and Curran, 2001). In contrast, heterozygous reeler mice have a normal gait but they exhibit memory deficits (Carboni *et al.*, 2004; Larson *et al.*, 2003).

In the cortex and hippocampus, it seems likely that VLDLR and ApoER2 mediate reelin signal transduction. Knockout mice lacking ApoR2 and VLDL exhibit normal hippocampal baseline synaptic activity but show a profound LTP deficit (Weeber *et al.*, 2002). Reelin, which in the adult mammalian brain is expressed in the proximity of cortical pyramidal neuron dendritic spines (Rodriguez *et al.*, 2000), augments LTP in hippocampal slices of wild-type mice but not in slices from VLDLR- and ApoER2-deficient mice (see Fig. 6 of Weeber *et al.*, 2002). Finally, support for a role for reelin in regulating the event-related increase of dendritic protein synthesis is suggested by reelin's ability to regulate protein synthesis in neurosome preparations (Dong *et al.*, 2003). The signal transduction pathway associated with this action is blocked by echistatin, a competitive integrin receptor antagonist, and thus, it may include the function of an integrin receptor located at postsynaptic dendritic sites (Dong *et al.*, 2003).

Taken together, these data suggest that reelin synthesized and secreted in abundance by cortical and hippocampal GABAergic interneurons (Costa *et al.*, 2001; Guidotti *et al.*, 2000; Liu *et al.*, 2001; Rodriguez *et al.*, 2000) plays a special role in the regulation of spine function at apical dendrites of telencephalic pyramidal neurons.

## VII. Is Reelin Expressed Only in a Selective Subpopulation of GABAergic Neurons?

In primate neocortices, the density and morphology of GABAergic neurons vary in different layers—from 20% to 30% in the deep cortical layers to nearly 100% in layer I (Rodriguez *et al.*, 2003). In human prefrontal cortex (Brodmann's areas 9 and 46), every GABAergic neuron expresses $GAD_{65}$ and/or $GAD_{67}$ but very likely not every GABAergic neuron synthesizes and stores reelin. As shown in Table I in layers I, II, and III, the number of $GAD_{65}$ and reelin mRNA positive neurons, as demonstrated by *in situ* hybridization histochemistry, is virtually identical. In contrast, in layers IV and V, approximately 30%, and in layer VI, approximately 50% of the GABAergic interneurons fail to express reelin mRNA. In layers I, II, and III, there is a marked decrease of reelin mRNA expression in the prefrontal cortex of SZ patients, whereas in these patients the decrease of reelin mRNA-positive neurons in layers IV, V, and VI is marginal (Veldic *et al.*, 2005). Although the subtypes of GABAergic interneurons (horizontal, bitufted, basket, or chandelier neurons) that express reelin in each cortical layer have not been identified, available data suggest the concept that GABAergic neurons can be divided into two families, those expressing reelin

**TABLE I** Neu-N Protein, $GAD_{65}$ and Reelin mRNA-Positive Neurons in Prefrontal Cortex, Brodmann's Area 9[a] (Positive Neurons/mm$^2$)

| *Layers* | *Neu-N protein* | *$GAD_{65}$ mRNA* | *Reelin mRNA* | *Reelin/$GAD_{65}$ (ratio)* |
|---|---|---|---|---|
| I | 428 ± 40 | 437 ± 22 | 410 ± 25 | 0.93 |
| II | 1230 ± 89 | 709 ± 44 | 660 ± 40 | 0.93 |
| III | 740 ± 22 | 330 ± 25 | 363 ± 38 | 1.1 |
| IV | 1140 ± 150 | 549 ± 35 | 412 ± 40 | 0.75 |
| V | 549 ± 60 | 366 ± 26 | 264 ± 20 | 0.72 |
| VI | 528 ± 52 | 330 ± 12 | 165 ± 18 | 0.50 |

[a]Postmortem tissues for this study were obtained from the Harvard Brain Tissue Resource Center McLean Hospital, Belmont, MA (The McLean 66 cohort). Values are the mean ± SD of 27 nonpsychiatric subjects. For demographic characteristics and for the methodology to perform the immunohistochemistry for Neu-N protein and *in situ* hybridization for $GAD_{65}$ and reelin mRNA detection (see Veldic *et al.*, 2005).

Neu-N, neuron-specific nuclear protein.

(the majority of interneurons in layers I, II, and III) and those in which reelin expression is minimal or fails to materialize. The latter neuronal population is primarily located in the deeper cortical layers V and VI.

Layers I, II, and III are enriched in horizontal, double bouquet, and Martinotti GABAergic interneurons. They provide axon terminals that synapse on distal dendritic spines or dendritic shafts expressed on pyramidal neurons or on the somata of other GABAergic interneurons (Somogyi *et al.*, 1998). Hence, a functional consequence of a reelin deficit in GABAergic neurons of layers I, II, and III may contribute to apical or basilar pyramidal neuron dendrite dystrophy, including a decrease in dendritic spines and a hypoplasia of cortical neuropil, as observed in SZ (Lewis *et al.*, 2005).

## VIII. *RELN* and *$GAD_{67}$* CpG Island Promoter Hypermethylation and Reelin and $GAD_{67}$ Expression Downregulation in SZ Patients

The reduction of prefrontal cortical reelin expression that occurs in GABAergic neurons, together with the downregulation of $GAD_{67}$ expression, are among the most consistent neuropathological findings in postmortem studies of SZ cortex (Knable *et al.*, 2004).

Several lines of evidence support the hypothesis that the expression deficit of reelin and $GAD_{67}$ detected in SZ brains cannot be explained by a *RELN* or $GAD_{67}$ gene haploinsufficiency (Costa *et al.*, 2003; Goldberger *et al.*, 2005). Converging evidence suggests that in SZ patients, the reduced reelin expression found in cortical GABAergic interneurons is related to the hypermethylation of its promoter (Abdolmaleky *et al.*, 2005; Grayson *et al.*, 2005). This hypermethylation is very likely mediated by the overexpression of DNMT1 (Veldic *et al.*, 2004, 2005) that is reported to occur in cortical GABAergic interneurons of these patients.

The increased methylation of *RELN* or $GAD_{67}$ promoters induced in mice by administering MET (see paragraph 11) is accompanied by an increased binding of methyl CpG binding domain (MBD) repressor proteins to the hypermethylated cytosines expressed in the promoters of the above-listed genes (Dong *et al.*, 2005). If the results obtained in mice are extrapolated to humans it can be suggested that the hypermethylation of *RELN* and $GAD_{67}$ promoters in cortical GABAergic neurons of SZ patients will recruit MBD repressor proteins and will bring about an abundant prevalence of a closed chromatin (heterochromatin) configuration in the vicinity of *RELN* and $GAD_{67}$ promoters (Costa *et al.*, 2003; Grayson *et al.*, 2005) (Fig. 1). Hence, the increased methylation of the *RELN* promoter establishes a clear mechanism for the reduced transcription of reelin mRNA in these patients.

## IX. Increased DNA-Methyltransferase-1 Expression in Cortical GABAergic Neurons of SZ Patients

To gain insight into the possible pathogenetic mechanisms operative in the *RELN* and $GAD_{67}$ promoter hypermethylation detected in the cortex of SZ patients, we studied the expression levels of DNMT mRNAs (DNMT1, DNMT3a, and DNMT3b) and their cognate proteins in cortical GABAergic neurons of SZ and nonpsychiatric subjects (NPS).

In the human brain, DNMT1 is the most abundant enzyme methylating hemimethylated cytosines expressed in CpG dinucleotides of gene promoters (Veldic *et al.*, 2004). In the cortex, this enzyme is almost exclusively expressed in GABAergic interneurons (Veldic *et al.*, 2004, 2005). In our study, DNMT1 mRNA expression was quantified by two methods: (1) nested RT-PCR of laser microdissected cortical neurons with an internal standard added to the PCR assay to correct for losses in this procedure, and (2) *in situ* hybridization histochemistry.

In NPS, DNMT1 mRNA, measured by *in situ* hybridization in the prefrontal cortex (Brodmann's areas 9 and 10), is preferentially expressed in GABAergic interneurons while its hybridization signals are consistently very faint and usually only sporadically detectable in pyramidal neurons (Veldic *et al.*, 2004, 2005). In SZ patients, the DNMT1 mRNA *in situ* hybridization signal is consistently faint and only sporadically visible in layers III, V, and VI pyramidal neurons. In contrast, it is strong and significantly increased in GABAergic interneurons of layers I, II, and III (Veldic *et al.*, 2004, 2005).

Similarly, DNMT1 mRNA measured by nested RT-PCR with internal standards increases by approximately threefold in layer I GABAergic interneurons (predominantly horizontal cells with only rare bitufted neurons) of SZ patients. In contrast, DNMT1 mRNA measured in layer V, which contains a prevalence of pyramidal neurons and only approximately 30% of GABAergic interneurons (basket and chandelier cells), failed to increase in SZ patients (Ruzicka *et al.*, 2005).

Based on these findings, it was of interest to investigate the mechanisms that could explain the higher level of DNMT1 expression in the GABAergic neurons of SZ patient cortices. Although an understanding of the regulation of DNMT1 expression in GABAergic neurons requires additional studies, analysis of the *DNMT1* gene reveals that the promoter of this gene is rich in consensi that can be targeted by several transcription factors (Campbell and Szyf, 2003; Slack *et al.*, 2001). We observed that nicotine (4.5 mg/kg s.c. twice a day for 5 days) administered to mice can decrease DNMT1 expression in layer I cortical GABAergic neurons, suggesting that these neurons may express nicotine acetylcholine receptors in their somata (Table II).

**TABLE II** Mode of Action of DNMT1 Inhibitors

| | *Drugs* | *Mechanism* |
|---|---|---|
| Direct | Zebularine | Noncompetitive[a] |
| | 5-Azacytidine | Noncompetitive[a] |
| | 5-Azadeoxycytidine | Noncompetitive[a] |
| | Procainamide | Competitive |
| Indirect | Hydralazine | Inhibits ERK |
| | Nicotine | Stimulation of nicotinic Ach receptors? |

[a]Intercalate into DNA in the place of cytosine. Acts only in S-phase cells.
Ach, acetylcholine.

## X. Relationship Between DNMT1 Overexpression and Reelin and $GAD_{67}$ Downregulation in GABAergic Neurons of SZ Patients

Thus far, the evidence we have collected strongly supports the view that SZ neuropathology includes a specific molecular dysfunction of cortical GABAergic neurons (Goldberger *et al.*, 2005; Guidotti *et al.*, 2000). We have found that this specific neuronal dysfunction is characterized by a selective DNMT1 overexpression in GABAergic cortical neurons of layers I, II, and III, which may be the cause of the hypermethylation of reelin, $GAD_{67}$, NMR2A receptor, $\alpha 7$ nicotinic receptor, and possibly other gene promoters, causing a subsequent reduction in the expression of the corresponding mRNAs (Costa *et al.*, 2001; Grayson *et al.*, 2005, 2006; Guidotti *et al.*, 2000, 2005; Martin *et al.*, 2004).

The suggestion that the hypermethylation of *RELN* promoter CpG islands is responsible for the reelin transcriptional downregulation detected in the GABAergic interneurons of SZ brains is supported by the studies of Chen *et al.* (2002), Mitchell *et al.* (2005), and Noh *et al.* (2005), which show that when the *reelin* gene is transcriptionally repressed, selective cytosines in the reelin promoter CpG islands are hypermethylated. Furthermore, the data suggest that this hypermethylation is restricted to a subset of cytosines in a region of the promoter, which is accompanied by transcription factors binding the RNA polymerase II complex (Grayson *et al.*, 2005).

An increase of brain *S*-adenosyl methionine (SAM) in mice treated with MET provides independent evidence that hypermethylation of *RELN* or $GAD_{67}$ promoters may elicit the reduction of reelin and $GAD_{67}$ expression in SZ patients (Dong *et al.*, 2005; Tremolizzo *et al.*, 2002, 2005). These results, evaluated with studies documenting a decrease of reelin and $GAD_{67}$ expression in cortex of SZ patients (Veldic *et al.*,

2004, 2005), strongly suggest that an epigenetic molecular pathology of cortical GABAergic interneurons related to DNMT1-mediated promoter hypermethylation is prominent in SZ morbidity.

## XI. Pharmacological Strategies to Reduce Reelin and $GAD_{67}$ Promoter Hypermethylation in SZ Patients

Based on the evidence that DNMT1 expression is increased in cortical GABAergic neurons of SZ patients, logical and theoretical considerations depicted in Fig. 1 suggest that a new approach for the treatment of SZ morbidity should address the hypermethylation of *RELN* and $GAD_{67}$ promoters expressed in GABAergic neurons. This approach may include: (1) inhibition of DNMT1 catalytic activity, (2) downregulation of DNMT1 expression, and (3) induction of DNA demethylation by long-term administration of HDAC inhibitors that are believed to induce this process (Detich *et al.*, 2003).

### A. DNA Methyltransferase 1 Inhibitors

Most of the inhibitors of DNMT1 catalytic activity available today are molecules that are incorporated into the DNA of proliferating cells (Table II) (Egger *et al.*, 2005). The prototypes in this group of drugs are 5-azacytidine and zebularine. Both nucleotide analogs are converted *in vivo* into deoxynucleotide triphosphate derivatives that are incorporated in the 5-position of the cytosine ring expressed in the CpG islands of the replicating DNA. These two drugs may be efficacious in the S-phase cell cycle where both work as powerful inhibitors of DNA methylation (Egger *et al.*, 2005). Unfortunately, these two inhibitors fail to act on nondividing cells and therefore are expected to be devoid of action in differentiated neurons.

A prospective DNA methylation inhibitor active in differentiated neurons is procainamide, a drug used to treat cardiac arrhythmias, which also inhibits DNA methylation. This compound is a nonnucleoside competitive inhibitor of DNA methylation (Scheinbart *et al.*, 1991) mediated by DNMT1 catalytic activity, which is also expected to be an effective inhibitor of DNA hypermethylation in neurons. We are now studying the potency of procainamide in inhibiting DNMT1-mediated hypermethylation of *RELN* and $GAD_{67}$ promoters in a mouse model of SZ induced by protracted MET treatment (1 g/kg twice daily) (Dong *et al.*, 2005; Tremolizzo *et al.*, 2002, 2005). The epigenetic nature of SZ pathology suggests that treatment with procainamide may downregulate this hypermethylation.

## B. Drugs That Downregulate DNMT1 Expression

The expression of several transcription factor consensi in the DNMT1 promoter (Bigey *et al.*, 2000; Campbell and Szyf, 2003; Slack *et al.*, 2001) suggests that this expression in neurons can be regulated by both environmental stimuli and neuroactive drugs. Therefore, we plan to test strategies (Table II) and/or procedures that either decrease DNMT1 expression or competitively reduce its catalytic activity.

Hydralazine, which is a pharmacological intervention used to treat hypertension, decreases DNMT1 expression and downregulates DNA methylation in T cells by inhibiting the ERK pathway (Deng *et al.*, 2003).

As mentioned earlier (Table II), nicotine is another drug that downregulates DNMT1 expression, suggesting that the abuse of nicotine by SZ patients may be an attempt to use nicotine to self-medicate the increase of DNMT1 expression in cortical GABAergic neurons.

## C. HDAC Inhibitors

A possible strategy for pharmacological intervention to normalize the reduced reelin or $GAD_{67}$ expression in cortical GABAergic neurons of SZ patients is to reduce their promoter hypermethylation by administering HDAC inhibitors. HDAC inhibitors hyperacetylating nucleosomal histone tails: (1) control DNMT1 accessibility to promoter DNA segments, or (2) induce DNA demethylase activity (Detich *et al.*, 2003) (Fig. 1). The possible success of such a strategy is supported by the report that VPA (used as an adjunctive with antipsychotics in the medication of SZ morbidity) given to animals in doses that increase acetylation of brain chromatin histones (Tremolizzo *et al.*, 2002, 2005), induces reelin and $GAD_{67}$ expression, thereby promoting DNA demethylation and thus facilitating the action of atypical antipsychotics.

The accessibility of DNA demethylase to DNA regions that are targets of DNMT1 induced DNA methylation depends on a higher order structural remodeling of chromatin and on the acetylation status of the core chromatin histone tails that are modulated by the balance of HAT and HDAC activities (Fig. 1).

Four major classes of HDAC inhibitors have been described, which are derivatives of: (1) hydroxamic acid, (2) short chain fatty acids, (3) cyclic tetrapeptides, and (4) benzamides (Table III). The hydroxamic acid derivative trichostatin A (TSA) is the most potent HDAC inhibitor available and *in vitro*, it inhibits HDACs in the nanomol/range. However, this compound does not readily cross the blood–brain barrier and when given systemically, cannot be effectively used to inhibit CNS HDACs. Suberoylanilide hydroxamic acid (SAHA) (see Table III for structure) is another hydroxamic acid derivative also active in micromole concentrations *in vitro* but it appears

**TABLE III** Structure and *In Vitro* Potency of Four Groups of Histone Deacetylase (HDAC) Inhibitors

| *Group and structure* | *Compounds* | In vitro $IC_{50}$ *range* |
|---|---|---|
| Hydroxamic acids | Trichostatin A SAHA (suberoyl anilide bishydroxamide) | nM μM |
| Short-chain fatty acids | Valproic acid | mM |
| Cyclic tetrapeptides | Apicidin | μM |
| Benzamides | MS-275 sulpiride | μM |

Modified with permission from De Ruijter *et al.* (2003). *Biochem J.* **15**, 737–749 © Biochemical Society.

to be a weak inhibitor of brain HDACs *in vivo* (De Ruijter *et al.*, 2003), presumably because of its short half-life and its low blood–brain barrier penetration. We obtained better results with apicidin and with the benzamide derivatives MS-275 and sulpiride. When these drugs are injected in mice, they are at least 10 times more potent than VPA in increasing brain acetyl H3 content, and with the exception of apicidin, they are well tolerated when injected repeatedly for several days.

Interestingly, sulpiride is a dopamine D2 and D3 receptor antagonist with a low extrapyramidal side effect liability and is used in Europe as an effective antipsychotic to treat SZ exacerbation episodes in chronic SZ patients (Munro *et al.*, 2004). Because of its strong HDAC inhibitory activity, its efficacy as an antipsychotic cannot be ascribed exclusively to the D2, D3 receptor function inhibition.

It was previously assumed that the HDACs expressed in the brain were approximately equally sensitive to different inhibitors of these enzymes. While this may be the case for TSA, indirect evidence suggests that this might not be the case for VPA and MS-275. For example, it has been reported that Class II HDACs are five times less susceptible to VPA inhibition than Class I HDACs (De Ruijter *et al.*, 2003). Furthermore, it has been reported that among the Class I HDACs, HDAC1 is most sensitive to MS-275, whereas HDAC3 and HDAC8 have significantly lower sensitivity (De Ruijter *et al.*, 2003). This information suggests that the development of new inhibitors targeted to specific HDACs combined with pertinent information on the selective brain tissue expression of various molecular forms of HDACs may allow the preparation of HDAC inhibitors tailored for pharmacological interventions to treat psychotic episodes in SZ and bipolar disorders.

## XII. The MET-Induced Epigenetic Mouse Model to Evaluate Prospective HDAC Inhibitors to be Used to Influence Epigenetic Mechanisms in Cortical GABAergic Neurons

In testing the potency and efficacy of HDAC inhibitors in reducing brain DNA promoter hypermethylation, a leading hypothesis is that an increase of histone tail covalent acetylation results in an inhibition of DNMT activity and/or a still hypothetical induction of DNA demethylase (Detich *et al.*, 2003), allowing an upregulation of those genes (including reelin and $GAD_{67}$) that became transcriptionally inhibited by epigenetic promoter hypermethylation in SZ brains overexpressing DNMT1 (Grayson *et al.*, 2005; Veldic *et al.*, 2004, 2005).

To establish whether HDAC inhibition can downregulate an experimentally induced reelin promoter hypermethylation, we elicited reelin promoter hypermethylation and reelin expression downregulation in mice by administering high dose regimens of MET (0.75–1 g/kg twice a day) for 2 weeks (Tremolizzo *et al.*, 2002, 2005). The injection of MET increases brain SAM levels (from $320 \pm 6.2$ to $470 \pm 24$ pmol/mg protein) and decreases the expression of the mRNAs encoding reelin and $GAD_{67}$ in the frontal cortex (Tremolizzo *et al.*, 2002, 2005). This MET action was associated with an increase in the number of 5′-methyl cytosines in the reelin promoter expressed in the mouse cortex. This hypermethylation model was then used to study whether the HDAC inhibitor VPA, in doses that favor brain histone tail acetylation, also reduces reelin promoter hypermethylation and facilitates reelin and $GAD_{67}$ expression. We measured the acetylation state of H3 and H4 by Western blot and immunochemistry technology. In mice receiving VPA, we found a dose-related increase (from 0.5 to 4 mmol/kg s.c.) in the expression of frontal cortex acetylated H3 tails and only a marginal increase of acetylated H4 tails. We have accumulated evidence that VPA, in doses that increase acetylation of H3 in interneurons, normalizes MET-induced reelin promoter hypermethylation and MET-induced reelin expression downregulation (Dong *et al.*, 2005; Tremolizzo *et al.*, 2002, 2005).

Because VPA is a weak HDAC inhibitor active in mmolar concentrations (Table III), it is possible that its pharmacological inhibition of DNA methylation could be mediated by mechanisms that are independent of the inhibition of nucleosomal histone core acetylation. To this end, we decided to further study histone acetylation, reelin, and $GAD_{67}$ promoter methylation in GABAergic neurons of vehicle and MET-treated mice, following administration of HDAC inhibitors that are chemically unrelated but more potent than VPA.

Testing the potency of different classes of HDAC inhibitors in increasing brain nucleosomal acetylated histone content, we observed that the benzamide sulpiride is 50- to 100-fold more potent than VPA in increasing acetylated H3 content in the frontal cortex, hippocampus, and striatum of mice (Simonini *et al.*, 2006).

Sulpiride is a particularly interesting atypical antipsychotic because of its relatively low extrapyramidal side effect liability (Munro *et al.*, 2004). Moreover, when coadministered with clozapine or other atypical antipsychotics (i.e., olanzapine), it leads to a substantial improvement in the positive and negative symptoms of SZ in patients resistant to treatment that includes only these atypical antipsychotics (Munro *et al.*, 2004). Sulpiride, administered to mice in doses of 30–60 μmol/kg, prevents MET-induced reelin and $GAD_{67}$ expression downregulation and also decreases the *RELN* and $GAD_{67}$ promoter hypermethylation elicited by MET (Simonini *et al.*, 2006).

Thus, using the MET-induced hypermethylation mouse model to evaluate VPA and structurally different and more selective and potent HDAC inhibitors, one may explore the interaction between certain classes of neuroleptics and specific HDAC inhibitors and establish whether neuroleptic association contributes to the regulation of DNA promoter methylation, histone acetylation, and the upregulation of reelin and $GAD_{67}$ mRNA expression elicited by the HDAC inhibitors.

## XIII. Conclusions

Evidence is accumulating that an epigenetic hypermethylation of *RELN* and $GAD_{67}$ promoters is part of the etiopathogenetic process that leads to their transcriptional inactivation and to the GABAergic neuronal functional deficit in SZ. This evidence encourages the development of new treatment procedures that can reverse the epigenetically induced reelin and $GAD_{67}$ transcriptional inactivation by acting on the dynamic interplay of chromatin remodeling processes, DNA promoter methylation, and histone covalent modifications.

Although the exact order in which these chromatin remodeling events occur in physiological or in pathological conditions is not certain, the data suggest that in GABAergic neurons, epigenetically repressed genes (i.e., *Reln* and $GAD_{67}$) can be reactivated pharmacologically by DNA methylation inhibitors or DNA-demethylation inducers, which favor the transition from heterochromatin to the euchromatin conformational state by removing promoter cytosine methylation (Fig. 1).

The more promising drugs to target epigenetic disorders of cortical GABAergic neurons in SZ are the HDAC inhibitors. Two of these drugs, namely VPA and sulpiride, are already known to be beneficial when administered in combination with atypical antipsychotics in patients resistant to antipsychotic monotherapy (Munro *et al.*, 2004; Wassef *et al.*, 2003).

The efficacy of sulpiride in augmenting clozapine's antipsychotic action has been attributed to the complementary inhibition of the DA receptor profile of these two drugs (Munro *et al.*, 2004). However, our experiments and the analogies of sulpiride action with that of VPA on HDAC activity, which modify reelin and $GAD_{67}$ expression, suggest that in the treatment of SZ symptomatology, their adjuvant action with atypical antipsychotics may be mediated via an epigenetic modification of GABAergic tone. It is also possible that by reversing the SZ-induced deficit of GABAergic neurotransmission impinging on monoaminergic neurons, VPA, and sulpiride reduce the firing rate of these neurons, thereby producing an actual reduction of monoamines at their receptors and in a complementary fashion increasing the monoaminergic antagonist action of atypical neuroleptics. Taken together, these results encourage the synthesis of new generations of HDAC inhibitors with different selectivities for the numerous HDAC families that are known to regulate cortical function.

If successful, an "epigenetic therapy" will shift the emphasis in SZ treatment from the use of drugs acting at membrane dopaminergic and other neurotransmitter receptors to drugs targeted to correct the putative chromatin remodeling disorders associated with SZ.

Considering that an epigenetic origin of cortical GABAergic dysfunction plays a role in SZ morbidity, the identification of pharmacological agents targeting the epigenetic origin of the GABAergic dysfunction opens a new approach to relieve GABAergic deficits in SZ without using direct $GABA_A$ or $GABA_B$ receptor agonists or antagonists.

## References

Abdolmaleky, H. M., Cheng, K. H., Russo, A., Smith, C. L., Faraone, S. V., Wilcox, M., Shafa, R., Glatt, S. J., Nguyen, G., Ponte, J. F., Thiagalingam, S., and Tsuang, M. T. (2005).

Hypermethylation of the reelin (RELN) promoter in the brain of schizophrenic patients: A preliminary report. *Am. J. Med. Genet. B Neuropsychiatr. Genet.* **134**, 60–66.

Adams, J. P., and Sweatt, J. D. (2002). Molecular psychology: Roles for the ERK MAP kinase cascade in memory. *Annu. Rev. Pharmacol. Toxicol.* **42**, 135–163.

Alarcon, J. M., Malleret, G., Tousani, K., Vronskaya, S., Ishii, S., Kandel, E. R., and Barco, A. (2004). Chromatin acetylation, memory, and LTP are impaired in $CBP^{+/-}$ mouse model for the cognitive deficit in Rubinstein-Taybi syndrome and its amelioration. *Neuron* **42**, 947–959.

Angus-Hill, M. L., Dutnall, R. N., Tafrov, S. T., Sternglanz, R., and Ramakrishnan, V. (1999). Crystal, structure of the histone acetyltransferase Hpa2: A tetrameric member of the Gcn5–related *N*-acetyltransferase superfamily. *J. Mol. Biol.* **294**, 1311–1325.

Battaglioli, E., Andres, M. E., Rose, D. W., Chenoweth, J. G., Rosenfeld, M. G., Anderson, M. E., and Mandel, G. (2002). REST repression of neuronal genes requires components of the hSWI/SNF complex. *J. Biol. Chem.* **277**, 41038–41045.

Bigey, P., Ramchandani, S., Theberge, J., Araujo, F. D., and Szyf, M. (2000). Transcriptional regulation of the human DNA methyltransferase (dnmt1) gene. *Gene* **242**, 407–418.

Campbell, P. M., and Szyf, M. (2003). Human DNA methyltransferase gene DNMT1 is regulated by the APC pathway. *Carcinogenesis* **24**, 17–24.

Carboni, G., Tueting, P., Tremolizzo, L., Sugaya, I., David, J., Costa, E., and Guidotti, A. (2004). Enhanced dizocilpine efficacy in heterozygous reeler mice relates to GABA turnover downregulation. *Neuropsychopharmacology* **46**, 1070–1081.

Chen, Y., Sharma, R. P., Costa, R. H., Costa, E., and Grayson, D. R. (2002). The epigenetic regulation of the human reelin promoter. *Nucleic Acids Res.* **30**, 2930–2939.

Cheung, P., Tanner, K. G., Cheung, W. L., Sassone-Corsi, P., Denu, J. M., and Allis, C. D. (2000). Synergistic coupling of histone H3 phosphorylation and acetylation in response to epidermal growth factor stimulation. *Med. Cell* **5**, 905–915.

Costa, E., Davis, J., Grayson, D. R., Guidotti, A., Pappas, G. D., and Pesold, C. (2001). Dendritic spine hypoplasticity and downregulation of reelin and GABAergic tone in schizophrenia vulnerability. *Neurobiol. Dis.* **8**, 723–742.

Costa, E., Grayson, D. R., and Guidotti, A. (2003). Epigenetic downregulation of GABAergic function in schizophrenia: Potential for pharmacological intervention? *Mol. Int.* 3(4), 220–229.

Crosio, C., Heitz, E., Allis, C. D., Borrelli, E., and Sassone-Corsi, P. (2003). Chromatin remodeling and neuronal response: Multiple signaling pathways induce specific histone H3 modifications and early gene expression in hippocampal neurons. *J. Cell Sci.* **116**, 4905–4914.

D'Arcangelo, G., Miao, G. G., Chen, S. C., Soares, H. D., Morgan, J. I., and Curran, T. (1995). A protein related to extracellular matrix proteins deleted in the mouse mutant reeler. *Nature* **374**, 719–723.

Davis, S., Vanhoutte, P., Pages, C., Caboche, J., and Laroche, S. (2000). The MAPK/ERK cascade targets both Elk-1 and cAMP response element-binding protein to control long-term potentiation-dependent gene expression in the dentate gyrus *in vivo*. *J. Neurosci.* **20**, 4563–4572.

De Ruijter, A. J., van Gennip, A. H., Caron, H. N., Kemp, S., and van Kuilenburg, A. B. (Ruijter 2003). Histone deacetylases (HDACs): Characterization of the classical HDAC family. *Biochem. J.* **15**, 737–749.

Deng, C., Lu, Q., Zhang, Z., Rao, T., Attwood, J., Yung, R., and Richardson, B. (2003). Hydralazine may induce autoimmunity by inhibiting extracellular signal-regulated kinase pathway signaling. *J. Arthritis Rheum.* **48**, 746–756.

Detich, N., Bovenzi, V., and Szyf, M. (2003). Valproate induces replication-independent active DNA demethylation. *J. Biol. Chem.* **278**, 27586–27592.

Dingledine, R. (1983). Excitatory amino acids: Modes of action on hippocampal pyramidal cells. *Fed. Proc.* **42**, 2881–2885.

Dong, E., Agis-Balboa, R. C., Simonini, M. V., Grayson, D. R., Costa, E., and Guidotti, A. (2005). Reelin and glutamic acid decarboxylase$_{67}$ promoter remodeling in an epigenetic MET-induced mouse model of schizophrenia. *Proc. Natl. Acad. Sci. USA* **102,** 12578–12583.

Dong, E., Caruncho, H., Liu, W. S., Smalheiser, N. R., Grayson, D. R., Costa, E., and Guidotti, A. (2003). A reelin-integrin receptor interaction regulates Arc mRNA translation in synaptoneurosomes. *Proc. Natl. Acad. Sci. USA* **100,** 5479–5484.

Drakew, A., Deller, T., Heimrich, B., Gebhardt, C., Del Turco, D., Tielsch, A., Forster, E., Herz, J., and Frotscher, M. (2002). Dentate granule cells in reeler mutants and VLDLR and ApoER2 knockout mice. *Exp. Neurol.* **176,** 12–24.

Egger, G., Liang, G., Aparicio, A., and Jones, P. A. (2005). Epigenetics in human disease and prospects for epigenetic therapy. *Nature* **429,** 457.

English, J. G., and Sweatt, J. D. (1997). A requirement for the mitogen-activated protein kinase cascade in hippocampal long term potentiation. *J. Biol. Chem.* **272,** 19103–19106.

Fanselow, M. S., Kim, J. J., Yipp, J., and DeOca, B. (1994). Differential effects of the *N*-methyl-D-aspartate antagonist DL-2–amino-5–phosphonovalerate on acquisition of fear of auditory and contextual cues. *Behav. Neurosci.* **108,** 235–240.

Freedman, L. (1999). Increasing the complexity of coactivation in nuclear receptor signaling. *Cell* **97,** 5–8.

Fromm, L., and Burden, S. J. (1998). Synapse specific and neuregulin induced transcription require an Ets site $GABP_{\alpha}/GABP_{\beta}$. *Gene Dev.* **12,** 3074–3083.

Garriga-Canut, M., Roopra, A., and Buckley, N. J. (2001). The basic helix-loop-helix protein, SHARP-1, represses transcription by a histone deacetylase-dependent and histone deacetylase-independent mechanism. *J. Biol. Chem.* **276,** 14821–14828.

Goldberger, C., Gourion, D., Leroy, S., Schurhoff, F., Bourdel, M. C., Leboyer, M., and Krebs, M. O. (2005). Population-based and family-based association study of 5′UTR polymorphism of the reelin gene and schizophrenia. *Am. J. Med. Neuropsychiatr. Genet.* **131,** 51–55.

Grayson, D. R., Jia, X., Chen, Y., Sharma, R., Mitchell, C., Guidotti, A., and Costa, E. (2005). Reelin promoter hypermethylation in schizophrenia. *Proc. Natl Acad. Sci. USA* **102,** 9341–9346.

Guan, Z., Kim, J. H., Lomvardas, S., Holick, K., Xu, S., Kandel, E. R., and Schwartz, J. H. (2003a). MAP kinase mediates both short-term and long-term synaptic depression in *aplysia. J. Neurosci.* **23,** 7317–7395.

Guan, Z., Giustetto, M., Lomvardes, S., Kim, J. H., Miniaci, M. C., Schwartz, J. H., Thanos, D., and Kandel, E. R. (2003b). Integration of long-term-memory-related synaptic plasticity involves bidirectional regulation of gene expression and chromatin structure. *Cell* **111,** 483–493.

Guidotti, A., Auta, J., Davis, J. M., DiGiorgi-Gerevini, V., Dwivedi, Y., Grayson, D. R., Impagnatiello, F., Pandey, G., Pesold, C., Sharma, R., Uzunov, D., and Costa, E. (2000). Decrease in reelin and glutamic acid decarboxylase$_{67}$ ($GAD_{67}$) expression in schizophrenia and bipolar disorder: A postmortem brain study. *Arch. Gen. Psychiatry* **57,** 1061–1069.

Guidotti, A., Auta, J., Davis, J. M., Dong, E., Grayson, D. R., Veldic, M., Zhang, X., and Costa, E. (2005). GABAergic dysfunction in schizophrenia: A new treatment target on the horizon. *Psychopharmacology (Berl.)* **180,** 191–205.

Harris, E. W., Ganong, A. H., and Cotman, C. W. (1984). Long-term potentiation in the hippocampus involves activation of *N*-methyl-D-aspartate receptors. *Brain Res.* **323,** 132–137.

Herz, J., and Beffert, U. (2000). Apolipoprotein E receptors: Linking brain development and Alzheimer's disease. *Nat. Rev. Neurosci.* **1,** 51–58.

Howell, B. W., Hawkes, R., Soriana, P., and Cooper, J. A. (1997). Neuronal position in the developing brain is regulated by mouse disabled-1. *Nature* **389,** 733–737.

Knable, M. B., Barci, B. M., Webster, M. J., Meador-Woodruff, J., and Torrey, E. F. (Stanley Neuropathology Consortium) (2004). Molecular abnormalities of the hippocampus in severe psychiatric illness: Postmortem findings from the Stanley Neuropathology Consortium. *Mol. Psychiatry* **9**, 609–620.

Korzus, E., Rosenfield, M. G., and Mayford, M. (2004). CBP histone acetyltransferase activity is a critical component of memory consolidation. *Neuron* **42**, 961–972.

Larson, J., Hoffman, J. S., Guidotti, A., and Costa, E. (2003). Olfactory discrimination learning deficit in heterozygous reeler mice. *Brain Res.* **971**, 40–46.

Levenson, J. M., and Sweatt, J. D. (2005). Epigenetic mechanisms in memory formation. *Nat. Rev. Neurosci.* **6**, 108–118.

Levenson, J. M., O'Riordan, K. J., Brown, K. D., Trinh, M. A., Molfese, D. L., and Sweatt, J. D. (2004). Regulation of histone acetylation during memory formation in the hippocampus. *J. Biol. Chem.* **279**, 40545–40559.

Lewis, D. A., Hashimoto, T., and Volk, D. W. (2005). Cortical inhibitory neurons and schizophrenia. *Nat. Rev. Neurosci.* **6**, 312–324.

Liu, W. S., Pesold, C., Rodriguez, M. A., Carboni, G., Auta, J., Lacor, P., Larson, J., Condie, B., Guidotti, A., and Costa, E. (2001). Downregulation of dendritic spine and glutamic acid decarboxylase$_{67}$ expressions in reelin haploinsufficient heterozygous reeler mouse. *Proc. Natl. Acad. Sci. USA* **98**, 3477–3482.

Lunyak, V. V., Burgess, R., Prefontaine, G. G., Nelson, C., Sze, S. H., Chenoweth, J., Schwartz, P., Pevzner, P. A., Glass, C., Mandel, G., and Rosenfeld, M. G. (2000). Corepressor-dependent silencing of chromosomal regions encoding neuronal genes. *Science* **298**, 1747–1752.

Martin, L. F., Kem, W. R., and Freedman, R. (2004). Alpha-7 nicotinic receptor agonists: Potential new candidates for the treatment of schizophrenia. *Psychopharmacology (Berl.)* **174**, 54–56.

Méjat, A., Ramond, F., Bassel-Duby, R., Khochbin, S., Olson, E. N., and Schaeffer, L. (2005). Histone deacetylase 9 couples neuronal activity to muscle chromatin acetylation and gene expression. *Nat. Neurosci.* **8**, 313–321.

Mitchell, C. P., Chen, Y., Costa, E., and Grayson, D. R. (2005). Histone deacetylase inhibitors decrease reelin promoter methylation *in vitro*. *J. Neurochem.* **93**, 483–492.

Monneret, C. (2005). Histone deacetylase inhibitors. *Eur. J. Med. Chem.* **40**, 1–13.

Morris, R. G., Anderson, E., Lynch, G. S., and Baudry, M. (1986). Selective impairment of learning and blockade of long-term potentiation by an *N*-methyl-D-aspartate receptor antagonist, AP5. *Nature* **319**, 774–778.

Munro, J., Matthiasson, P., Osborne, S., Travis, M., Purcell, S., Cobb, A. M., Launer, M., Beer, M. D., and Kerwin, R. (2004). Amisulpride augmentation of clozapine: An open non-randomized study in patients with schizophrenia partially responsive to clozapine. *Acta Psychiatr. Scand.* **110**, 292–298.

Niu, S., Renfro, A., Quattrocchi, C. C., Sheldon, M., and D'Arcangelo, G. (2004). Reelin promotes hippocampal dendrite development through the VLDLR/ApoER2–DAB1 pathway. *Neuron* **41**, 71–84.

Noh, J. S., Sharma, R. P., Veldic, M., Salvacion, A. A., Jia, X., Chen, Y., Costa, E., Guidotti, A., and Grayson, R. (2005). DNA methyltransferase 1 regulates reelin mRNA expression in mouse primary cortical cultures. *Proc. Natl. Acad. Sci. USA* **102**, 1749–1754.

Orphanides, G., and Reinberg, D. (2000). RNA polymerase II elongation through chromatin. *Nature* **404**, 471–475.

Pesold, C., Impagnatiello, F., Pisu, M. G., Uzunov, D. P., Costa, E., Guidotti, A., and Caruncho, H. J. (1998). Reelin is preferentially expressed in neurons synthesizing gamma-aminobutyric acid in cortex and hippocampus of adult rats. *Proc. Natl. Acad. Sci. USA* **95**, 3221–3226.

Rice, D. A., and Curran, T. (2001). Role of the reelin signaling pathway in central nervous system development. *Annu. Rev. Neurosci.* **24**, 1005–1039.

Rodriguez, M. A., Pesold, C., Liu, W. S., Kriho, V., Guidotti, A., Pappas, G. D., and Costa, E. (2000). Colocalization of integrin receptors and reelin in dendritic spine postsynaptic densities of adult nonhuman primate cortex. *Proc. Natl. Acad. Sci. USA* **97**, 3550–3555.

Rodriguez, M. A., Caruncho, H. J., Costa, E., Pesold, C., Liu, W. S., and Guidotti, A. (2003). In Patas monkey, glutamic acid decarboxylase67 and reelin mRNA coexpression varies in a manner dependent on layers and cortical areas. *J. Comp. Neurol.* **451**, 279–288.

Rossel, M., Loulier, K., Feuillet, C., Alonso, S., and Carroll, P. (2005). Reelin signaling is necessary for a specific step in the migration of hindbrain efferent neurons. *Development* **132**, 1175–1185.

Ruzicka, W. B., Costa, E., and Guidotti, A. (2005). Cortical GABAergic interneurons sampled from schizophrenia brains with laser assisted microdissection (LAM) overexpress DNA methyltransferase1 (DNMT1) mRNA. *Neuroscience* (Abstract 912.3).

Sanes, J. R., and Lichtman, J. W. (2001). Induction, assembly, and maintenance of a postsynaptic apparatus. *Nat. Rev. Neurosci.* **2**, 791–805.

Schaeffer, L., Duclert, N., Huchet-Dymanus, M., and Changeux, J. P. (1998). Implication of a multisubunit Ets related transcription factor in synaptic expression of the nicotinic acetylcholine receptor. *EMBO J.* **17**, 3078–3090.

Schaeffer, L., de Kerchove d'Exaerde, A., and Changeux, J. P. (2001). Targeting transcription to the neuromuscular synapse. *Neuron* **31**, 15–22.

Schalch, T., Duda, S., Sargent, D. F., and Richmond, T. J. (2005). X-ray structure of a tetranucleosome and its implications for the chromatin fibre. *Nature* **436**, 138–141.

Scheinbart, L. S., Johnson, M. A., Gross, L. A., Edelstein, S. R., and Richardson, B. C. (1991). Procainamide inhibits DNA methyltransferase in a human T cell line. *J. Rheumatol.* **18**, 530–534.

Schmechel, D. E., Saunders, A. M., Strittmatter, W. J., Crain, B. J., Hulette, C. M., Joo, S. H., Pericak-Vance, M. A., Goldgaber, D., and Roses, A. D. (1993). Increased amyloid beta-peptide deposition in cerebral cortex as a consequence of apolipoprotein E genotype in late-onset Alzheimer's disease. *Proc. Natl. Acad. Sci. USA* **90**, 9649–9653.

Sheldon, M., Rice, D. S., D'Arcangelo, G., Yoneshima, H., Nakajima, K., Mikoshiba, K., Howell, B. W., Cooper, J. A., Goldowitz, D., and Curran, T. (1997). Scrambler and yotari disrupt the disabled gene and produce a reeler-like phenotype in mice. *Nature* **389**, 730–733.

Simonini, M. V., Camargo, M. L., Dong, E., Maloku, E., Veldic, M., Costa, E., and Guidotti, A. (2006). The benzamide MS-275 is a potent long-lasting brain region-selective inhibitor of histone deacetylases. *Proc. Natl. Acad. Sci. USA*, **103**, 1587–1592.

Slack, A., Pinard, M., Araujo, F. D., and Szyf, M. (2001). A novel regulatory element in the dnmt1 gene that responds to co-activation by Rb and c-Jun. *Gene* **268**, 87–96.

Somogyi, P., Tamas, G., Lujan, R., and Buhl, E. H. (1998). Salient features of synaptic organisation in the cerebral cortex. *Brain Res. Rev.* **26**, 113–135.

Sananbenesi, F., Fisher, A., Schrick, C., Spiess, J., and Radolovic, J. (2002). Phosphorylation of hippocampal Erk-1/2, Elk-1, and p90–Rsk-1 during contextual fear conditioning: Interactions between Erk-1/2 and Elk-1. *Mol. Cell Neurosci.* **21**, 463–476.

Stahl, S. M., and Grady, M. M. (2004). A critical review of atypical antipsychotic utilization: Comparing monotherapy with polypharmacy and augmentation. *Curr. Med. Chem.* **11**, 313–327.

Tremolizzo, L., Carboni, G., Ruzicka, W. B., Mitchell, C. P., Sugaya, I., Tueting, P., Sharma, R., Grayson, D. R., Costa, E., and Guidotti, A. (2002). An epigenetic mouse model for molecular and behavioral neuropathologies related to schizophrenia vulnerability. *Proc. Natl. Acad. Sci. USA* **99**, 17095–17100.

Tremolizzo, L., Doueiri, M. S., Dong, E., Grayson, D. R., Pinna, G., Tueting, P., Rodriguez-Menendez, V., Costa, E., and Guidotti, A. (2005). Valproate corrects a methionine-induced schizophrenia neuropathology in mice. *Biol. Psychiatry* **57**, 500–509.

Trommsdorff, M., Gotthardt, M., Hiesberger, T., Shelton, J., Stockinger, W., Nimpf, J., Hammer, R. E., Richardson, J. A., and Herz, J. (1999). Reeler/disabled-like disruption of neuronal migration in knockout mice lacking the VLDL receptor and ApoE receptor 2. *Cell* **97**, 689–701.

Turner, B. M. (2002). Cellular memory and the histone code. *Cell* **111**, 285–291.

Varga-Weisz, P., and Becker, P. (1998). Chromatin-remodeling factors: Machines that regulate? *Curr. Opin. Cell Biol.* **10**, 346–353.

Veldic, M., Caruncho, H. M., Liu, W. S., Davis, J., Satta, R., Grayson, D. R., Guidotti, A., and Costa, E. (2004). DNA-methyltransferase 1 mRNA is selectively overexpressed in telencephalic GABAergic interneurons of schizophrenia brains. *Proc. Natl. Acad. Sci. USA* **101**, 348–353.

Veldic, M., Guidotti, A., Maloku, E., Davis, J. M., and Costa, E. (2005). In psychosis, cortical interneurons overexpress DNA-methyltransferase 1. *Proc. Natl. Acad. Sci. USA* **102**, 2152–2157.

Ware, M. L., Fox, J. W., Gonzales, J. L., Davis, N. M., Lambert de Rouvroit, C., Russo, C. J., Chua, S. C., Jr., Goffinet, A. M., and Walsh, C. A. (1997). Aberrant splicing of a mouse disabled homolog, mdab1, in the scrambler mouse. *Neuron* **19**, 239–249.

Wassef, A., Baker, J., and Kochan, L. D. (2003). GABA and schizophrenia: A review of basic science and clinical studies. *J. Clin. Psychopharmacol.* **23**, 601–640.

Weeber, E. J., Beffert, U., Jones, C., Christian, J. M., Forster, E., Sweatt, J. D., and Herz, J. (2002). Reelin and ApoE receptors cooperate to enhance hippocampal synaptic plasticity and learning. *J. Biol. Chem.* **277**, 39944–39952.

**Eugene Roberts**

Director, Department of Neurobiochemistry, Emeritus
Beckman Research Institute, City of Hope Medical Center
Duarte, California 91010

# GABAergic Malfunction in the Limbic System Resulting from an Aboriginal Genetic Defect in Voltage-Gated $Na^+$-Channel SCN5A is Proposed to Give Rise to Susceptibility to Schizophrenia

## I. Chapter Overview

A genetic defect in habituation in schizophrenic patients results from malfunction in the limbic system of the brain, which is correctable by administration of propranolol but not by phenothiazines. I propose that disturbances in communication patterns among subunits of the limbic system, which largely are coordinated by activities of the GABAergic system, result from mutation of the *SCN5A* gene that uniquely codes for the major voltage-gated $Na^+$ channel in the limbic system. Therapeutic problems in large-scale clinical use of propranolol may arise because the *SCN5A* gene also codes for the major $Na^+$ channel in the heart; and appropriate use of propranolol requires maintenance of a careful balance between achieving behavioral improvement and occurrence of cardiac insufficiency. Conditions for use of propranolol or similarly effective substances are being sought that maximize the former and minimize the latter.

*Advances in Pharmacology, Volume 54*

1054-3589/06 $35.00
DOI: 10.1016/S1054-3589(06)54006-2

## II. Introduction

Even at a time of comparative paucity of knowledge of nervous system function 40 years ago, long before the currently explosive developments of molecular biology, I had faith that integration of the information coming at an accelerating rate from the various pertinent disciplines eventually would make possible the comprehension of the continuity that exists "from the molecule to the couch" (Roberts, 1966a,b; Roberts and Matthysse, 1970). It was probably for this reason that I was invited to a prestigious conference "Prospects for Research on Schizophrenia," held from May 9 to 11, 1971, sponsored by the Neuroscience Program at MIT, a summary report of which was published by Kety and Matthysse (1972). Researchers concerned with psychology, physiology, genetics, pharmacology, and biochemistry of schizophrenia were invited together with a group of basic scientists. The wealth of information new to me was overwhelming. Upon return home, I isolated myself for a period of time to try to assimilate it. I then sent the result of my effort to the organizers of the conference, who were preparing a report of the conference. One of their stated purposes had been "to evoke interest on the part of neuroscientists in the problem of schizophrenia." My effort was rewarded in the introduction to their report with the following:

> The thoughtful speculative essay by Roberts is evidence that this was achieved by one neuroscientist. Although it was written afterward, the underlying ideas germinated at the Work Session, and it seemed appropriate to include the essay as an Appendix. Let us hope that the Work Session kindled as strong and productive interest in the problem of schizophrenia among other participants.

Although my essay was entitled "An hypothesis that there is a defect in the GABA system in schizophrenia," it set the pattern for subsequent multidisciplinary, multifactorial approaches to schizophrenia and other cognitive disorders. It was not meant to replace one or another hypothesis. Single neural or transmitter systems cannot be evaluated in isolation. An effect on one reverberates in others as well. Interactional models are more useful than preoccupation with only one. I now would like to add to the existing mix consideration of a key role for voltage-gated $Na^+$ channels.

The data in the literature and the discussion at the above meeting seemed to be in agreement that the maladaptive functioning characteristic of schizophrenic disorders could arise when there are *defects of genetic origin in some primary aspects of central nervous system (CNS) coordination*. The biochemical, pharmacological, and physiological data available on nervous system function at that time suggested to me that a defect in the function of the widely distributed system of inhibitory neurons utilizing GABA as neurotransmitter might be a key system underlying schizophrenia and related cognitive disorders (Roberts, 1972). The conjecture originally was supported by the finding that GABA levels were vastly greater than levels of the biogenic amines in every brain region in which they were reported. There were more marked differences in concentrations of the biogenic amines from one brain region to another than in the case of GABA. Thus for 11 brain regions the ratio of the highest to the lowest level of GABA was 4.7 while the ratio for dopamine, norepinephrine, and serotonin were 267, 51, and 17, respectively. GABA levels were high everywhere but in only some regions were there found to be relatively high levels of one or two of the biogenic amines. How GABAergic and dopaminergic interactions might be wedded was suggested in a report (Yee *et al.*, 2005): "Employing knock-out mice with an absence of a $\alpha 3$ subunit-containing $GABA_A$ receptor induces a hyperdopaminergic phenotype including a severe deficit in sensorimotor gating, a common feature among psychiatric conditions including schizophrenia." A direct bridge from the highly manipulated mouse experiments to the naturally occurring cognitive deficits of human schizophrenia does not yet exist.

Over the years, I have engaged in considerations related to problems of epilepsy, schizophrenia, Huntington's disease, multiple sclerosis, senile dementia of the Alzheimer's type, autism, hepatic coma, neural regeneration, and addiction to alcohol and other drugs. Each time I embarked on such a study, in countercurrent fashion, I passed whatever knowledge was available to me at that time against what was known of the particular disease process in order to determine whether or not there would be an aspect on which I could hang my scientific hat. In the study of the above conditions, with few exceptions no ready handles appeared. The exceptions of which I was aware consisted largely of symptoms that mimic some aspects of the above disorders produced by dietary deficiencies, intake of drugs or toxic substances, or an easily correctable clinical condition. Provided that truly irreversible changes had not taken place, such symptoms often could be ameliorated by correcting the deficiency by cessation of exposure to certain exogenous agents or their intake or by a simple therapeutic maneuver. For example, convulsive seizures in otherwise normal infants with a simple dietary deficiency of vitamin $B_6$, induced by feeding a commercial infant formula from which the vitamin was inadvertently omitted, were completely eliminated almost immediately after the intramuscular injection of pyridoxine, presumably because of an extremely rapid conversion of the injected pyridoxine to the coenzymatically active pyridoxal phosphate, the association of the latter with a suboptimally functional glutamic acid decarboxylase (GAD) in nerve terminals of inhibitory nerves, accelerated synthesis of GABA therein, and the release of GABA from the terminals onto postsynaptic receptor sites. The consequent desynchronization resulting from the reinstitution of normal neural inhibition prevented the paroxysmal discharges of groups of neurons whose firing was causing the seizures. Paranoid schizophrenia-like symptoms sometimes associated with amphetamine intake often can be cured by stopping the drug. Hallucinations and psychotic behavior in uremic individuals may be reversed by renal dialysis. Hallucinations accompanying high fever or sensory isolation may disappear with normalization of body temperature and sensory input, respectively. Some consequences of spinal cord injury may be attenuated by early treatment with anti-inflammatory drugs or free radical-trapping agents or by administration of substances that decrease activity of hyperactive macrophages (Guth *et al.*, 1994). In instances such as those cited above, it is possible to help the system *self-organize* into a more normal state of function.

The above are trivial solutions to a few disease-mimetic instances. In the case of schizophrenia and other cognitive disorders, the situation generally appeared to be much more complicated; and we were wandering in the wilderness of complexities of the CNS without being able definitively to come to terms with all relevant problems at structural, metabolic, and/or molecular levels. This may be because the conceptual frameworks and information bases with which we operated often were inadequate. I believe that we must strive constantly to establish valid, commonly shared core positions from which to view meaningful phenomena of major human interest such as memory, consciousness, various aspects of normal and abnormal behavior, neurological disease, aging, and so on, and the molecular and submolecular events that constantly are taking place at the level of excitable membranes. To whatever extent they are pertinent to a given problem, our studies must make use of the methods and knowledge of the physical, chemical, and biological sciences and of any other applicable disciplines. This does not mean that we should be paralyzed into inactivity by a need to study all of the factors involved simultaneously or that huge research groups with a variety of experts in different disciplines should be assembled to work on every problem. Rather, it suggests that we should maintain an awareness of multiple factors while studying one or only a few which seem to be most pertinent at a particular time. Above all, as scientists and scholars, we should remain open to serendipitous observations and not be pigeonholed by so-called expertise, previous research experience, currently held beliefs, or considerations related to patentability and profitability.

Ingenious manipulation of structures and uses of substances arrived at unexpectedly or empirically can lead to great and rapid therapeutic progress, which, in turn, can give rise to new tools for study of basic biological mechanisms. For example, although for some time there has been much information about the glutamatergic and GABAergic transmitter systems, respectively, few widely clinically useful drugs based on this knowledge had been devised to date. On the other hand, curiosity about the analgesic and antispastic properties of baclofen, a failed GABA-mimetic in classical $GABA_A$ $Cl^-$ channel conductance paradigms, led to the discovery of $GABA_B$ receptors that are coupled to $K^+$ channels and to many new therapeutic possibilities (Bowery *et al.*, 1990). In this current chapter it will be recounted how a report of the use of unprecedentedly high doses of propranolol to reduce the dangerously high blood pressure and tachycardia of a patient suffering from acute variegate porphyria accompanied by psychotic symptoms (Atsmon and Blum, 1978; Atsmon *et al.*, 1972) eventually led me to the suggestion that in schizophrenia a major genetic defect might be traceable to the abnormal operation of a particular type of voltage-gated $Na^+$ channel.

## III. Levels of Concern

One of the keystones of a useful research strategy and a realistic interpretation of experimental results is recognition of the level at which one is working and knowledge of the overall structure of the framework at that level. In the discussion that follows I draw heavily on previous integrative efforts either directly or with emendations.

### A. The Organism in its Environment

The organism is a hedonic optimizer (Fig. 1). In its waking condition, it seeks the optimal state of well-being, which is associated with comfort, pleasure, ease, satisfaction, absence of anxiety and boredom, and so on. Displacement from such a state, the set points for the detection of which are variable, may result in feelings of anxiety, discomfort, boredom, or pain. Continual changes taking place in the external environment and in the internal metabolism generally act counter to the maintenance or achievement of a hedonic state and tend to displace the organism away from it.

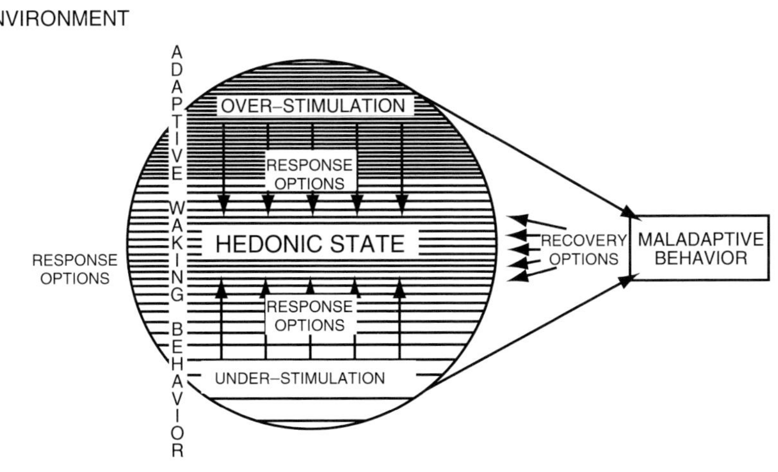


**FIGURE 1** A hedonic "homing" model for an organism in its environment.

If stimulus input is too small, too rapid, or too great in intensity for the organism to handle, maladaptive responses might take place that eventually might lead to the actual destruction of the organism. If the organism survives, return to an adaptive behavioral pattern may occur through new learning and/or simplifying or increasing the complexity of the environmental input. Intervention is possible with drugs, hormones, surgical techniques, electroshock, and so forth. Psychotherapeutic approaches may be effective, particularly those that disclose the existence and encourage the use of previously unused potentially adaptive behavioral options. The effect of any therapeutic approach must be evaluated at this level of organization for which evaluation valid quantitative measurements of efficacy of treatment must be sought.

An awake organism continually scans with specialized receptors its multisensory environment, internally and externally, for physical and chemical changes (Fig. 2). At any particular time, the changing pattern in the perceived environment is the stimulus for the organism. A novel effective *stimulus pattern* activates receptors in a unique fashion, that is, the types and numbers of receptors activated, and their sequences, intensities, and rates of activation result in receptor and neural activation patterns that are different

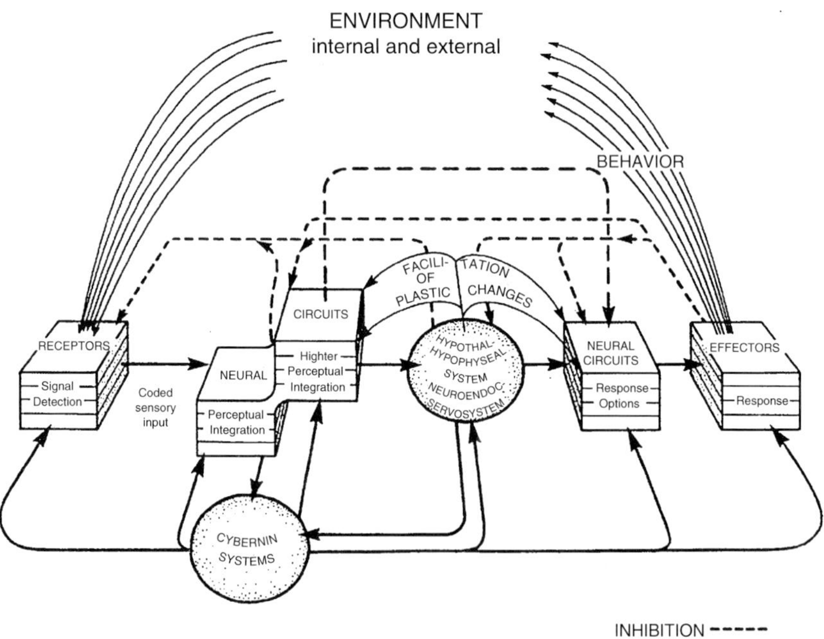


**FIGURE 2** A model for behavior showing the major systems involved in informational transactions.

from any experienced previously by the organism. Release occurs of neural circuits, which may be considered to consist of cascades of serially aligned neuronal assemblies in which coded patterns of information entering from sensory transducers are progressively refined by the reduction of redundancy and the selection of particular features (Fig. 2). The transformations of coded patterns in different neural sectors are achieved to a considerable extent by negative feedback loops that exist between and within the sectors, and their temporal and spatial integration is achieved by activity of neural command centers such as the cerebellar cortex, hippocampus, basal ganglia, thalamus, and association cortex. The "hard-wired" neuronal elements of the throughput and command neuronal circuits, the blueprints for the construction of whose framework largely are inherited by the organism, are surrounded by local-circuit neurons whose specific commitments may be made during development, as well as later in life, and which not only participate in virtually all phases of information processing but also may undergo plastic changes that may be involved in long-term retention of experience. Communication between neural elements takes place largely through synaptic and gap junctions on a millisecond or submillisecond timescale.

Work on information processing in the sensory pathways, as exemplified by findings in the visual system, shows that the nervous system can abstract from the unanalyzed stimulation impinging on the receptor qualities of the perceived objects that are more relevant for behavior than the unprocessed signal itself. Thus, similarity and contrast, onset and termination of stimuli, motion, and geometrical shape are singled out for perceptual attention. A still higher level of perceptual integration takes place before the organism can respond adaptively to the pattern of sensory input. The stimulus pattern is brought into relation with memories of past stimuli and their consequences (associative integration) and with the drive state of the organism (emotional integration). In other words, stimulus patterns similar to the one at hand are called up from memory storage and a decision is made as to whether or not the stimulus presents opportunities for need satisfaction or a potential threat to survival. The highest order of perceptual integration and executive decision in human beings now is believed by many to take place in the prefrontal cortex. The result of the impingement and the processing of information is behavior, some reaction of the organism to the environment and/or action upon the environment.

During early stages of the response of an organism to displacement from the hedonic state (Fig. 1), there is maximal desynchronization of firing within and between neural regions in the CNS (Fig. 2). The behavior observed initially is of the "alarm" type indigenous to the species being studied. For a period after the first experience with a particular stimulus pattern, more primary sensory neural circuits are active than when subsequently the stimulus intensity is being reduced by effective behavior.

As problem solving proceeds, the degree of asynchrony is reduced as a result of decreased environmental inputs and inhibitory feedbacks from neural activity in other brain regions. Eventually, neural activity in brain regions irrelevant to the solution of the problem at hand is reduced essentially to basal levels (Fig. 3).

The net effect of a maximal development of connectivities upon the experience of an organism with a particular new stimulus set is the establishment of a facilitated system of information flow, different at least in some respects from any present in the organism before. With continued experience in a given situation, after the first moment of stimulation the activation of the minimal number of neural circuits and the minimal release of hormones and cybernins (see Section V) is accompanied by behavior that approaches the maximal efficiency and adaptability attainable by the organism under the circumstances.

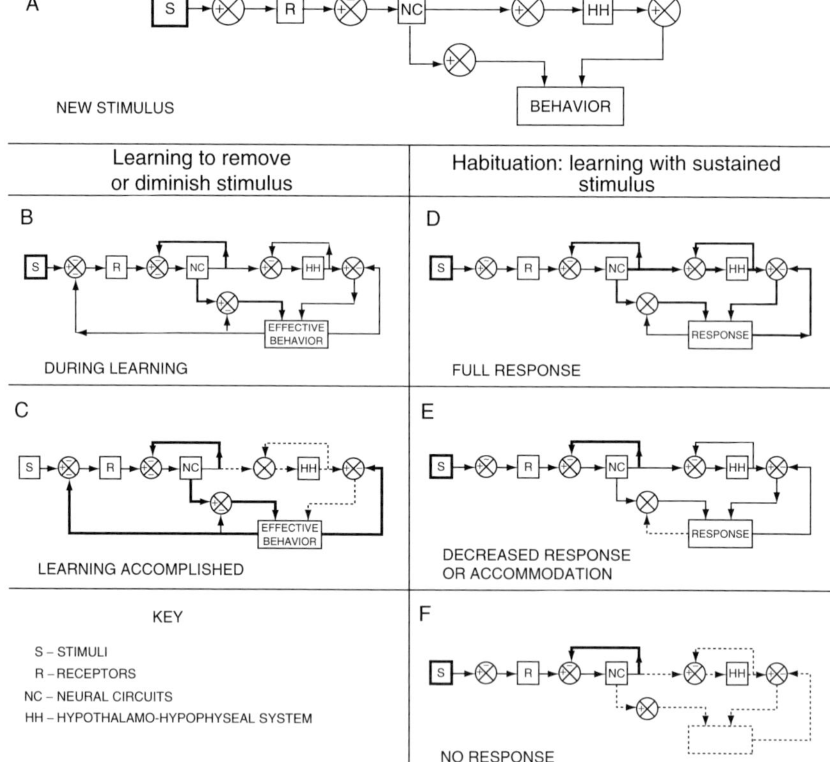


**FIGURE 3** Learning and habituation: patterns of reactions to stimuli during development of connectivities.

## B. Responses of the Organism to Stimulus Patterns: Action or Habituation

Upon exposure to a particular stimulus pattern, the subsequent course of the behavioral responses is determined by whether or not the behavior can lead to removal or modification of the stimulus (Fig. 3B and C) or whether circumstances are such that a meaningless stimulus, for example, sound, becomes less effective (Fig. 3D–F). In the former case the intensity of the stimulus is decreased by the initial behavior of the organism (avoiding a dangerous or noxious situation, obtaining food, water, or sexual satisfaction, and so on) and each reoccurrence of the stimulus set affords opportunity for the organism to achieve behavior which is more effective in terms of responding more appropriately and is more efficient and economical in terms of use of the resources of the organism (Fig. 3B and C). The learning process is accompanied by increases in connectivities in those neural pathways that set into action appropriate combinations of effectors (behavior). Also, increases occur in connectivities of those associations from the neural circuits that feed back and inhibit the receptor signaling systems and of those associations from the effectors that exert inhibitory feedback effects on the neural circuits in the CNS, which activate them. At least some of the effector organs liberate or remove substances in such a manner that the changes in concentrations of these substances in the blood constitute inhibitory feedback signals to hormone-secreting cells activated by the stimulus. The net effect upon continued experience of an organism with a particular stimulus pattern is the establishment of a cybernetic system, different at least in some respects from any present in the organism before, in which after the first moment of stimulation, the activation of the minimal number of neural circuits and the minimal release of hormones and cybernins would be accompanied by behavior that would approach the maximal efficiency attainable by the organism under the circumstances.

Although the same general type of reasoning as above may be applied to the situation in which the organism cannot act on the environment to change or modify the stimulus (Fig. 3D–F), there are important differences. When no possibility exists of achieving a new coordinated behavioral (or effector) pattern appropriate to the stimulus, the behavior observed initially for as long as any overt responses to the stimulus can be observed, is of the "alarm" type indigenous to the species studied. For a period after the first experience with the stimulus, more primary sensory neural circuits are active than would be the case if the stimulus intensity could be reduced by effective behavior. As a result, more neural circuits develop strong negative feedback connectivities with the receptor signaling systems and, in the limiting case, a state is achieved in which the particular stimulus pattern to which the organism is exposed evokes some activity in the CNS but there is no overt behavioral response and little or no apparent activation the hypothalamo-hypophyseal (HH) endocrine and neural responses (Fig. 3F). From the point of view of the organism this would be the most effective way of dealing with such a situation.

Thus, under normal circumstances there is an initial focus on the stimulus, that is, *orienting* toward it, and then ignoring it when it is determined to be inconsequential, that is, *habituating* to it. A clear-cut example of observations of habituation in man can be cited in which simultaneous recordings were made of the EEG from the occipital and motor regions, the skin galvanic response, muscle tension, eye movements, and respiration. At first presentation of a tactile stimulation there was a generalized response, all of the recordings showing activation. After 24 presentations of the stimulus, the only response recorded was a brief change in EEG in the motor region. Similar results were obtained with proprioceptive stimuli (Sokolov, 1960).

Experiments were performed with cats in which there were chronically implanted electrodes in the following areas: visual and auditory cortex, mesencephalic reticular formation, superior colliculus, amygdala, posterior hippocampus, lateral geniculate, and anterior hippocampus. When the animals were first exposed to flickering light of a given frequency, responses with the frequency of the light stimulus were observed in all of the areas in stimulus, and the responses decreased markedly in all areas. After 20 days there was virtually no longer any evidence of following in the visual cortex, brain stem reticular formation, and hippocampus and even in the lateral geniculate body in which originally there was continuous frequency-specific following of a relatively high amplitude, only occasional small residual bursts of very low amplitude were observed (John and Killam, 1959).

Inhibitory feedback pathways to various sensory receptors come from regions in the brain stem, thalamus, and cortex, which operate in such a manner as to decrease the amount of sensory information reaching the latter. Thalamic and cortical inhibitory pathways restrict the effects of activation at lower levels, and cortical feedback to thalamic regions acts as a final brake on the degree of cortical activation elicited by sensory stimulation. Inhibitory feedback from cortical areas undoubtedly plays an important part in establishment of feedback connectivities during learning and habituation (Fig. 2). In the case of well-established habituations (Fig. 3F), the feedback connectivities at the subcortical levels might become sufficiently powerful so that eventually there is little or no activation of the pertinent cortical regions by the stimulus, and consequently no detectable participation of the cortex in the inhibitory processes necessary for the maintenance of a particular habituation.

*There now is much compelling evidence in the literature to suggest that disturbances in habituation may be major causative factors leading to the cognitive defects of schizophrenia.*

## IV. The Hypothalamo-Hypophyseal System

The environment acting through the receptors on neural circuits in the CNS has an effect on the neuroendocrine servosystem or the HH system, a part of the central visceromotor system, which in turn has important influences on behavior, particularly at times when a new environmental setting requires the organism to develop new ways of adjustment (Fig. 2). The key to the HH is in the hypothalamus, which plays a central role in the coordination of physiological processes within the organism so that a relative constancy of the steady states (homeostasis) within the organism is maintained at all times.

The HH system has a controlling role in the release of pituitary hormones that have antidiuretic and oxytocic effects (posterior pituitary) as well as controlling effects on the function of the anterior pituitary, adrenal, and thyroid glands and the gonads. The hypothalamus also sends impulses to the adrenal and pancreas via conduction systems originating in the mesencephalon, thus playing a governing role in the secretion of epinephrine, norepinephrine, insulin, thyroxin and a variety of steroids, for example, cortisone, dehydroepiandrosterone, pregnenolone, and so forth. Neural pathways from the hypothalamus participate in the regulation of respiration, shivering, piloerection, sweating, heart rate, vasomotor changes in peripheral organs, gut motility and secretion, dilation of the pupil, the widening of the bronchioles, and so on. Other projections from the hypothalamus connect with the thalamus and cerebral cortex and ascending impulses into these regions are thought to be involved in the maintenance of the alert state. Thus, the hypothalamus is strategically situated to exert a major influence upon practically all those effector systems that are qualified to adjust and preserve the constancy of the internal environment. There are many inputs to it both from forebrain structures and from the brain stem, and in many neurons of the hypothalamus there is convergence of several sensory modalities. In addition, some neurons in the hypothalamus are remarkably sensitive to changes in osmotic pressure, glucose concentration, insulin, $pO_2$, $pCO_2$, steroid hormones, or temperature. The imperfection of the blood–brain barrier in the hypothalamus makes nerve cells in this region much more sensitive to humoral influences than are those in most other regions of the CNS. Changes in levels of most blood constituents appear to exert effects on some specialized neurons in the hypothalamus.

The HH receives inputs from the amygdala representing the emotionally significant aspects of the total stimulus pattern, external and internal, and summates them. When the response to the signal (arousal level), $L$, is greater than a preprogrammed optimal value $L_0$, drive level and/or intensity and complexity of environmental stimuli are too high, whereas when the arousal level is less, they are too low. The neural representation of the HH signal may be the frequency of discharge of neurons in a certain hypothalamic nucleus, or a more complicated index, such as the degree of correlation between discharge times of pairs of neurons taken at random from a given hypothalamic nucleus, in other words, an index of the degree of synchrony. The HH may initiate two kinds of restorative processes when the deviation from $L_0$ and/or the rate of change of deviation from $L_0$ exceeds a certain value. In the first place, it generates a signal that causes the organism to act according to the response options already available. These options are stored as fully programmed, hierarchically arranged, integrated sequences of behavior in various parts of the nervous system (including the hypothalamus), ready to go into effect when released, but usually held in check by tonic inhibitory GABAergic interneurons. These behavioral sequences are normally in a state of inhibition, except perhaps for occasional spontaneous release that gives rise to a low background of unstimulated display of behavior. The HH releasing signal inhibits these inhibitory interneurons nonspecifically, resulting in the release of whatever behavior patterns are "prepotent," that is, at the top of the hierarchy of options at that time. In addition to this behavior-releasing function, the HH causes neurohumoral changes to take place, which facilitate plastic change throughout the CNS. In other words, through increasing local circulation and, therefore, glucose and oxygen availability and through secretion of hormones and growth factors, it puts the organism in a condition of optimal readiness to learn new adaptive behaviors. Thus, it has both a short- and long-range function in restoring the state of well-being and enhancing future adaptive capacity.

## V. The Cybernins

Some neurons, such as those that release GABA, acetylcholine, glutamate, aspartate, and glycine, probably largely are involved in direct point-to-point information transmittal. In other words, release of transmitter from the presynaptic endings of such neurons affects postsynaptic sites in such a way that, within approximately a millisecond, excitatory or inhibitory information is transmitted to postsynaptic sites, recognized, and the signaling substance removed. There are other groups of neurons, such as those that release catecholamines, serotonin, a variety of peptides, prostaglandins, and possibly other substances, which current evidence suggests may act chiefly by liberating their characteristic substances more generally into whole regions that contain various neuronal elements as well as glial cells and blood vessels. These substances may exert relatively long-lasting effects on blood flow and capillary permeability as well as more direct metabolic and trophic effects on the cellular elements, possibly setting the gain on the efficacy of individual synapses, on specific types of synapses, or on all of the synapses in a given region. Their effects may be exerted at many functional loci, such as transmitter synthesis, the postsynaptic control of total ion channel open time after transmitter impingement, and the setting of windows on which of the total range of potential firing frequencies may be employed by given neurons or groups of neurons. These effects are exerted by a large variety of cascading molecular mechanisms.

Such neurons, as mentioned above, furnish the "oil" required for the neuronal machinery to function smoothly. That is, the effects of the neurons releasing such substances may be analogous to that of squirting oil into inadequately lubricated but intact machinery, the parts of which will not function properly if sufficient oil is not furnished or if they are over oiled. However, the oil is not part of the actual machinery. I suggest that in many instances in which they act in the CNS, the catecholamines, serotonin, neurally released peptides, and prostaglandins serve to optimize regional nervous system activity in relation to functional demands without themselves necessarily being involved in specific point-to-point information transmittal. It was proposed to call such substances cybernins, according to the suggestion of Roger Guillemin (1977). For example, immunocytochemical, isotope labeling, and physiologic experiments are compatible with the suggestion that norepinephrine neurons in rat brain largely perform global, hormone-like functions, although they also may participate in typical synaptic relationships.

An inappropriate balance between availability and distribution of such cybernins may result in gross malfunction of the CNS as found in Parkinson's and Huntington's diseases or schizophrenia. It is striking that when the substantia nigra is stimulated, physiologically recorded signals in the corpus striatum do not seem to be greatly altered when the nigrostriatal neurons are destroyed by 6-OH-dopamine or when the action of dopamine is blocked completely by large doses of haloperidol. Also, the spontaneous firing rates of cells in the caudate nucleus are not altered by dopamine-depleting lesions of the nigrostriatal pathway. This suggests that the physiologically relevant signals are carried by fibers of nondopaminergic nigral neurons and that the effects of dopamine released from the dopaminergic fibers are not informational in the strictest sense of the word, as suggested above. A phenomenon related to the above is described in many anecdotal accounts about parkinsonian patients, obviously suffering from defective functioning of nigrostriatal dopaminergic neurons, who can fully mobilize normal and adaptive physical activity in an emergency but who relapse into the typically inactive parkinsonian state as soon as the emergency is over. The above and the therapeutic effects of exogenously supplied levodopa in parkinsonism are compatible with the suggestion that the neuronal "hard-wired" circuitry in the neostriatum is potentially available and that the dopaminergic neurons furnish dopamine, the "oil" required for the neuronal machinery to function smoothly. In contrast, it seems likely that relative overactivity of the dopamine and/or the noradrenergic systems in particular brain regions is associated with psychotic and cognitive disorders and that the favorable action of neuroleptic drugs and propranolol in some of these conditions probably is attributable, in part, to their damping of the effects of these systems, possibly by frequency-dependent nerve block (see later).

The cybernin and neurotransmitter systems can be considered as entities having somewhat different, but complementary, functions in the CNS. They are mutually interactive in all instances and in all neural regions. The main idea is that when an organism perceives that a problem exists, the stimuli reflecting the problem release both throughput, HH, and cybernin circuits simultaneously, the latter helping maintain a general state of readiness at the outset. Once the nature of the problem is assessed in the CNS, internal decisions are reached with regard to which brain regions and what specific circuitry within these regions would be most likely to be employed in the solution of the problem. Then the cybernin systems are instructed to focus onto elements of the pertinent neural machinery, liberating their chemical facilitators and modulators, as though sprayed from an oil gun, to ready specific neural components for appropriate action. This sets the stage for rapid recovery from the activity and for those plastic changes to take place, which would make it possible for the organism to solve the same or similar problems more expeditiously in the future. This action of cybernins gives the temporarily functionally favored regions priority on the available oxygen and nutrient supplies and adjusts the cyclic nucleotide levels so that appropriate neural and glial membrane sensitivities and permeabilities would be maintained. Various intracellular metabolic cascades are adjusted to keep transmitter synthesis, release, and inactivation and general housekeeping reactions going at rates commensurate with the functional requirements. The cybernins also act in such a way as to decrease activities and shunt oxygen and nutrients away from those cerebral regions and circuits not germane to the solution of the particular problem at hand. *There is constant interactional adjustment between the throughput circuitry and the cybernin neurons and HH systems, largely via inhibitory and disinhibitory actions of GABAergic interneurons, so that the entire system, through gradually diminishing oscillations, would "home" in on the optimal functional state. Disease states occur when such a system goes out of the range in which cybernetic adjustment can take place in a self-organizing manner.*

## VI. A Failed Therapeutic Adventure

In the late 1960s and early 1970s I was a member of the research committee of the California State Mental Health Commission, whose job was to oversee clinical and basic research activities in eight well-run and felicitously located mental hospitals throughout the state—a truly model program. I was busy scanning the environment for possibilities of new antipsychotic drugs for treatment of patients with chronic schizophrenia, who constituted a majority of the patient population. This seemed to me to be a matter of great urgency because of physically undesirable and psychologically adverse effects of the drugs then in use. Immunological disorders were detected in some patients. The unpredictable appearance of irreversible neurological damage in the form of the so-called tardive dyskinesias in many patients receiving tranquilizing drugs raised the frightening specter of the accumulation of a population of individuals who were both psychotic and permanently neurologically disabled.

It was at that time that I became aware of the work of two Israeli internists, Ilana Blum and Abraham Atsmon, of the Beilinson Medical Center in Tel Aviv who had decided to use extremely high doses of propranolol in a last-ditch effort to reduce the dangerously high blood pressure and bradycardia of a female patient with variegate porphyria who also was showing acute psychotic behavior (Atsmon *et al.*, 1972). Large doses of chlorpromazine and Demerol were not helpful. It was decided to use propranolol because it was a widely employed agent effective in reduction of heart rate and blood pressure. During treatment with the latter, there was a sudden cessation of a variety of characteristic symptoms of porphyria and a complete clearance of neurological and psychotic manifestations in the patient. Careful extension of these studies to nonporphyric psychotic patients subsequently was carried out, first in Israel and then elsewhere, often with observation of marked improvement in symptoms related to schizophrenia (Atsmon and Blum, 1978). Relatively large-scale studies carried out at Friern Hospital in London confirmed, refined, and amplified the original results reported by Atsmon and Blum (Yorkston *et al.*, 1978a).

Curious and skeptical, I visited both groups *in situ* and engaged in lengthy discussions with the respective teams. I was impressed by their competence and sincerity. Upon return, I convinced Peter Amacher, then director of the conference program of the Kroc Foundation, to host a conference based on these findings, to which were invited some distinguished research psychiatrists and neuropharmacologists in addition to the groups from Tel Aviv and London. An account of the conference was published (Roberts and Amacher, 1978).

Throughout the proceedings, emphasis was placed on the detailed discussion of the clinical results and assessment of the validity of the findings. This was particularly critical because, up to the time of the conference, the studies that had been reported were open ones and, therefore, were subject to all of the usual criticisms directed at such studies. The urgency of applying the practical, empirical findings, if valid, to human psychotic disorders greatly outweighed the immediate necessity of elucidating the exact mechanisms of the antipsychotic action of propranolol. By the time of the meeting, the Yorkston group had completed the first controlled double-blind study that showed a highly significant ameliorative effect with propranolol in carefully diagnosed schizophrenic patients.

The group consensus at the meeting was that the results were of sufficient promise for the work to be rapidly accelerated to determine definitively the clinical utility of the propranolol approach. The conference, at the Kroc Foundation, was followed by meetings held at the City of Hope National Medical Center and at the University of Southern California School of Medicine. Both latter meetings were attended by large numbers of interested members of the medical and scientific communities from California and other Southwestern states. There, too, the work was subjected to critical and extensive discussion with very positive consensus. Hope was expressed that many patients might benefit from application of the material presented. Although since that time 156 papers have appeared (PubMed) that have dealt with propranolol and schizophrenia in one way or another, no widely useful approaches in treatment have been devised.

In the intervening 27 years, the widespread use of the original neuroleptics and a second generation of related antipsychotic drugs has continued unabated with unimproved results. Much to my chagrin, a report that appeared last week analyzing results of a multicenter study of 1493 patients with schizophrenia at 57 US sites concluded that "the majority of patients in each (drug) group discontinued their assigned treatment owing to inefficacy or intolerable side effects or for other reasons" (Lieberman *et al.*, 2005).

The failure to pursue effectively the propranolol work might be because of inability to obtain funds to perform sufficient numbers of controlled studies employing the appropriate precautions in the use of propranolol such as those recommended by Yorkston *et al.* (1978b). This, also may, in part, be attributable to the lack of financial interest of drug companies because of nonpatentability of the technology and the high profitability of their continued sale of old remedies. Other important factors may be that use of propranolol requires the careful monitoring of individual patients by physicians who are well-schooled in internal medicine and clinical pharmacology and that the fiscal structure of current medical practice precludes this kind of care for mental patients.

My own thoughts and activities turned elsewhere because I considered that my role as catalyst had been fulfilled and because the excellent California mental health system was virtually completely dismantled during the period of 1967–1974. Many chronic schizophrenic patients swelled the ranks of the homeless in the major urban centers and continue to do so. However, my scientific interest in propranolol and schizophrenia has continued unabated. The considerations to be discussed in the following sections may serve to help put a new face on the subject.

## VII. Linkage of Propranolol Cognitive Effects with Correction of a Limbic System Defect that Results in Failure of Habituation in Schizophrenia (See Gruzelier, 1978)

Similarities have been noted between the behavioral *effects* of propranolol and the behavioral *functions* of the amygdala. The amygdala and the hippocampus exert modulatory controls over the hypothalamus and thereby affect the regulation of the visceroautonomic system, which plays a key role in emotional expression and in learning and conditioning processes. An example of this control is reflected in the autonomic orienting response and its rate of habituation. This can be demonstrated in the laboratory by observing the electrodermal response, often termed the GSR, to a pure tone of moderate intensity and watching it diminish with each successive tone presentation. Amygdalectomized monkeys do not show these processes of first orienting to the sound and then habituating to it. They show one of two patterns—either they fail to exhibit responses at all or their responses fail to extinguish as the sound is repeated. Hippocampal damage in monkeys also results in deficits of habituation. Schizophrenics display electrodermal orienting patterns similar to those of amygdalectomized monkeys. "Evidence from many sources points to the involvement of temporal-limbic processes in schizophrenia .... It is conceivable that the efficacy of propranolol in schizophrenia results through the restoration of temporal-limbic functions, such as those of the amygdala and hippocampus" (Gruzelier, 1978).

The above hypothesis was tested in an elegant study of the electrodermal orienting and habituation responses of a suitable control population and of untreated schizophrenics and of schizophrenics treated either with propranolol or phenothiazines.

At all times the subjects sat in a sound-attenuated room. Briefly, skin conductance responses were measured to 1000 Hz tones (70 dB/s) presented 13 times at intervals varying between 20 and 40 s. Skin conductance was measured from bipolar placements on the distal phalanges of the first and second finger of each hand. Appropriately designed and calibrated equipment was used in measurement and recording of the results. A positive response was operationally defined as occurring between 0.8 and 5 s after stimulus onset. A minimum criterion for a response was judged to be a 1 mm deflection. Three successive failures to respond was the criterion set as failure of habituation to have taken place.

Among the normal controls (Fig. 4A), all but two subjects gave orienting responses, and of the responders three were slow in habituating and five failed to habituate at all. In the case of the schizophrenic patients studied (Fig. 4B), most of these were nonresponders and those who were responders were slow habituators or did not habituate at all. Phenothiazines did not

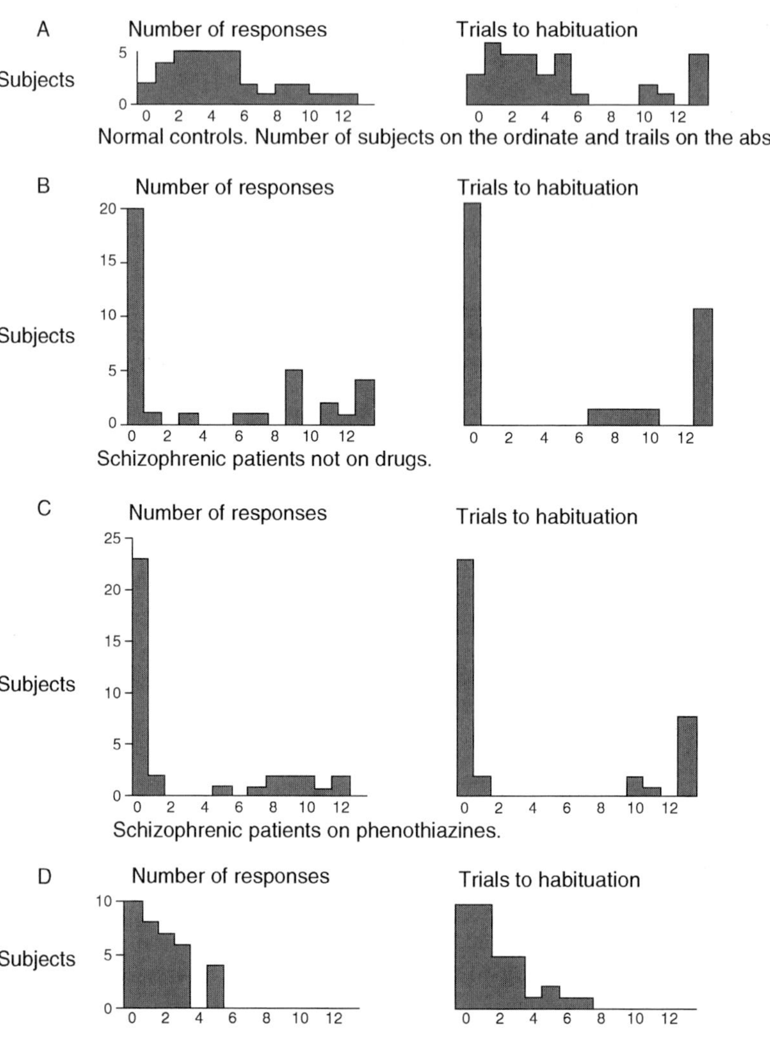


**FIGURE 4** Orienting responses and habituation in normal controls and in untreated schizophrenics and in those receiving either phenothiazines or propranolol.

correct the failure to orient or the slowness in habituating (Fig. 4C). However, propranolol treatment (Fig. 4D) reduced nonresponders to approximately half the number found with untreated schizophrenic patients or those on phenothiazines, and there were no nonhabituators among the responders. Amazingly, propranolol reinstated the orienting response in some previously nonresponders and increased the rate of habituation in responders, even above that observed in the nonschizophrenic controls.

To my knowledge, propranolol is the only substance known that improves schizophrenic symptoms and also corrects a defect in limbic system function that probably is related to the disease—failure of habituation.

## VIII. Susceptibility to Schizophrenia may Result from Mutation of the $Na^+$ Channel-Coding *SCN5A* Gene, Which Occurs at Uniquely High Levels in Neural Components of the Limbic System

There is constant interaction among all of the excitatory and inhibitory influences, which impinge on the membranes of neurons. Many factors determine, at a particular time, whether or not the spatially and temporally summated effects of excitatory and disinhibitory inputs are sufficient to reduce the membrane potential to the critical level at which the all-or-none propagation of a spike discharge takes place along the axon or in nonspiking neurons to reduce the membrane potential to an extent that would result in an increase in transmitter release from its terminals above the resting level. Even in the absence of spike generation or of any transmitter release, local depolarizations or hyperpolarizations of neuronal membranes may exert transient and/or long-range effects on properties of neurons by changing the local properties of the membrane regions at which they occur. Most neurons in their normal environments in intact organisms are members of neuronal groupings or circuits and have largely ceded their autonomy while becoming participants in an integrated neural community.

Depolarization of excitable membranes results in increases in their permeability to cations, largely $Na^+$ ions. It is the voltage-dependent flow of $Na^+$ ions that is largely responsible for the rapid membrane depolarization that initiates action potentials in neurons and other types of excitable cells. Although there is diffuse expression of the several $Na^+$ ion channel $\alpha 1$ subunits throughout the brain, there is a remarkably restricted regional distribution of the mRNA coded by *SCN5A* genes in tissue of the limbic system (Hartmann *et al.*, 1999). Very low levels of the SCN5A transcripts were detected in the hippocampal formation as well as in other brain regions. Interestingly, the *SCN5A* gene also is the major $Na^+$ channel coding gene expressed in cardiac muscle, mutations in the human gene resulting in various pathophysiological defects, among which is the long QT syndrome, which is characterized by prolonged myocardial depolarization with episodic tachyarrythmias and idiopathic ventricular fibrillation. *SCN5A* mutant phenotypes also may be associated with epileptiform phenomena (Meisler *et al.*, 2002; Noebels, 2002). Mutations in $Na^+$ channel genes and use or disuse dependent changes in transcriptional and translational patterns within individual neurons or groups of communicating neurons have opened a vast new field of study of so-called channelopathies (Bock and Goode, 2002).

> The restricted pattern of SCN5A expression contrasts with the diffuse expression of other sodium-channel genes, predicting a role in regulating excitability and synchronization specifically within these circuits. SCN5A-positive regions comprise a synaptically linked pathway from the piriform cortex and bed nucleus of the stria terminalis to all subdivisions of the amygdaloid nuclei complex, and reciprocal connections from the septofimbrial and septohypothalamic nuclei to the hippocampus and hypothalamus. The heavily labeled septum receives a major topographic input from the hippocampus and projects back to the region via cholinergic and GABAergic neurons of the medial septum. The lateral septum is also a major relay of hippocampal output to hypothalamic nuclei and may integrate endocrine responses with emotional behaviors. Our data suggest that SCN5A regulates signals linking diverse functions, including olfactory perception, attention, spatial memory, and autonomic responses. These circuits show prominent intrinsic oscillations (Hartmann *et al.*, 1999).

Gross failure in limbic system function, for whatever reason, would lead rapidly to the demise of an organism. Less severe malfunctions of the limbic system—whether one looks at neuropathological, physiological, neurochemical, or behavioral aspects—would result in preclusion of some options ordinarily available to an organism to achieve adaptive responses. Incoordination in communication may be occurring to some extent at all times among subunits of the limbic system but are being compensated for by the adjustments of neural feedback and modulator systems. This is believed to be the case when the voltage-gated $Na^+$ channels are coded for by the commonly occurring normal variant of the *SCN5A* gene. However, a mutation of the *SCN5A* gene may give rise to formation of $Na^+$ channels that are sufficiently dysfunctional so that compensatory adjustments become inadequate when the system is pushed by stress to high levels of functional demands. Then social, behavioral, and physiological responses of an affected individual become maladaptive, as observed in schizophrenia and in a variety of other cognitive disorders.

Regardless of whether the sensory input is too great or too small (Fig. 1), some neurons, either inhibitory or excitatory, are firing at rates that are *relatively* too great for those of other members of the system or subsystem of which they are a part to allow the whole functional unit to achieve a cybernetically effective balance. There now are many links of abnormal voltage-gated $Na^+$ channels to seizure-like activity in local and global nervous system activity.

The best strategy to correct such imbalances might be to decrease the firing rates of the *relatively overheated* neurons by frequency-dependent $Na^+$ channel blockade, which could allow the system to self-organize into a normal functional mode. Substances which act in this fashion are described as local anesthetics. Propranolol is one of the most potent members of this group.

## IX. Recyberneticizing Substances and Mechanisms of Their Action

In the study of any pathologic phenomenon, one aim is to identify the rate-limiting steps, bottlenecks, so to speak, at which the tools at hand may enable one to choke off the spread of the manifestations of the pathologic state. Often the best strategy is to try to focus on key events as close to the origin of the problem as possible because the consequential, ever-widening ripples at every point of advance of the pathologic process create subsidiary problems that often are unpredictable and may eventually require additional therapies far removed from the original problem. There are multiple causations and many overt manifestations of incordinated nervous system function. What do all of them have in common? The most apparent common denominator is that neurons, which are normally involved as individuals or as members of small groups in highly specific aspects of information processing in a particular neural sector, first begin to fire abnormally frequently when engaged in performing their regular assignments and then engage other neurons in the sector in a series of nonsense communications in a manner irrelevant to their role in overall adaptive information processing. Eventually this may lead to self-sustaining abnormal discharges in adjacent and even distant neural sectors with various behavioral consequences occurring.

### A. Several Substances with Anticonvulsant Action also Produce Frequency-Dependent Nerve Block (Bernhard and Bohm, 1965; Courtney *et al.*, 1978a,b; Hille, 1977)

Perhaps the most general approach that might be applicable to the treatment and/or prevention of abnormal discharges in the nervous system would be to affect the conductile properties of those nerves that generate action potentials in such a way as to set a ceiling on the frequencies with which they could fire. It has been known for some time that local anesthetics exert their action by producing a conduction block in peripheral nerves by blocking transmembrane sodium current. In addition, quite aside from knowledge of their mechanisms of action, local anesthetics have been used to prevent or abort a variety of seizures in animals and in man, suppressing spike generation in cortical epileptic foci and even afterdischarges in electrically stimulated isolated brain slabs. The nerve blocking action of local anesthetics is frequency selective. An example of such action is illustrated in Fig. 5. An untreated desheathed frog sciatic nerve can follow a 40 Hz stimulus without spike attenuation (Fig. 5A). Figure 5B shows that mepivacaine, a local anesthetic as is propranolol, at a concentration of 1 mM, attenuated the compound action potential only slightly when the nerve was stimulated infrequently but that almost all excitability was blocked

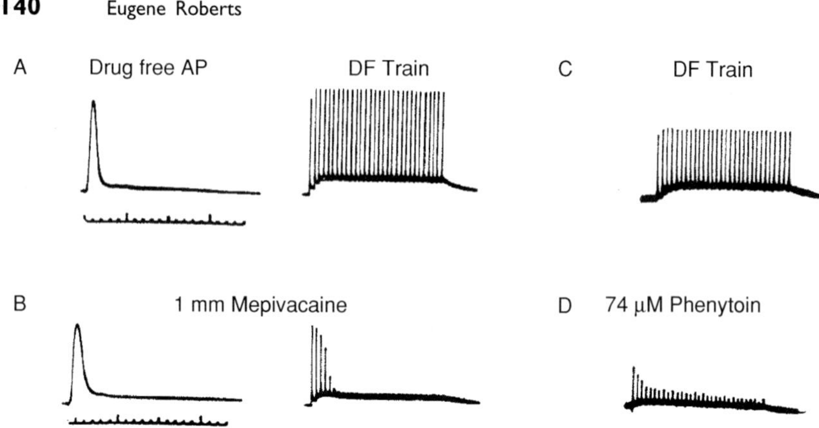


**FIGURE 5** Frequency-dependent nerve block by a local anesthetic and anticonvulsant. (A) Left: compound action potential recorded from desheathed frog sciatic nerve preparation. (A) Right: 40 Hz train of stimulated action potentials photographed on much slower time base, showing that drug-free preparation can follow a 40 Hz stimulus without spike attenuation. (B) Similar set of records to those in (A) but with local anesthetic treatment producing frequency-dependent conduction block. (C) 40 Hz train record in another drug-free preparation. (D) Frequency-dependent conduction block produced by treatment with phenytoin. Time calibration: 1 ms/division on leftmost traces and 50 ms/division on other (train) records. Spike amplitude: about 30 mV recorded across a sucrose gap. (Figure kindly furnished by Dr. K. R. Courtney.)

when the nerve was stimulated at a rate of 40/s. A similar result was obtained when the experiment was performed in the presence of an even lower concentration of phenytoin (0.074 mM) (Fig. 5D). Similarly, phenobarbital was found to produce a frequency-dependent nerve block in this preparation.

The differential blockade by local anesthetics of sensory impulses in preference to motor impulses possibly may be attributable to the fact that neurons bringing peripheral signals into the CNS (e.g., pain signals) may often fire with higher frequencies than those dealing with motor functions. Frequency-dependent conduction block may play an important role in the analgesia associated with the actions of local anesthetics. However, without actual relevant measurement, little can be inferred about specific central actions from studies of peripheral nerves, since frequencies of firing of neurons in circuits released in the CNS subsequent to primary afferent activation may be very different from those of their inputs.

Frequency-dependent nerve block by local anesthetics has been shown in voltage clamp experiments to be attributable to a blockade of the $Na^+$ channels responsible for generation of the action potential. There appears to be a preferential, reversible binding of these drugs to some structural component of open sodium channels and, therefore, the efficacy of blockade of nerve excitability by these substances is greatly enhanced when a nerve is firing rapidly in comparison with that observed when the frequency of firing is low. The degree of block depends on the rate of opening of sodium channels. Substances that exert such effects also have been found to have antiarrhythmic pharmacologic effects. Phenytoin has widespread therapeutic use as an antiarrhythmic drug as well as an anticonvulsant. Several antiarrhythmic drugs, including propranolol, have been shown to block myocardial excitability in a frequency-dependent manner, an action probably contributing importantly to their antifibrillatory efficacy.

## X. Problems in Therapy with Racemic Propranolol

Atsmon and Blum (1978) described the yoking of antipsychotic and cardiovascular effects of racemic propranolol in schizophrenic patients:

> Each patient's behavior, pulse rate, and blood pressure were monitored every 1 to 3 h. When behavior became markedly more normal or when the pulse rate dropped to 58–64 and/or the blood pressure fell to about 90/60, the daily dose was kept constant. In patients in whom treatment was successful, changes in these three parameters generally occurred at approximately the same time. In those patients in whom mental symptoms did not improve, dosage was adjusted largely according to the pulse rate and/or blood pressure criteria. Once the patient had become "stabilized," i.e., pulse rate about 60/min, blood pressure about 90/60 mm Hg, and improved mental symptoms, we kept the dosage schedule constant. Generally, however, after a few days both pulse rate and blood pressure started to rise slowly and the patient's mental condition deteriorated. We called this phenomenon 'escape.' When this happened, we increased the dose of the drug until stabilization was achieved again, generally within 1–2 days. This process of 'escape' with a requirement for higher doses of propranolol occurred several times. Therefore, the dose at which stabilization was achieved initially was nearly always markedly less than the final one at which the patient remained stabilized. From this point on the amount of drug did not have to change for many months (Atsmon and Blum, 1978).

Propranolol enters from the blood readily into both heart and brain. Ingenuity is challenged in attempting to devise methods for attenuating its entry into heart, while allowing it to be fully effective on brain function. Hope is offered by the finding that one of the optical isomers of propranolol, (+)propranolol (Howe and Shanks, 1966), has much weaker caradiovascular effects than the racemic mixture or the (−)propranolol isomer (Barrett and Cullum, 1968), while facilitating habituation of the orienting response reflex and amelioration of psychotic dysfunction in schizophrenic patients (Gruzelier *et al.*, 1979; Hirsch *et al.*, 1980).

## XI. The GABA System and Schizophrenia

The efficient operation of the nervous system diagrammed in Fig. 2 requires a coordination of neural activity that can determine from birth, or even before, the capacity of an individual to prevent the too-frequent firing of preprogrammed circuits of behavioral options spontaneously or maladaptively and to maintain within physiological limits the rates of operation of continuously needed neural circuits, such as those required for heart function, respiration, maintenance of blood pressure, and so on, under a variety of environmental circumstances. When gross malfunctions of the coordination of inhibitory and excitatory neuronal systems are found at birth, there may result lethal effects either through generalized seizures or cessation of operation of some vital function or, alternatively, some obviously severe neurological dysfunctions may occur.

GABA neurons play key roles at all levels, from setting the gain on the sensitivity of sensory receptors to coordinating the function of the systems involved in perceptual integration and in reaching the decisions with regard to which neural circuits should be released for use at a particular time. For example, an individual who has a paucity or defective function of horizontal GABA neurons in layer IV of the motor cortex might be expected to be more susceptible than other individuals to the occurrence of grand mal seizures. If such a problem should exist in the region of the globus pallidus, postural control would be expected to be defective. An inadequate GABA system in those regions of the hypothalamus dealing with food intake might cause an individual to have hyperphagia or anorexia nervosa. Inadequately functional GABA neurons in the dorsal horn of the spinal cord might result in an inordinately great sensitivity to tactile and thermal stimulation and pain and inadequate spatial and temporal discrimination of the stimuli. Visual perception and integration might be faulty in an individual with a defect in GABA function in the retina.

What happens when there is a relatively small, but continuous, degree of incoordination between the GABA system and other transmitter systems because for some reason the inhibitory GABA neurons have a considerably lower or higher than normal effectiveness upon their recipient neurons? The defect may be restricted to a local brain region, may include several regions, or may be global throughout the CNS, depending on a variety of hereditary and/or developmental factors. Under relatively simple environmental conditions, the nervous system in such an individual could function in an apparently adequately adaptive manner, which to an observer might appear to be well within the normal range. As the complexity and intensity of environmental inputs is increased, there would be a correlated increase of disinhibitory influences acting upon the GABA neurons, largely via the monoaminergic systems. If the capacities of the monoaminergic systems to deliver their characteristic transmitters are normal, then under conditions of environmental stress, which are considered for most to be within the normal adaptive range, imbalances often might arise. Thus, if special limbic system regions are affected, greater than normal degrees of changes in responses might be observed in emotional reactivity, pain sensitivity, heart and respiratory functions, blood pressure, galvanic skin response, insulin secretion, liberation of gastric acid, motility of colon, and so forth. Herein may lie one of the bases for psychosomatic medicine. Those systems in the nervous system that are most poorly controlled will tend to break down under stress and to produce peripheral symptoms that express such a breakdown. Almost everyone has an Achilles heel. This reflection of the physiological breaking point starts from a relatively poorly compensated region in the CNS. In this regard it is interesting that there are families in which there is a common maladaptive response to stress. There are families in which members tend to respond to stress with gastrointestinal symptoms, cardiac problems, skin outbreaks, respiratory ailments, and so on, which suggests that there may be strong hereditary factors involved, although learning factors cannot be entirely eliminated in most instances.

Viral and bacterial infections, dietary deficiencies and imbalances, cardiovascular, metabolic, and endocrine disorders, anoxia, various types of space-occupying lesions and traumata, and toxins may by themselves cause pathological changes that produce schizophrenia-like symptoms or they may predispose genetically susceptible, but apparently normally operating individuals, to exhibit schizophrenic disorder.

Primary analysis of sensory data takes place in the limbic system, the results of which are fine-tuned by thalamo–cortical interactions and finally passed on to the prefrontal cortex for executive action, without the permission of which habituation cannot take place. Consistent with the above formulation are experiments in rats in which small bilateral frontal lesions of the cerebral cortex prevented habituation (decrease in acceleration of heart rate) both to successive exposure to a given experimental setting and to repeated cooling of the tail, while unilateral frontal or occipito-parietal lesions of the cortex did not affect the habituation pattern (Glaser and Griffen, 1962). However, a completely normal prefrontal cortex cannot make the right decisions if the processed information being fed to it comes from a faulty source such as a limbic system with a mutant tissue-selective $Na^+$ channel gene. GABA neurons and those dealing with other transmitters in the limbic system would all be abnormal since they would have defective $Na^+$ channels. But this would not be the case elsewhere in the nervous system, at least at the outset of the disease. Therefore the weak link in an individual genetically susceptible to schizophrenia may be said to lie in the limbic system.

Technology now available makes it possible to compare the rates of mutation of the *SCN5A* gene in schizophrenic and normal individuals. Such work now is in progress and the results will determine whether or not the premise of the present chapter is in the right direction.

## Acknowledgments

The author gratefully acknowledges the essential and enthusiastic participation of Ruth Roberts in the preparation of this manuscript.

## References

Atsmon, A., and Blum, I. (1978). The discovery. *In* "Propranolol and Schizophrenia" (E. Roberts and P. Amacher, Eds.), *Kroc Foundation Series* **10**, 5–38. Alan R. Liss, Inc., New York.

Atsmon, A., Blum, I., Steiner, M., Latz, A., and Wijsenbeek, H. (1972). Further studies with propranolol in psychotic patients. *Psychopharmacologia (Berlin)* **27**, 249–254.

Barrett, A. M., and Cullum, V. A. (1968). The biological properties of the optical isomers of propranolol and their effects on cardiac arrhythmias. *Br. J. Pharmacol.* **34**, 43–55.

Bernhard, C. G., and Bohm, E. (1965). "Local Anaesthetics as Anticonvulsants." Almqvist and Wiksell, Stockholm.

Bock, G., and Goode, J. A. (Eds.) (2002). Sodium channels and neuronal hyperexcitability. *Novartis Found. Symp.* **241**, 1–244.

Bowery, N. G., Bittiger, H., and Olpe, H.-R. (Eds.) (1990). "$GABA_B$ Receptors in Mammalian Function." John Wiley & Sons, Chichester.

Courtney, K. R. (1975). Mechanism of frequency-dependent inhibition of sodium currents in frog myelinated nerve by the lidocaine derivative GEA 968. *J. Pharmacol. Exp. Ther.* **195**, 225–236.

Courtney, K. R., Kendig, J. J., and Cohen, E. N. (1978a). Frequency-dependent conduction block: The role of nerve impulse pattern in local anesthetic potency. *Anesthesiology* **48**, 111–117.

Courtney, K. R., Kendig, J. J., and Cohen, E. N. (1978b). The rates of interaction of local anesthetics with sodium channels in nerve. *J. Pharmacol. Exp. Ther.* **207**, 594–604.

Glaser, E. M., and Griffin, J. P. (1962). Influence of the cerebral cortex on habituation. *J. Physiol. (London)* **160**, 429–445.

Gruzelier, J. H. (1978). 3D. Propranolol acts to modulate autonomic orienting and habituation processes in schizophrenia. *In* "Propranolol and Schizophrenia" (E. Roberts and P. Amacher, Eds.), *Kroc Foundation Series* **10**, 99–118. Alan R. Liss, Inc., New York.

Gruzelier, J. H., Hirsch, S. R., Weller, M., and Murphy, C. (1979). Influence of D- or DL-propranolol and chlorpromazine on habituation of phasic electrodermal responses in schizophrenia. *Acta Psychiatr. Scand.* **3**, 241–248.

Guillemin, R. (1977). Peptides in the Brain, The New Endocrinology of the Neuron. *Nobel Lecture, Physiology or Medicine.*

Guth, L., Zhang, Z., and Roberts, E. (1994). Key role for pregnenolone in combination therapy that promotes recovery after spinal cord injury. *Proc. Natl. Acad. Sci. USA* **91**, 12308–12312.

Hartmann, H. A., Colom, L. V., Sutherland, M. L., and Noebels, J. L. (1999). Selective localization of cardiac SCN5A sodium channels in limbic regions of rat brain. *Nat. Neurosci.* **2**, 593–595.

Hille, B. (1977). Local anesthetics: Hydrophilic and hydrophobic pathways for the drug-receptor reaction. *J. Gen. Physiol.* **69**, 497–515.

Hirsch, S. R., Manchanda, R., and Weller, M. P. (1980). Dextro-propranolol in schizophrenia. *Prog. Neuropsychopharmacol.* **6**, 633–637.

Howe, R., and Shanks, R. G. (1966). Optical isomers of propranolol. *Nature* **210**, 1336–1338.

John, E. R., and Killam, K. F. (1959). Electrophysiological correlates of avoidance conditioning in the cat. *J. Pharmacol. Exp. Ther.* **125**, 252–274.

Kety, S. S., and Matthysse, S. (Eds.) (1972). Prospects for research on schizophrenia. *Neurosci. Res. Program Bull.* **10**, 370–507.

Lieberman, J. A., Stroup, T. S., McEvoy, J. P., Swartz, M. S., Rosenheck, R. A., Perkins, D. O., Keefe, R. S., Davis, S. M., Davis, C. E., Lebowitz, B. D., Severe, J., and Hsiao, J. K., and Clinical Antipsychotic Trials of Intervention Effectiveness (CATIE) Investigators (2005).

Effectiveness of antipsychotic drugs in patients with chronic schizophrenia. *N. Engl. J. Med.* **353**, 1209–1223.

Manchanda, R., and Weller, M. P. (1980). Dextro-propranolol in schizophrenia. *Prog. Neuropsychopharmacol.* **6**, 633–637.

Meisler, M. H., Kearney, J. A., Sprunger, L. K., MacDonald, B. T., Buchner, D. A., and Escayg, A. (2002). Mutations of voltage-gated sodium channels in movement disorders and epilepsy. *Novartis Found. Symp.* **241**, 72–81.

Noebels, J. L. (2002). Sodium channel gene expression and epilepsy. *Novartis Found. Symp.* **241**, 109–120.

Roberts, E. (1966a). The synapse as a biochemical self-organizing micro-cybernetic unit. *Brain Res.* **1**, 117–166.

Roberts, E. (1966b). Models for correlative thinking about brain, behavior, and biochemistry. *Brain Res.* **2**, 109–144.

Roberts, E. (1972). An hypothesis suggesting that there is a defect in the GABA system in schizophrenia: An essay. *Neurosci. Res. Program Bull.* **10**, 468–482.

Roberts, E., and Amacher, P. (Eds.) (1978). "Propranolol and Schizophrenia," *Kroc Foundation Series* **10**. Alan R. Liss, Inc., New York.

Roberts, E., and Matthysse, S. (1970). Neurochemistry: At the crossroads of neurobiology. *Annu. Rev. Biochem.* **39**, 777–820.

Sokolov, E. N. (1960). Neuronal models and the orienting reflex. *In* "The Central Nervous System and Behavior" (M. A. B. Brazier, Ed.), Transactions of Third Conference. Josiah Macy Jr. Foundation, New York.

Yee, B. K., Keist, R., von Boehmer, L., Studer, R., Benke, D., Hagenbuch, N., Dong, Y., Malenka, R. C., Frischy, J.-M., Bluethmann, H., Feldon, J., Möhler, H., *et al.* (2005). A schizophrenia-related sensorimotor deficit links a3-containing $GABA_A$ receptors to a dopamine hyperfunction. *Proc. Natl. Acad. Sci. USA* **102**, 17154–17159.

Yorkston, N. J., Zaki, S. A., and Havard, C. W. H. (1978a). Propranolol in the treatment of schizophrenia: An uncontrolled study with 55 adults. *In* "Propranolol and Schizophrenia" (E. Roberts and P. Amacher, Eds.), *Kroc Foundation Series* **10**, 39–67. Alan R. Liss, Inc., New York.

Yorkston, N. J., Zaki, S. A., and Havard, C. W. H. (1978b). Some practical aspects of using propranolol in the treatment of schizophrenia. *In* "Propranolol and Schizophrenia" (E. Roberts and P. Amacher, Eds.), *Kroc Foundation Series* **10**, 83–97. Alan R. Liss, Inc., New York.

**Robert L. Macdonald*,†,‡, Jing-Qiong Kang*, Martin J. Gallagher*, and Hua-Jun Feng***

*Department of Neurology
Vanderbilt University
Nashville
Tennessee 37232

†Department of Molecular Physiology
Vanderbilt University
Nashville
Tennessee 37232

‡Department of Biophysics and Pharmacology
Vanderbilt University
Nashville
Tennessee 37232

# $GABA_A$ Receptor Mutations Associated with Generalized Epilepsies[1]

## I. Chapter Overview

Idiopathic generalized epilepsies (IGEs) are characterized by absence, myoclonic, and/or primary generalized tonic-clonic seizures in the absence of structural brain abnormalities and are thought to have a genetic basis. Here we review mutations in $GABA_A$ receptor $\gamma 2$, $\alpha 1$, and $\delta$ subunits that have been associated with different IGE syndromes. These mutations have been shown to alter $GABA_A$ receptor gating, expression, and/or trafficking of the receptor to the cell surface, all pathophysiological mechanisms that result in reduced GABA-evoked currents that in neurons would cause neuronal disinhibition and thus predispose affected patients to manifest seizures.

[1] This is a revised and updated version of an article entitled "$GABA_A$ receptor epilepsy mutations" that appeared in *Biochem. Pharmacol.* **68**, 1497–1506 (2004).

*Advances in Pharmacology, Volume 54*
1054-3589/06 $35.00
DOI: 10.1016/S1054-3589(06)54007-4

## II. GABA$_A$ Receptors

GABA$_A$ receptors are the primary mediators of fast inhibitory synaptic transmission in the central nervous system (CNS) and have been repeatedly documented to play a critical role in animal models of seizures (Banerjee *et al.*, 1998; Chang *et al.*, 1996; Cohen *et al.*, 2003; Evans *et al.*, 1994; Feng *et al.*, 2001; Kapur and Macdonald, 1997; Karle *et al.*, 1998; Poulter *et al.*, 1999). Mutations associated with IGEs have also been identified in human GABA$_A$ receptor genes (Fig. 1) (Hirose *et al.*, 2005; Mulley *et al.*, 2003). This review will focus on the described human GABA$_A$ receptor channel epilepsy mutations.

GABA$_A$ receptors are formed by pentameric assembly of multiple subunit subtypes ($\alpha$1–6, $\beta$1–3, $\gamma$1–$\gamma$3, $\delta$, $\epsilon$, $\pi$, $\theta$, and $\rho$–3). The most common GABA$_A$ receptors contain two $\alpha$ subunits, two $\beta$ subunits, and a $\gamma$ or $\delta$ subunit (Baumann *et al.*, 2001, 2002b; Chang *et al.*, 1996). GABA$_A$ receptors form chloride ion channels, and GABA$_A$ receptor currents can be modulated by a number of positive and negative allosteric regulators, including barbiturates, benzodiazepines (BZDs), and neurosteroids, bicuculline,

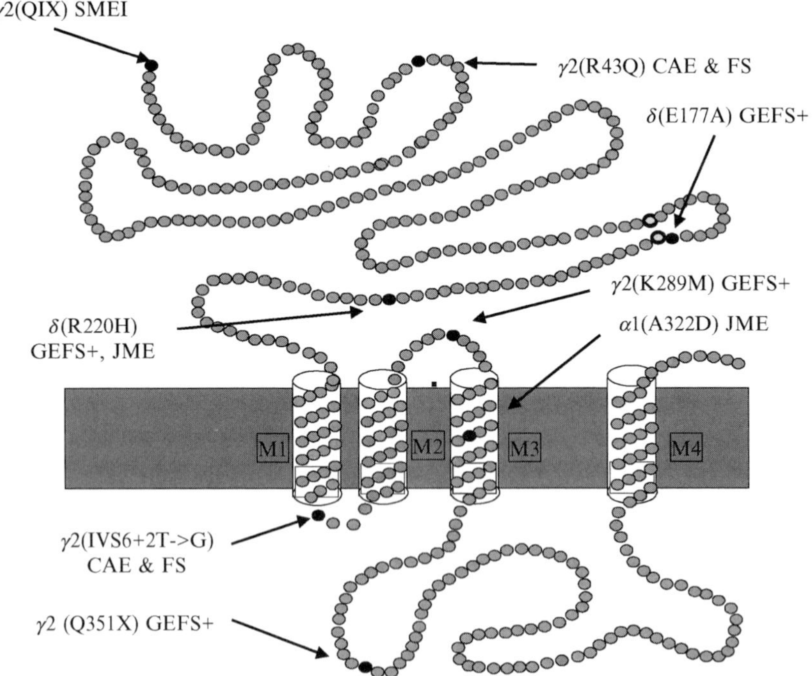


**FIGURE 1** Diagram of the GABA$_A$ receptor subunit topology, showing the location of epilepsy mutations.

picrotoxin, and zinc. $GABA_A$ receptors mediate both phasic, inhibitory synaptic transmission and tonic, perisynaptic inhibition.

## III. $GABA_A$ Receptor Epilepsy Genes

$GABA_A$ receptor mutations associated with IGEs have been reported in $\gamma2$, $\delta$, and $\alpha1$ subunits (Fig. 1). The $\gamma2$ subunit mutations include $\gamma2$(R43Q) associated with febrile seizures (FS) and childhood absence epilepsy (CAE) (Wallace *et al.*, 2001), $\gamma2$(K289M) associated with generalized epilepsy with febrile seizures plus (GEFS+) (Baulac *et al.*, 2001), $\gamma2$(Q351X) associated with GEFS+ (Harkin *et al.*, 2002), $\gamma2$(QIX) associated with severe myoclonic epilepsy of infancy (SMEI) (Hirose *et al.*, 2004), and $\gamma2$(IVS6 + 2T $\rightarrow$ G) associated with GEFS+ (Kananura *et al.*, 2002). The $\alpha1$ subunit mutation, $\alpha1$(A322D), is associated with juvenile myoclonic epilepsy (JME) (Cossette *et al.*, 2002). Two $\delta$ subunit variants, $\delta$(R220H) and $\delta$(E177A) were identified as susceptibility genes associated with GEFS+ and JME (Dibbens *et al.*, 2004).

### A. $GABA_A$ Receptor $\gamma2$(K289M) Subunit Mutation

A family with an autosomal dominant generalized epilepsy similar to GEFS+ was shown to have a mutation in the $GABA_A$ receptor $\gamma2$ subunit, $\gamma2$(K289M), (Baulac *et al.*, 2001) that is located in the short extracellular loop between transmembrane domains M2 and M3 (M2–M3 loop) (Fig. 1), a region implicated in the gating of ligand-gated ion channels (Campos-Caro *et al.*, 1996; Kash *et al.*, 2003; Lynch *et al.*, 1997; Miyazawa *et al.*, 2003). Recordings from oocytes expressing homozygous $\alpha1\beta2\gamma2$(K289M) receptors revealed smaller amplitude currents relative to wild-type receptor current amplitudes (Baulac *et al.*, 2001).

We reinvestigated the effects of this mutation (Bianchi *et al.*, 2002) in transfected HEK293T cells using a rapid application, concentration jump technique (open tip application rise time ~400 μs) to apply GABA (Hinkle *et al.*, 2003) for long (400 ms or 6 s) or brief (2–5 ms) durations and the excised outside-out patch clamp recording technique to determine the effects of these mutations on the pharmacological and biophysical properties of transient macropatch and single channel wild-type $\alpha1\beta3\gamma2$L and mutant $\alpha1\beta3\gamma2$L(K289M) $GABA_A$ receptor currents (Fig. 2). Wild-type $\alpha1\beta3\gamma2$L $GABA_A$ receptor macropatch currents evoked by 400-ms applications of 1-mM GABA were large (~500 pA) (Fig. 2A and E), desensitized with two time constants (~7.5 and 130 ms) (Fig. 2B and C), and deactivated biphasically with a weighted time constant of ~200 ms (Fig. 2F). Homozygous $\alpha1\beta3\gamma2$L(K289M) currents evoked by 400-ms applications of 1-mM GABA had unchanged current amplitude, rate of activation (Fig. 2D), and rate of desensitization (Fig. 2B and C) but had faster deactivation (~100 ms) (Fig. 2F). Currents evoked by brief applications of 1-mM GABA had reduced weighted current deactivation rates (~70 ms compared to ~35 ms in

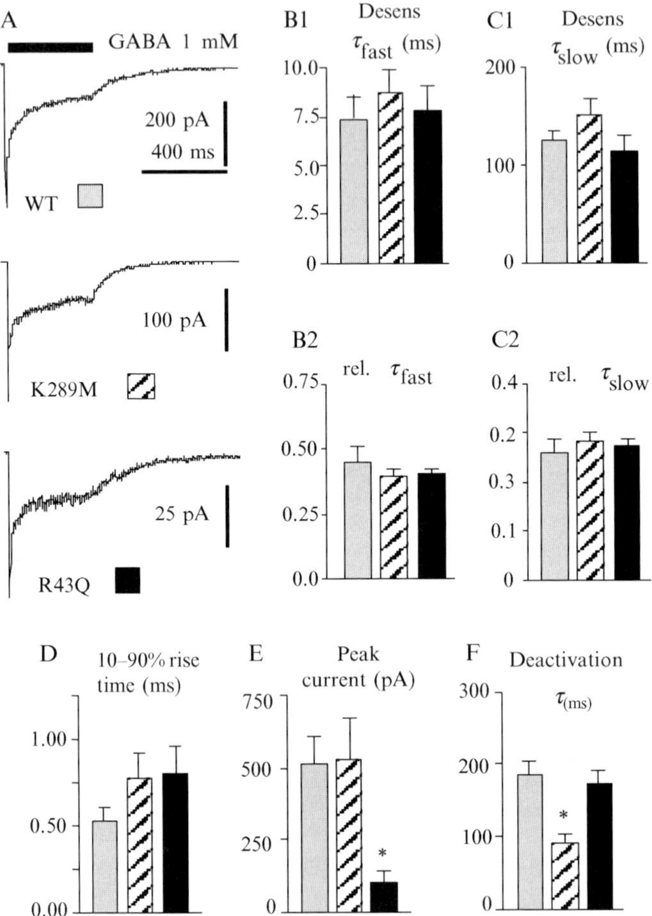


**FIGURE 2** Wild-type $\alpha1\beta3\gamma2L$ and mutant $\alpha1\beta3\gamma2L$(K289M) and $\alpha1\beta3\gamma2L$(R43Q) $GABA_A$ receptor macroscopic current kinetic properties. (A) Representative currents evoked by 400-ms jumps into 1-mM GABA from wild-type $\alpha1\beta3\gamma2L$ or mutated $\alpha1\beta3\gamma2L$(K289M) and $\alpha1\beta3\gamma2L$(R43Q) receptors. The time scale (top) trace applies to all three traces. (B, C) The $\gamma2L$(K289M) subunit mutation did not alter either the fast (B1) or slow (C1) time constants of desensitization, or their relative contributions (B2, C2). (D) The current rise times (10–90%) were not significantly altered by the mutations. (E) $\alpha1\beta3\gamma2L$(R43Q) but not $\alpha1\beta3\gamma2L$(K289M) receptors had significantly smaller peak current amplitudes (*, $p < 0.01$). (F) The current deactivation rate was significantly faster for $\alpha1\beta3\gamma2L$(K289M) but not $\alpha1\beta3\gamma2L$(R43Q) receptors (*, $p < 0.001$). Taken from Bianchi *et al.* (2002) with permission.

control) (Fig. 3A1, A2, and B). Single channel currents from homozygous $\alpha 1\beta 3\gamma 2$(K289M) receptors had mean open times that were one-fourth as long as wild-type $\alpha 1\beta 3\gamma 2$L receptor currents, consistent with its faster whole cell current deactivation time. Brief, rapid GABA applications to excised macropatches evoke currents that are similar to inhibitory post synaptic currents (IPSCs) (Haas and Macdonald, 1999; Jones and Westbrook, 1995), and thus reduction of the duration of rapid GABA-evoked current by the $\gamma 2$L(K289M) mutation suggests that it results in reduced IPSC duration, thus producing disinhibition that may lead to epilepsy.

The structural basis for the mutation-induced acceleration of deactivation and reduced single channel mean open times is unclear, but it has been suggested that the N-terminal domain of cys-loop receptors interacts with

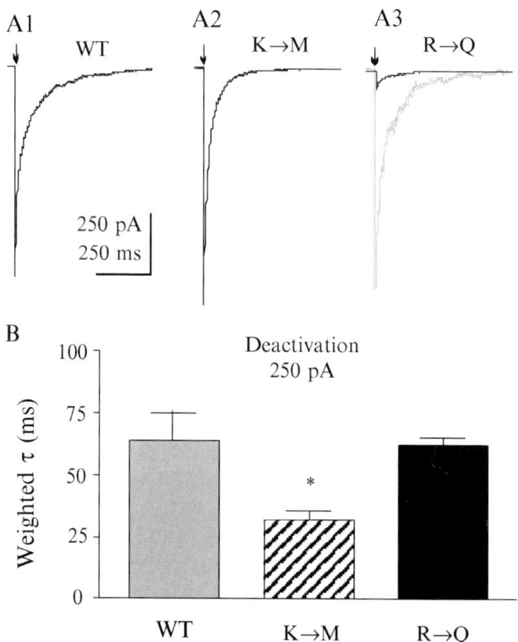


**FIGURE 3** Brief wild-type $\alpha 1\beta 3\gamma 2$L and mutant $\alpha 1\beta 3\gamma 2$L(K289M) and $\alpha 1\beta 3\gamma 2$L(R43Q) GABA$_A$ receptor currents. (A) Representative currents in response to brief (<5 ms) pulses of GABA (1 mM) illustrate deactivation rates of $\alpha 1\beta 3\gamma 2$L (A1), $\alpha 1\beta 3\gamma 2$L(K289M) (A2), and $\alpha 1\beta 3\gamma 2$L(R43Q) (A3) receptor currents. Scale bars are applicable to all three black traces. The black trace in (A3) is expanded tenfold (gray trace) for comparison of deactivation current time course. (B) Weighted deactivation time constants are depicted for wild-type and mutated channels and were significantly faster for $\alpha 1\beta 3\gamma 2$L(K289M) receptor currents (hatched bar; *, $p < 0.05$) than wild type. The $\alpha 1\beta 3\gamma 2$L(R43Q) receptor deactivation rate (solid bar) was not different than that of wild-type receptors (gray bar). Taken from Bianchi *et al.* (2002) with permission.

M2 and the M2–M3 loop during channel gating (Brejc *et al.*, 2001; Smit *et al.*, 2001) and that $GABA_A$ receptor $\alpha$ subunit loops 2 and 7 interact with a lysine residue in the M2–M3 loop to couple GABA binding to gating (Kash *et al.*, 2003). Although the $\gamma$2L subunit does not appear to be directly in the binding–gating transduction pathway, it may modify other properties of the receptor channel such as deactivation.

## B. $GABA_A$ Receptor $\gamma$2(R43Q) Subunit Mutation

A missense mutation in the N-terminal extracellular domain of the $\gamma$2 subunit, $\gamma$2(R43Q), was reported in affected individuals of a large family having both CAE and FS (Wallace *et al.*, 2001) (Fig. 1). In *Xenopus* oocytes $\alpha1\beta2\gamma2$(R43Q) $GABA_A$ receptors had no differences in GABA $EC_{50}$, current amplitude, or desensitization, but were insensitive to enhancement by the BZD diazepam. Subsequently, we reported that the $\gamma$2(R43Q) mutation did not alter BZD sensitivity, rate of activation, desensitization, or deactivation but did reduce peak current amplitude of $\alpha1\beta3\gamma2$(R43Q) receptor currents (Fig. 2) (Bianchi *et al.*, 2002). Importantly, when currents were evoked by brief applications of 1-mM GABA, the weighted current deactivation rate was unchanged but current amplitude was reduced (Fig. 3A1, A3, and B). Using similar techniques, another study reported that the mutation increased the rate of desensitization and slowed deactivation and slightly reduced BZD sensitivity (Bowser *et al.*, 2002). The basis for these different effects of the $\gamma$2(R43Q) mutation are unclear.

We explored the basis for the effect of the $\gamma$2(R43Q) mutation on peak current amplitude (Kang and Macdonald, 2004). We used tethered constructs consisting of a single cDNA encoding a $\beta$2 subunit connected through a polyglutamine linker to an $\alpha$1 subunit; functional receptors cannot be formed when the $\beta$–$\alpha$ construct is expressed alone but only when it is expressed with an untethered $\beta$, $\gamma$, or $\delta$ subunit (Baumann *et al.*, 2001, 2002b). Using this method of "forced assembly," we expressed either $\alpha\beta$ receptors ($\beta$–$\alpha$ construct with free $\beta$2 subunit) or $\alpha\beta\gamma$ receptors ($\beta$–$\alpha$ construct with free $\gamma$2 subunit) without generating a mixture of the two receptor types. We found that heterozygous and homozygous $\alpha1\beta2\gamma$2S(R43Q) receptors expressed using forced or free assembly had similar reductions in current amplitude (Fig. 4A and B). Heterozygous $\alpha1\beta2\gamma$2S(R43Q) and $\beta2$-$\alpha1\gamma$2L(R43Q) receptor peak current amplitudes were significantly smaller than those of wild type but were significantly larger than those of homozygous peak current amplitudes (Fig. 4C).

The reduction of GABA peak currents in $\gamma$2(R43Q) subunit-containing receptors results from reduced surface expression of receptor protein (Fig. 5). We constructed fusion proteins in which DNA encoding enhanced yellow fluorescent protein (YFP) was inserted between amino acids four and five of the mature $\gamma$2 subunit ($\gamma$2-YFP) for use as an epitope tag and for

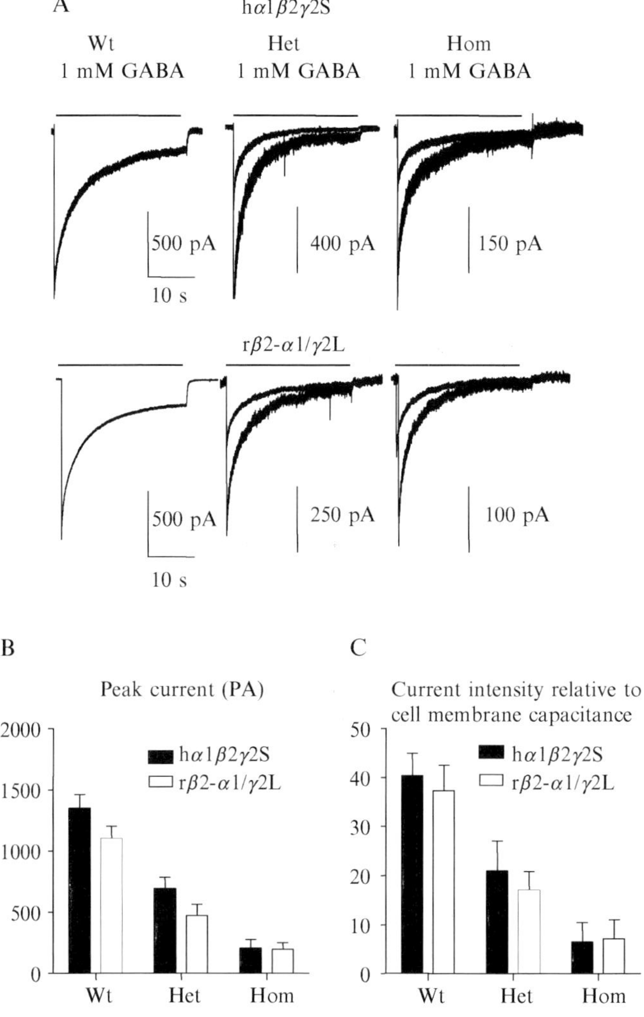


**FIGURE 4** Heterozygous and homozygous $\alpha1\beta2\gamma2S$(R43Q) receptors had reduced current amplitudes. (A) Representative traces of human $\alpha1\beta2\gamma2S$ (free assembly) or rat $\beta2$-$\alpha1\gamma2L$ (forced assembly) (Wt), heterozygous (Het), and homozygous (Hom) receptor currents were obtained from HEK293T cells. Cells were voltage-clamped at −50 mV. GABA (1 mM) was applied for 28 s. Currents are shown to scale (dark traces) and normalized to Wt currents (gray traces). The time scale for the first trace applies to all traces. Peak amplitudes (B) and relative current intensities (C) of Het and Hom $\alpha1\beta2\gamma2S$(R43Q) and $\beta2$-$\alpha1\gamma2L$(R43Q) receptor currents were significantly reduced with both free and forced assembly. Modified from Kang and Macdonald (2004).

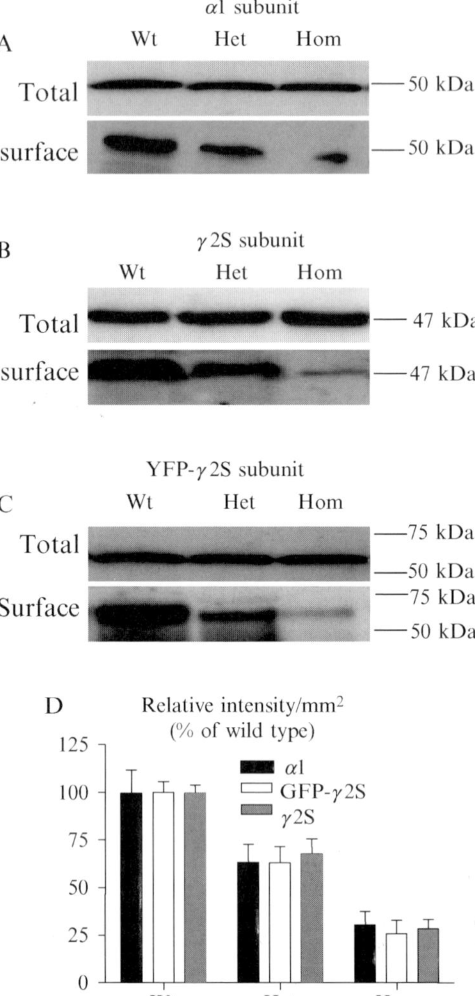


**FIGURE 5** Heterozygous and homozygous h$\alpha1\beta2\gamma2$S(R43Q) receptors had reduced surface expression. (A, B, C) Cells were transfected with wild type (Wt), heterozygous (Het), or homozygous (Hom) $\alpha1\beta2\gamma2$S(R43Q) receptors (A, C) or $\alpha1\beta2\gamma2$S(R43Q)-YFP receptors (B) and were biotinylated and immunoblotted with antibodies against the $\alpha1$ subunit (A), GFP (B), or the $\gamma2$ subunit (C). In (A), (B), and (C), Het and Hom $\alpha1\beta2\gamma2$S(R43Q) receptors revealed similar whole cell protein expression (total) but reduced subunit protein expression on the cell surface (surface). (D) The optical absorbance of the Western blots was quantified. Expression of Het or Hom $\alpha1\beta2\gamma2$S(R43Q) receptors resulted in similar levels of total whole cell protein expression (not shown) but reduced cell surface protein expression (surface) compared to Wt receptors. In each group, heterozygous protein intensities were lower than wild-type intensities but higher than of homozygous intensities. Modified from Kang and Macdonald (2004).

fluorescence microscopy experiments. HEK293T cells were transfected with wild-type, heterozygous and homozygous $\alpha1\beta2\gamma2S$ or $\alpha1\beta2\gamma2S$-YFP receptors, and the amount of total and surface membrane bound $\alpha1$, $\gamma2S/\gamma2S$-YFP subunit protein was determined. In both heterozygous and homozygous receptors, the $\gamma2S$(R43Q) mutation reduced the surface expression of the $\alpha1$, $\gamma2S$, or $\gamma2S$-YFP subunit proteins but did not alter the amount of total expression of each of these subunits (Fig. 5).

The surface and intracellular distribution of $\alpha1\beta2\gamma2S$-YFP receptors was then determined using confocal microscopy by colabeling with fluorescent ER marker, pECFP-ER, and membrane selective dye FM4–64 to mark the plasma membrane. In live COS-7 cells, a significant portion of wild-type $\alpha1\beta2\gamma2S$-YFP receptor fluorescence had a smooth distribution in addition to some clusters that were detected both on the surface and in intracellular compartments (Fig. 6A, Wt). Heterozygous and homozygous expression of $\alpha1\beta2\gamma2S$(R43Q)-YFP receptors also resulted in cell surface and intracellular fluorescence (Fig. 6A, Het and Hom), but homozygous and heterozygous $\alpha1\beta2\gamma2S$(R43Q)-YFP cell surface fluorescence was reduced relative to wild type (Fig. 6B). Thus, the reduced surface expression of mutant $\alpha1\beta2\gamma2S$ (R43Q) receptors was a consequence of receptor ER retention due to impaired protein assembly, folding, and/or trafficking.

## C. GABA$_A$ Receptor $\gamma2$(Q351X) Subunit Mutation

A $\gamma2$ subunit mutation, Q351X, localized in the intracellular loop between M3 and M4 (Fig. 1) was identified in a family with GEFS+, which introduced a premature translation-termination codon (PTC) at residue Q351. With homozygous expression in oocytes, GABA sensitivity was abolished, suggesting that the GABA$_A$ receptors were nonfunctional. When this mutation was further analyzed by using a green fluorescent protein (GFP)-tagged $\gamma2$ subunit (Harkin *et al.*, 2002), it was found that the receptor, although possibly assembled, did not exhibit surface expression but was retained in the ER. Thus, the $\gamma2$(Q351X) mutation would be expected to reduce surface expression of functional GABA$_A$ receptor complexes, leading to decreased GABAergic inhibition and presumably increased excitatory activity. However, patients with the $\gamma2$(Q351X) mutation are heterozygous, not homozygous, for this mutation, and the combination of effects of neurons expressing both wild-type and mutant $\gamma2$ subunits could differ from a simple summation of the effects of expressing wild-type or mutant $\gamma2$ subunit individually.

The cellular fate of the truncated protein is unknown. It is possible that the truncated $\gamma2$ subunit is simply subject to proteasomal degradation due to ER quality control. Alternatively, the truncated protein may be able to assemble with the $\alpha$ and $\beta$ subunits and cotraffick with the wild-type receptor, thus causing a dominant negative action to retain both wild-type and

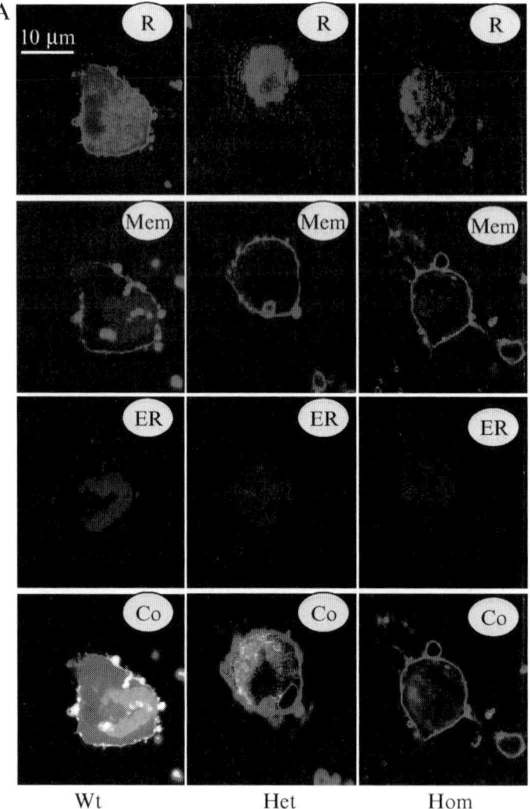


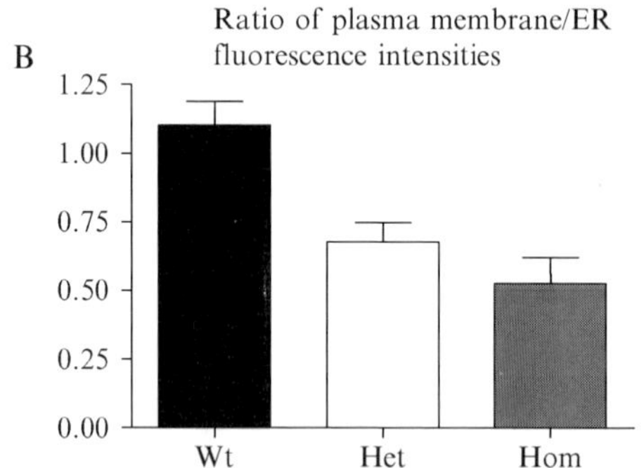


**FIGURE 6** Heterozygous and homozygous $\alpha1\beta2\gamma2S$(R43Q) receptors were retained in the ER. (A) COS-7 cells were cotransfected with human $\alpha1\beta2\gamma2S$-YFP wild type (Wt) or $\alpha1\beta2\gamma2S$ (R43Q)-YFP heterozygous (Het) or homozygous (Hom) receptors with enhanced CFP-tagged ER marker and labeled with FM4–64 membrane marker. R, receptor; Mem, membrane; ER, endoplasmic reticulum; and Co, colocalized image. Wt $\alpha1\beta2\gamma2S$-YFP receptors were primarily in the cell membrane. Het $\alpha1\beta2\gamma2S$(R43Q)-YFP receptors were found in both the membrane and intracellular compartments. Hom $\alpha1\beta2\gamma2S$(R43Q)-YFP receptors were primarily found in

mutant receptors in the downstream trafficking itinerary and result in abnormal cleavage and/or degradation through the lysosome pathway.

Cellular mRNA quality control mechanisms may affect $\gamma 2$(Q351X) subunit expression. Genetic mutations producing PTCs can result in C-terminally truncated proteins that can produce dominant negative inhibition of full-length proteins, thus potentially harming the cells. Quality control checkpoints during gene expression are required to maintain a low level of aberrant gene products and prevent them from interfering with the functioning of the cell. On the posttranscriptional level, nonsense mediated decay (NMD), or mRNA surveillance, recognizes and specifically degrades aberrant mRNAs in which the open reading frame is truncated due to the presence of a PTC (Lejeune and Maquat, 2005; Maquat, 2004). The position of the PTC relative to the position of a downstream intron is the primary determinant of whether the PTC elicits NMD. PTCs that are followed by an intron, which is located more than 50–55-nt downstream, generally elicit NMD, and thus, NMD does not likely play a substantial role in the expression of $\gamma 2$(Q351X) subunits, which contain the PTC in the terminal exon of the *GABRG2* gene. Therefore, the $\gamma 2$(Q351X) mutation likely produces a truncated $\gamma 2$ subunit protein in patients.

## D. GABA$_A$ Receptor $\gamma 2$(QIX) Subunit Truncation Mutation

NMD is more likely to affect the expression of another epilepsy mutation, $\gamma 2$(QIX). A $\gamma 2$ subunit mutation that introduced a PTC, QIX, between the signal peptide and mature peptide was identified in a family with SMEI (Hirose *et al.*, 2004). The functional consequence of the mutation is unknown. The mutation may produce haploinsufficiency, since the $\gamma 2$(QIX) mutation would prevent production of full-length protein and also trigger NMD (see the earlier section), thus preventing the production of a signal peptide. Haploinsufficiency occurs when an individual who is heterozygous for a certain gene mutation or hemizygous at a particular locus, often due to a deletion of the corresponding allele, is clinically affected because a single copy of the normal gene is incapable of providing sufficient protein for normal function.

Assuming that mRNA transcription for each gene is the same and due to the $2\alpha 2\beta 1\gamma 2S$ pentameric stoichiometry of GABA$_A$ receptors, there should be an extra copy of the $\gamma 2S$ subunit. If the $\gamma 2$(QIX) mutation resulted in

---

intracellular compartments with minimal localization on the cell surface. Both Het and Hom receptors had a fluorescence pattern that was similar in distribution to that of the ER fluorescence pattern. (B) The relative membrane/ER fluorescence intensity ratios for Het and Hom receptors were significantly reduced compared with that for the Wt receptors. Modified from Kang and Macdonald (2004). (See Color Insert.)

NMD and if the mutant $\gamma 2S$ subunit does not interfere with transcription of the wild-type $\gamma 2S$ subunit at the mRNA level, theoretically, there would be sufficient wild-type $\gamma 2S$ subunit to form a normal complement of functional wild-type $\alpha 1\beta 2\gamma 2S$ receptors and no epilepsy would result. However, in the case report, both twins carrying the mutation were diagnosed with SMEI, while the father with the *de novo* mutation was apparently healthy. What are the underlying molecular mechanisms of this early truncation in heterozygous patients? Since conventional study with intronless cDNA constructs would not trigger activation of NMD, this method of study is nonphysiological. Future studies in which heterologous cells are transfected with cDNA constructs that contain the $\gamma 2S$(QIX) subunit cDNA interrupted with the cDNA encoding the appropriate intron (a minigene construct) or with knock-in animals may elucidate the underlying molecular pathology.

## E. GABA$_A$ Receptor $\gamma 2$(IVS6 + 2T → G) Subunit Truncation Mutation

A splice-site mutation in the $\gamma 2$ subunit has been identified in a family with CAE and FS (Kananura *et al.*, 2002) (Fig. 1). The effect of this mutation on GABA$_A$ receptor function is unknown but was predicted to lead to a nonfunctional protein through exon skipping. The point mutation in the gene leads to a splice-donor site mutation in intron 6 (IVS6 + 2T → G), resulting in production of a truncated $\gamma 2$ subunit protein. This mutation has been identified in a family that presented with clinical CAE and FS. To date, electrophysiological experiments to study the effects of this mutation have not been reported. Due to the site of the putative truncation (just upstream of M1), it is questionable whether a GABA$_A$ receptor subunit that contains this mutation would be expressed and incorporated into a functional GABA$_A$ receptor. In addition, the predicted exon skipping would result in a new PTC at the 5th and 7th exon junction site. Thus, it is very likely that this prematurely terminated codon may also trigger NMD, thus eliminating the expression of mutant protein at mRNA level. Therefore, the underlying mechanism for this splice donor site mutation may also be due to haploinsufficiency.

## F. GABA$_A$ Receptor $\alpha 1$(A322D) Subunit Mutation

An $\alpha 1$ subunit mutation, $\alpha 1$(A322D), was reported to be associated with an autosomal dominant JME. The mutation introduces a negatively charged aspartate into the middle of the M3 transmembrane helix of the $\alpha 1$ subunit (A322D) (Cossette *et al.*, 2002). It could be predicted that such a nonconserved mutation in a transmembrane domain would destabilize helix formation and alter $\alpha 1$ subunit folding and pentamer assembly. In fact, we demonstrated that when coexpressed with wild-type $\beta 2$ and $\gamma 2$ subunits, the

$\alpha$1(A322D) mutation reduced both total (94 ± 6%) and surface (97 ± 3%) $\alpha$1 subunit expression and had an intermediate effect with "heterozygous" 1:1 $\alpha$1:$\alpha$1(A322D) subunit expression (44 ± 13% total protein expression reduction, 78 ± 10% surface protein expression reduction) (Gallagher *et al.*, 2004). In accordance with the reduction of protein expression, peak GABA-evoked currents were reduced by 94% in $\alpha$1(A322D)$\beta$2$\gamma$2 receptors (Cossette *et al.*, 2002; Fisher, 2004; Gallagher *et al.*, 2004) and by 50% in "heterozygous" $\alpha$1$\alpha$1(A322D)$\beta$2$\gamma$2 receptors. It is of note that the effect of the $\alpha$1(A322D) mutation on $\alpha$1 subunit trafficking substantially differed from that of the $\gamma$2(R43Q) mutation, which reduced surface, but not total $\gamma$2 subunit expression.

We determined that ER associated degradation (ERAD) is a prominent mechanism by which the $\alpha$1(A322D) mutation reduces $\alpha$1 subunit protein expression (Gallagher *et al.*, 2005). Evidence for this conclusion was obtained from three sets of experiments. First, the $\alpha$1(A322D) subunit reduced total $\alpha$1 subunit protein expression by about the same amount when it was expressed alone or when coexpressed with $\beta$2 and $\gamma$2 subunits (Fig. 7A), thus demonstrating that the mutation reduces $\alpha$1 subunit expression before subunit oligomerization. Second, while $\alpha$1$\beta$2$\gamma$2 receptors contained evidence of both mature, Golgi-associated, low-mannose N-linked glycosylation as well as immature, ER-associated high-mannose N-linked glycosylation, $\alpha$1(A322D)$\beta$2$\gamma$2 receptors contained essentially only ER-associated glycosylation (Fig. 7B), consistent with a posttranslational trafficking arrest and sequestration in the ER. Third, subcellular localization by confocal microscopy of YFP-tagged $\alpha$1 and $\alpha$1(A322D) subunits demonstrated that wild-type $\alpha$1-YFP$\beta$2$\gamma$2 receptors were present both on the cell surface as well as in the ER while mutant $\alpha$1(A322D)-YFP$\beta$2$\gamma$2 receptors were only detected in the ER (Fig. 8) (Gallagher *et al.*, 2005; Krampfl *et al.*, 2005). These three lines of evidence show that total $\alpha$1(A322D) subunit protein expression is reduced after biosynthesis but prior to subunit oligomerization and that the residual $\alpha$1(A322D) subunit protein is associated with the ER. These results imply that a substantial fraction of the mutant $\alpha$1(A322D) subunit is eliminated by ERAD. The removal of the $\alpha$1(A322D) subunit by ERAD is similar to that of another misfolded, disease-associated protein, the cystic fibrosis transporter regulator (Amaral, 2004).

Although most of the mutant $\alpha$1(A322D) subunit protein is eliminated by ERAD prior to assembly with $\beta$2 and $\gamma$2 subunits, some does not degrade, and thus it was of interest to determine the assembly and function of GABA$_A$ receptors that contain $\alpha$1(A322D) subunits. Most GABA$_A$ receptors contain two $\alpha$-subunits that are positioned asymmetrically within the pentamer; one $\alpha$ subunit is located between two $\beta$ subunits ($\alpha_{\beta\alpha\beta}$) (Baumann *et al.*, 2001, 2002b) and the other between a $\beta$ and $\gamma$ subunit ($\alpha_{\beta\alpha\gamma}$) (Fig. 9A) (Baumann *et al.*, 2002a). Thus, the autosomal dominant mutation, $\alpha$1(A322D), would be

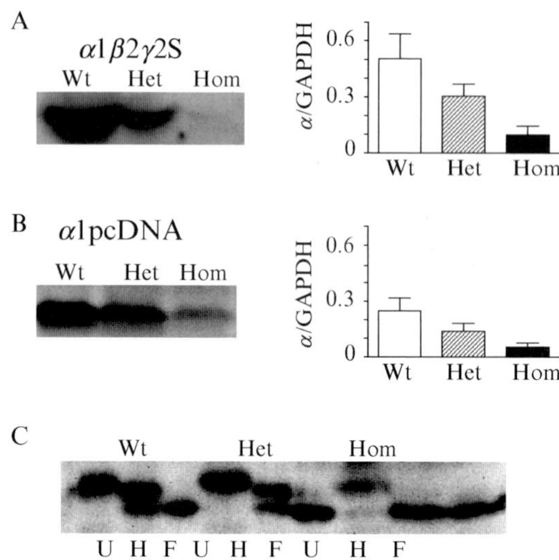


**FIGURE 7** The JME α1(A322D) mutation reduced α1 subunit expression before receptor oligomerization and lacked Golgi-associated N-linked glycosylation. (A, B) Cells were transfected with α1 subunits (2 μg) and either 2 μg of both β2 and γ2S subunits (A) or 4 μg of empty pcDNA3.1 vector. (B) Whole cell lysates were fractionated on 10% SDS-PAGE gels and Western blots were probed with antibodies directed to the α1 subunit and glyceraldehydes-3-phosphate dehydrogenase (GAPDH), which controlled for the amount of protein loaded on the gel. The fraction of the α1 subunit band relative to GAPDH was quantified and depicted to the right of the gel. (C) Cells were transfected with wild type (Wt, α1β2γ2), heterozygous (Het, α1α1(A322D)β2γ2), or homozygous (Hom, α1(A322D)β2γ2) receptors. Cellular lysates (2.5 mg/ml) were left undigested (U), or digested with endoglycosidase-H (endo-H, H), or peptide-N-glycosidase F (PNGaseF, F). The digestion products were fractionated via 12.5% SDS-PAGE, which was stained by Western blot with an antibody directed against the α1 subunit. Because Wt, Het, and Hom receptors differ in α1 subunit expression (A), the lysates were loaded on the gel in the ratios 8 mg:15 mg:50mg::Wt:Het:Hom to balance the amount the α1 subunit on the gel. The α1 subunits from undigested lysates from Wt, Het, and Hom receptors migrated at 50 kDa, and those digested with PNGaseF migrated at 46 kDa. Following endo-H digestion, Wt and Het subunits migrated in two bands at 48.4 (endo-H resistant) and 46 kDa (endo-H sensitive), but Hom α1 subunits migrated in a single endo-H sensitive band at 46 kDa. Modified from Gallagher *et al.* (2005).

expected to produce four different $GABA_A$ receptor pentameric assemblies: α1β2α1β2γ2 (wild type), α1β2α1(A322D)β2γ2 ($Het_{\beta\alpha\beta}$), α1(A322D)β2α1β2γ2 ($Het_{\beta\alpha\gamma}$), and α1(A322D)β2α1(A322D)β2γ2 (homozygous). To selectively produce either $Het_{\beta\alpha\beta}$ or $Het_{\beta\alpha\gamma}$ receptors without generating a binomial mixture of receptors, we made α1(A322D) mutations in tethered concatamers in which a single cDNA that encoded either the γ2 subunit linked to the β2 subunit linked to the α1 subunit or the β2 subunit linked to the α1 subunits. A mutation in the β2–α1 concatamer (β2–α1(A322D))

A

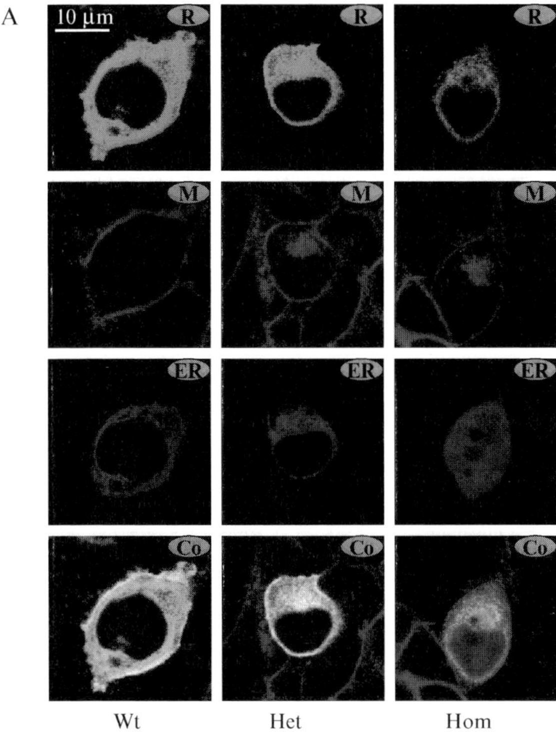


B

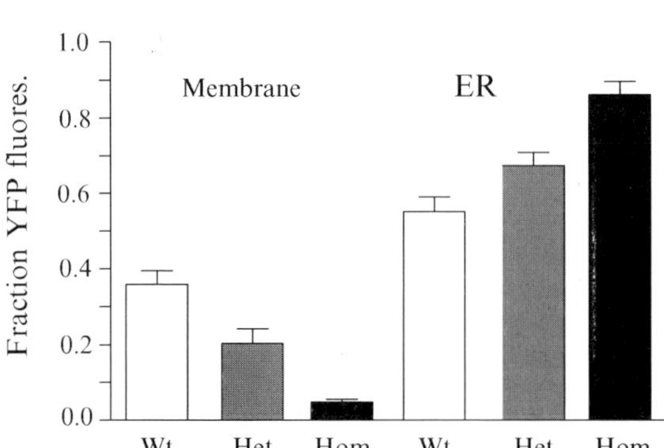


**FIGURE 8** The JME α1(A322D) mutation colocalized to the ER cells were transfected with the ER marker, CFP-ER (ER, blue) and either wild type (Wt, α1-YFPβ2γ2S), heterozygous (Het, α1-YFPα1(A322D)-YFPβ2γ2S) or homozygous (Hom, α1(A322D)-YFPβ2γ2S) receptors (R, green) and stained with the membrane marker, FM 4–64 (M, red). The majority of all receptors colocalized (Co) with the ER (cyan). Only wild-type and heterozygous α1-YFP subunit colocalized with the plasma membrane marker (yellow). The fraction of total wild type, heterozygous, and homozygous α1-YFP that colocalized to the ER or membrane is graphed. Modified from Gallagher *et al.* (2005). (See Color Insert.)

coexpressed with wild-type $\gamma$2-$\beta$2-$\alpha$1 concatamer produced the Het$_{\beta\alpha\gamma}$ receptor and the $\gamma$2-$\beta$2-$\alpha$1(A322D) concatamer coexpressed with the $\beta$2–$\alpha$1 concatamer produced the Het$_{\beta\alpha\beta}$ receptor. The Het$_{\beta\alpha\beta}$ receptor mean peak current amplitude was less than wild type (35%), but Het$_{\beta\alpha\gamma}$ receptors had essentially no detectable GABA-evoked currents (Fig. 9B–E) (Gallagher *et al.*, 2004). In addition, there was an asymmetric difference in $\beta$2–$\alpha$1 protein expression with Het$_{\beta\alpha\gamma}$ receptors having approximately 72% of the $\beta$2–$\alpha$1 expression as Het$_{\beta\alpha\beta}$ receptors (not shown). These results indicate that not only does the $\alpha$1(A322D) mutation cause $\alpha$1 subunit degradation by

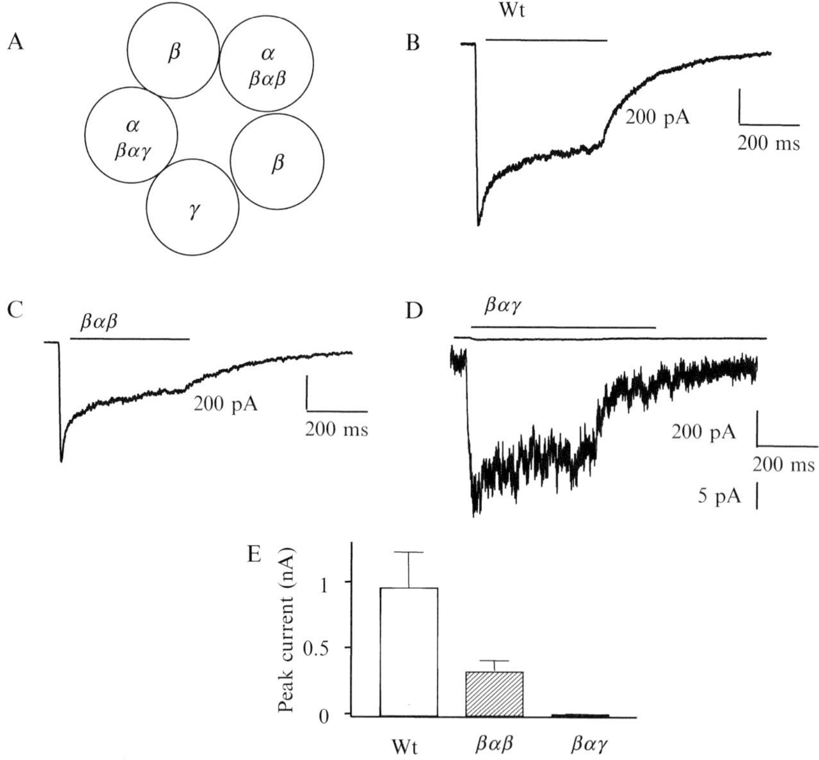


**FIGURE 9** The JME $\alpha$1(A322D) mutation was asymmetrical. (A) $\alpha\beta\gamma$ receptor subunits are arranged (as viewed from the synapse) in the counterclockwise sequence $\gamma$-$\beta$-$\alpha$-$\beta$-$\alpha$. (B–D) Sample current traces are depicted from (B) wild type (Wt), (C) Het$_{\beta\alpha\beta}$, or (D) Het$_{\beta\alpha\gamma}$ receptors. The gray trace in (D) is shown in an expanded scale to display the time course of the current. (E) Mean peak currents of wild-type concatamer receptors ($n = 20$) were larger than those of Het$_{\beta\alpha\beta}$ ($n = 17, p < 0.05$), which were substantially larger than those from Het$_{\beta\alpha\gamma}$ concatameric receptors ($n = 8, p < 0.01$). Modified from Gallagher *et al.* (2004).

ERAD prior to subunit oligomerization, but that it also reduces the production of functional $Het_{\beta\alpha\gamma}$ receptors and essentially precludes the production of functional $Het_{\beta\alpha\gamma}$ receptors.

## G. $GABA_A$ Receptor $\delta$ Subunit Susceptibility Variants for Complex Epilepsies

Although the monogenic mutations provide useful models for the pathogenesis of epilepsy syndromes, they only account for a small portion of IGE syndromes. This suggests that most of the idiopathic epilepsies are polygenic requiring additive actions of a set of susceptibility genes. We reported the first $GABA_A$ receptor susceptibility gene, *GABRD*, for IGEs (Dibbens *et al.*, 2004). Two putative missense mutations in *GABRD* were identified: $\delta$(E177A) was detected in a small GEFS+ family, and $\delta$(R220C) was detected in a second small GEFS+ family. Both mutations were heterozygously associated with epilepsy in these kindreds. In addition, a polymorphic allele, $\delta$(R220H), is associated with JME patients but is also found in the general population. All of these variants are localized in the N-terminus of the $\delta$ subunit. The $\delta$(E177A) variant is adjacent to one of the invariant cysteines that form a disulfide bond, an important feature for cys-loop receptors. The $\delta$(R220H) and $\delta$(R220C) variants are localized about in the middle between the $\delta$(E177A) variant and the entrance to the first transmembrane domain (M1). The effects of these variants on $GABA_A$ receptor function were examined by recording human $\alpha1\beta2\delta$ receptors expressed in HEK293T cells. The GABA $EC_{50}$s of $\alpha1\beta2\delta$(E177A), $\alpha1\beta2\delta$(R220H), and $\alpha1\beta2\delta$(R220C) receptors were not significantly altered compared to wild-type receptors. In the presence of saturating concentration of GABA, the current amplitudes of heterozygous or homozygous $\alpha1\beta2\delta$(R220C) receptors were not significantly different from those of wild-type receptors. However, compared to the wild-type receptors, the current amplitudes of heterozygous or homozygous $\alpha1\beta2\delta$(E177A) receptors were significantly smaller (Fig. 10). The current amplitudes of heterozygous or homozygous $\alpha1\beta2\delta$(R220H) receptors were also significantly reduced compared to those of wild-type receptors (Fig. 11). Single channel recordings demonstrated that the reduced peak currents of both the $\alpha1\beta2\delta$(E177A) and $\alpha1\beta2\delta$(R220H) receptors could be attributed to reduced mean channel open times (Feng *et al.*, 2004). Given that the $\delta$(R220H) variant is present in both the JME kindred and the general population and that the $\delta$(E177A) variant does not segregate monogenically with epilepsy in a large family, we proposed that both of these variants are susceptibility genes for IGEs (Dibbens *et al.*, 2004). Since $\delta$ subunit-containing $GABA_A$ receptors are involved in tonic inhibition, we suggested that alteration of tonic, perisynaptic inhibition may contribute to the some IGEs.

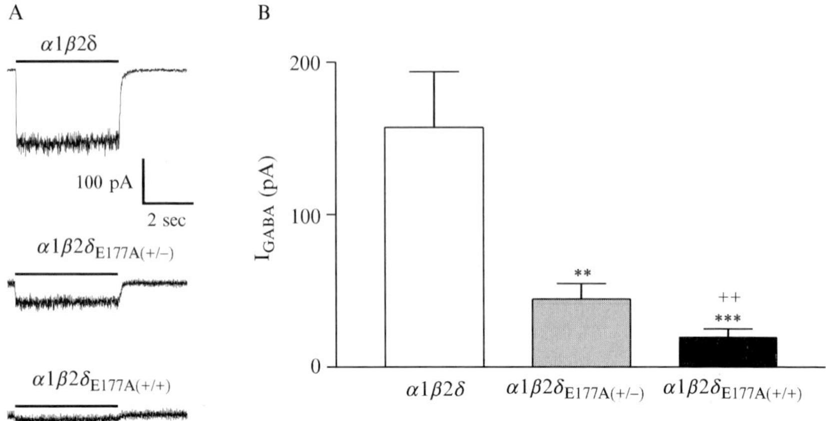


**FIGURE 10** The GEFS+ $\delta$(E177A) variant reduced $\alpha 1\beta 2\delta$ current amplitudes. (A) Typical examples of whole cell currents evoked by 1-mM GABA from wild-type $\delta$ subunit-, heterozygous (+/−), or homozygous (+/+) $\delta$(E177A) variant subunit-containing $GABA_A$ receptors. (B) Incorporation of either heterozygous or homozygous $\delta$(E177A) variant into $GABA_A$ receptors resulted in reduction of maximal GABA currents. Compared to wild-type receptors ($n = 39$), the maximal currents were significantly decreased for heterozygous ($n = 18$) or homozygous ($n = 25$) $\delta$(E177A) variant subunit-containing receptors. The maximal currents were also significantly different between heterozygous and homozygous $\delta$(E177A) variant subunit-containing receptors. Modified from Dibbens *et al.* (2004). ** $p < 0.01$ compared with wild-type receptors; *** $p < 0.001$; ++ $p < 0.01$ compared with Het receptors.

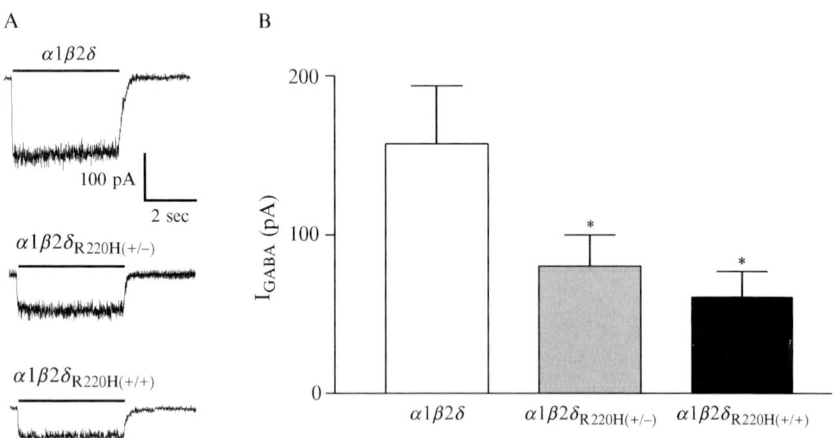


**FIGURE 11** The JME $\delta$(R220H) polymorphism reduced $\alpha 1\beta 2\delta$ current amplitudes. (A) Typical examples of the whole cell currents evoked by 1-mM GABA from wild-type $\delta$ subunit-, heterozygous (+/−), or homozygous (−/−) $\delta$(R220H) polymorphic subunit-containing $GABA_A$ receptors. (B) Incorporation of either heterozygous or homozygous $\delta$(R220H) variant into $GABA_A$ receptors resulted in reduction of maximal GABA currents. Compared to wild-type receptors ($n = 39$), the maximal currents were significantly decreased for heterozygous ($n = 33$),

## IV. Conclusions

The studies reviewed here demonstrate that GABA$_A$ receptor subunit mutations associated with IGEs alter GABA$_A$ receptor channel gating, expression, or trafficking when expressed in mammalian cell lines. The primary basis for the decreased whole cell current and increased rate of current deactivation of GABA$_A$ receptors containing the $\gamma$2(K289M), $\delta$(E177A), and $\delta$(R220H) mutations was explained by reduced mean single channel open times. In contrast, the primary mechanistic basis for the reduction in whole cell current for GABA$_A$ receptors containing $\alpha$1(A322D), $\gamma$2(R43Q), and $\gamma$2(Q351X) mutant subunits was decreased GABA$_A$ receptor subunit cell surface expression. While the "gating" and "trafficking" mutants appear to produce different defects in GABA$_A$ receptor function, the mechanisms are actually somewhat overlapping. The $\gamma$2(K289M), $\delta$(E177A), and $\delta$(R220H) mutations all produce some defects in receptor trafficking (Feng, Kang and Macdonald, unpublished), and the $\alpha$1(A322D) and $\gamma$2(Q351X) subunit mutations were associated with altered current kinetic properties (Gallagher *et al.*, 2004; Kang and Macdonald, unpublished). Furthermore, the mechanisms by which their gating, expression, and/or trafficking is reduced are unknown. Given their position in the interior of the subunit proteins, it is likely that the $\alpha$1(A322D) and $\gamma$2(Q351X) subunit mutations inhibit proper protein folding and assembly: the $\alpha$1(A322D) mutation by disruption a transmembrane helix and the $\gamma$2(Q351X) mutation by truncation of the C-terminus before the transmembrane domain. Misfolded GABA$_A$ receptor subunit proteins do not assemble properly in the ER and are then degraded (Barnes, 2000). We demonstrated that the reduction of expression of total $\alpha$1(A322D) subunit-containing receptors is consistent with ERAD (Gallagher *et al.*, 2005). In contrast to the $\alpha$1(A322D) mutation, a nonconservative missense mutation that inserts a negative charge in a transmembrane domain, and the $\gamma$2(Q351X) subunit mutation that inserts a PTC, the $\gamma$2(R43Q) subunit mutation is a simple missense mutation within an extracellular loop. Thus, it is not surprising that the $\gamma$2(R43Q) subunit does not reduce total $\gamma$2 subunit expression. However, it is of considerable interest to determine how the $\gamma$2(R43Q) mutation reduces receptor expression on the cell surface. One possibility may involve reduced $\gamma$2(R43Q) subunit oligomerization with other GABA$_A$ receptor subunits. Klausberger *et al.* (2000, 2001a,b) identified domains in the GABA$_A$ receptor subunits' N-termini near $\gamma$2(R43) that are critical for receptor oligomerization. Another possibility is that the $\gamma$2(R43Q) mutation may perturb a cell

or homozygous ($n = 21$) $\delta$(R220H) variant subunit-containing receptors. No significant difference in maximal currents was observed between heterozygous and homozygous $\delta$(R220H) variant subunit-containing receptors. * $p < 0.05$ compared with wild-type receptors. Modified from Dibbens *et al.* (2004).

surface trafficking signal similar to that identified in the nicotinic acetylcholine receptor (Wang *et al.*, 2002); such a mechanism may be responsive to pharmacological manipulation.

One of the most intriguing questions surrounding the IGE mutations is how can the mutations that severely disrupt $\gamma 2$ subunit expression ($\gamma 2$(QIX), $\gamma 2$(Q351X), and $\gamma 2$(IVS6 + 2T $\rightarrow$ G)) result in epilepsy? The $\gamma 2$(QIX) and $\gamma 2$(IVS6 + 2T $\rightarrow$ G) mutations likely result in NMD and thus should result in minimal to no mutant subunit production. This implies that the resultant seizures would be due to haploinsufficiency. However, the stoichiometry of $GABA_A$ receptors is $2\alpha 2\beta 1\gamma$, implying that half as much $\gamma 2$ subunit protein would be required to assemble $GABA_A$ receptors. Furthermore, initial attempts to determine the functional consequences of deletion of a single allele have not provided clear evidence for haploinsufficiency. When $\alpha 1\beta 2\gamma 2$ receptors were expressed in HEK293T cells by transfecting with an $\alpha 1$:$\beta 2$:$\gamma 2$ 1:1:0.5 cDNA ratio to mimic the effect of two $\alpha 1$ and $\beta 2$ subunit genes and only one $\gamma 2$ subunit gene, current amplitudes were not reduced relative to wild-type $\alpha 1\beta 2\gamma 2$ currents obtained by transfection with an $\alpha 1$:$\beta 2$:$\gamma 2$ 1:1:1 cDNA ratio (Kang and Macdonald, unpublished). The results may be due to the fact that the overexpression of transiently transfected $\gamma 2$ subunit protein in HEK293T cells has compensated the loss of protein of another half gene dose while in neurons, the protein expression level is not enough to compensate the loss. Alternatively, these results imply that these severe mutations do not simply produce a loss of function via haploinsufficiency but produce a dominant negative effect on the wild-type receptors by unknown mechanisms.

Finally, all the studies reviewed here were performed in heterologous expression systems. The effects of the mutations on expression, trafficking, and biophysical properties in neurons are unknown. Not only could neurons assemble $GABA_A$ receptors with different current kinetic properties and expression profiles than are seen in cell lines but neurons also target receptors to different neuronal compartments including somata and dendrites and to synaptic, perisynaptic, and extrasynaptic locations. It is entirely possible that wild-type and mutant receptors are trafficked differently to these neuronal compartments, a defect that would not be detected in mammalian expression systems. In addition, virtually all neurons express multiple subtypes of $GABA_A$ receptor subunits. It is possible that, unlike fibroblasts, neurons may compensate for a $GABA_A$ receptor subunit mutation by upregulating other $GABA_A$ receptor subunit subtypes, thus creating compensatory receptors with different properties. Thus, the ultimate goal of understanding the consequences of $GABA_A$ receptor epilepsy mutations is to characterize their actions following heterozygous expression in relevant neurons, and ultimately to study their effects on the properties of CNS networks that are involved in producing IGEs such as at the thalamocortical circuit.

## References


Amaral, M. D. (2004). CFTR and chaperones: Processing and degradation. *J. Mol. Neurosci.* 23, 41–48.

Banerjee, P. K., Tillakaratne, N. J., Brailowsky, S., Olsen, R. W., Tobin, A. J., and Snead, O. C., III (1998). Alterations in GABA$_A$ receptor alpha 1 and alpha 4 subunit mRNA levels in thalamic relay nuclei following absence-like seizures in rats. *Exp. Neurol.* **154**, 213–223.

Barnes, E. M., Jr. (2000). Intracellular trafficking of GABA$_A$ receptors. *Life Sci.* **66**, 1063–1070.

Baulac, S., Huberfeld, G., Gourfinkel-An, I., Mitropoulou, G., Beranger, A., Prud'homme, J. F., Baulac, M., Brice, A., Bruzzone, R., and LeGuern, E. (2001). First genetic evidence of GABA$_A$ receptor dysfunction in epilepsy: A mutation in the gamma2-subunit gene. *Nat. Genet.* **28**, 46–48.

Baumann, S. W., Baur, R., and Sigel, E. (2001). Subunit arrangement of gamma-aminobutyric acid type a receptors. *J. Biol. Chem.* **276**, 36275–36280.

Baumann, S. W., Baur, R., and Sigel, E. (2002a). Forced subunit assembly in alpha 1beta 2gamma 2 GABA$_A$ receptors: Insight into the absolute arrangement. *J. Biol. Chem.* **277**, 46020–46025.

Baumann, S. W., Baur, R., and Sigel, E. (2002b). Forced subunit assembly in alpha 1beta 2gamma 2 GABA$_A$ receptors: Insight into the absolute arrangement. *J. Biol. Chem.* **277**, 46020–46025.

Bianchi, M. T., Song, L., Zhang, H., and Macdonald, R. L. (2002). Two different mechanisms of disinhibition produced by GABA$_A$ receptor mutations linked to epilepsy in humans. *J. Neurosci.* **22**, 5321–5327.

Bowser, D. N., Wagner, D. A., Czajkowski, C., Cromer, B. A., Parker, M. W., Wallace, R. H., Harkin, L. A., Mulley, J. C., Marini, C., Berkovic, S. F., Williams, D. A., Jones, M. V., *et al.* (2002). Altered kinetics and benzodiazepine sensitivity of a GABA$_A$ receptor subunit mutation [gamma 2(R43Q)] found in human epilepsy. *Proc. Natl. Acad. Sci. USA* **99**, 15170–15175.

Brejc, K., van Dijk, W. J., Klaassen, R. V., Schuurmans, M., van Der, O. J., Smit, A. B., and Sixma, T. K. (2001). Crystal structure of an ACh-binding protein reveals the ligand-binding domain of nicotinic receptors. *Nature* **411**, 269–276.

Campos-Caro, A., Sala, S., Ballesta, J. J., Vicente-Agullo, F., Criado, M., and Sala, F. (1996). A single residue in the M2-M3 loop is a major determinant of coupling between binding and gating in neuronal nicotinic receptors. *Proc. Natl. Acad. Sci. USA* **93**, 6118–6123.

Chang, Y., Wang, R., Barot, S., and Weiss, D. S. (1996). Stoichiometry of a recombinant GABA$_A$ receptor. *J. Neurosci.* **16**, 5415–5424.

Cohen, A. S., Lin, D. D., Quirk, G. L., and Coulter, D. A. (2003). Dentate granule cell GABA$_A$ receptors in epileptic hippocampus: Enhanced synaptic efficacy and altered pharmacology. *Eur. J. Neurosci.* **17**, 1607–1616.

Cossette, P., Liu, L., Brisebois, K., Dong, H., Lortie, A., Vanasse, M., Saint-Hilaire, J. M., Carmant, L., Verner, A., Lu, W. Y., Wang, Y. T., and Rouleau, G. A. (2002). Mutation of GABRA1 in an autosomal dominant form of juvenile myoclonic epilepsy. *Nat. Genet.* **31**, 184–189.

Dibbens, L. M., Feng, H. J., Richards, M. C., Harkin, L. A., Hodgson, B. L., Scott, D., Jenkins, M., Petrou, S., Sutherland, G. R., Scheffer, I. E., Berkovic, S. F., Macdonald, R. L., *et al.* (2004). GABRD encoding a protein for extra- or peri-synaptic GABA$_A$ receptors is a susceptibility locus for generalized epilepsies. *Hum. Mol. Genet.* **13**, 1315–1319.

Evans, M. S., Viola-McCabe, K. E., Caspary, D. M., and Faingold, C. L. (1994). Loss of synaptic inhibition during repetitive stimulation in genetically epilepsy-prone rats (GEPR). *Epilepsy Res.* **18**, 97–105.

Feng, H. J., Naritoku, D. K., Randall, M. E., and Faingold, C. L. (2001). Modulation of audiogenically kindled seizures by gamma-aminobutyric acid-related mechanisms in the amygdala. *Exp. Neurol.* **172**, 477–481.

Feng, H. J., Song, L., and Macdonald, R. L. (2004). Susceptibility genes of $GABA_A$ receptor $\delta$ subunit for human generalized epilepsies have defective channel gating. *Epilepsia* **45**(Suppl. 7), 11.

Fisher, J. L. (2004). A mutation in the $GABA_A$ receptor alpha1 subunit linked to human epilepsy affects channel gating properties. *Neuropharmacology* **46**, 629–637.

Gallagher, M. J., Song, L., Arain, F., and Macdonald, R. L. (2004). The juvenile myoclonic epilepsy $GABA_A$ receptor alpha1 subunit mutation A322D producesasymmetrical, subunit position-dependent reduction. *J. Neurosci.* **24**, 5570–5578.

Gallagher, M. J., Shen, W., Song, L., and Macdonald, R. L. (2005). Endoplasmic reticulum retention and associated degradation of a $GABA_A$ receptor epilepsy mutation that inserts an aspartate in the M3 transmembrane segment of the alpha 1 subunit. *J. Biol. Chem.* **280**, 37995–38004.

Haas, K. F., and Macdonald, R. L. (1999). $GABA_A$ receptor subunit gamma2 and delta subtypes confer unique kinetic properties on recombinant $GABA_A$ receptor currents in mouse fibroblasts. *J. Physiol.* **514**(Pt. 1), 27–45.

Harkin, L. A., Bowser, D. N., Dibbens, L. M., Singh, R., Phillips, F., Wallace, R. H., Richards, M. C., Williams, D. A., Mulley, J. C., Berkovic, S. F., Scheffer, I. E., and Petrou, S. (2002). Truncation of the $GABA_A$-receptor gamma2 subunit in a family with generalized epilepsy with febrile seizures plus. *Am. J. Hum. Genet.* **70**, 530–536.

Hinkle, D. J., Bianchi, M. T., and Macdonald, R. L. (2003). Modifications of a commercial perfusion system for use in ultrafast solution exchange during patch clamp recording. *Biotechniques* **35**, 472–474, 476.

Hirose, S., Fukuma, G., Kanaumi, T., Ueno, S., Ishii, A., Haga, Y., Hamachi, A., Yonetan, M., Itho, M., Takashima, S., Kaneko, S., and Mitsudome, A. (2004). Severe myoclonic epilepsy in infancy (SMEI) resulting from *SCN1A* and *GABRG2* mutations inherited from non SMEI parents. *Am. J. Hum. Genet.* Supplement.

Hirose, S., Mitsudome, A., Okada, M., and Kaneko, S. (2005). Genetics of idiopathic epilepsies. *Epilepsia* **46**(Suppl. 1), 38–43.

Jones, M. V., and Westbrook, G. L. (1995). Desensitized states prolong $GABA_A$ channel responses to brief agonist pulses. *Neuron* **15**, 181–191.

Kananura, C., Haug, K., Sander, T., Runge, U., Gu, W., Hallmann, K., Rebstock, J., Heils, A., and Steinlein, O. K. (2002). A splice-site mutation in GABRG2 associated with childhood absence epilepsy and febrile convulsions. *Arch. Neurol.* **59**, 1137–1141.

Kang, J., and Macdonald, R. L. (2004). The $GABA_A$ receptor gamma2 subunit R43Q mutation linked to childhood absence epilepsy and febrile seizures causes retention of alpha1beta2gamma2s receptors in the endoplasmic reticulum. *J. Neurosci.* **24**, 8672–8677.

Kapur, J., and Macdonald, R. L. (1997). Rapid seizure-induced reduction of benzodiazepine and Zn2+ sensitivity of hippocampal dentate granule cell $GABA_A$ receptors. *J. Neurosci.* **17**, 7532–7540.

Karle, J., Woldbye, D. P., Elster, L., Diemer, N. H., Bolwig, T. G., Olsen, R. W., and Nielsen, M. (1998). Antisense oligonucleotide to $GABA_A$ receptor gamma2 subunit induces limbic status epilepticus. *J. Neurosci. Res.* **54**, 863–869.

Kash, T. L., Jenkins, A., Kelley, J. C., Trudell, J. R., and Harrison, N. L. (2003). Coupling of agonist binding to channel gating in the $GABA_A$ receptor. *Nature* **421**, 272–275.

Klausberger, T., Fuchs, K., Mayer, B., Ehya, N., and Sieghart, W. (2000). $GABA_A$ receptor assembly: Identification and structure of gamma(2) sequences forming the intersubunit contacts with alpha(1) and beta(3) subunits. *J. Biol. Chem.* **275**, 8921–8928.

Klausberger, T., Ehya, N., Fuchs, K., Fuchs, T., Ebert, V., Sarto, I., and Sieghart, W. (2001a). Detection and binding properties of GABA$_A$ receptor assembly intermediates. *J. Biol. Chem.* **276**, 16024–16032.

Klausberger, T., Sarto, I., Ehya, N., Fuchs, K., Furtmuller, R., Mayer, B., Huck, S., and Sieghart, W. (2001b). Alternate use of distinct intersubunit contacts controls GABA$_A$ receptor assembly and stoichiometry. *J. Neurosci.* **21**, 9124–9133.

Krampfl, K., Maljevic, S., Cossette, P., Ziegler, E., Rouleau, G. A., Lerche, H., and Bufler, J. (2005). Molecular analysis of the A322D mutation in the GABA receptor alpha-subunit causing juvenile myoclonic epilepsy. *Eur. J. Neurosci.* **22**, 10–20.

Lejeune, F., and Maquat, L. E. (2005). Mechanistic links between nonsense-mediated mRNA decay and pre-mRNA splicing in mammalian cells. *Curr. Opinion in Cell Biol.* **17**, 309–315.

Lynch, J. W., Rajendra, S., Pierce, K. D., Handford, C. A., Barry, P. H., and Schofield, P. R. (1997). Identification of intracellular and extracellular domains mediating signal transduction in the inhibitory glycine receptor chloride channel. *EMBO J.* **16**, 110–120.

Maquat, L. E. (2004). Nonsense-mediated mRNA decay: Splicing, translation and mRNP dynamics. *Nature Reviews* **5**, 89–99.

Miyazawa, A., Fujiyoshi, Y., and Unwin, N. (2003). Structure and gating mechanism of the acetylcholine receptor pore. *Nature* **424**, 949–955.

Mulley, J. C., Scheffer, I. E., Petrou, S., and Berkovic, S. F. (2003). Channelopathies as a genetic cause of epilepsy. *Curr. Opin. Neurol.* **16**, 171–176.

Poulter, M. O., Brown, L. A., Tynan, S., Willick, G., William, R., and McIntyre, D. C. (1999). Differential expression of alpha1, alpha2, alpha3, and alpha5 GABA$_A$ receptor subunits in seizure-prone and seizure-resistant rat models of temporal lobe epilepsy. *J. Neurosci.* **19**, 4654–4661.

Smit, A. B., Syed, N. I., Schaap, D., van Minnen, J., Klumperman, J., Kits, K. S., Lodder, H., van der Schors, R. C., van Elk, R., Sorgedrager, B., Brejc, K., Sixma, T. K., *et al.* (2001). A glia-derived acetylcholine-binding protein that modulates synaptic transmission. *Nature* **411**, 261–268.

Wallace, R. H., Marini, C., Petrou, S., Harkin, L. A., Bowser, D. N., Panchal, R. G., Williams, D. A., Sutherland, G. R., Mulley, J. C., Scheffer, I. E., and Berkovic, S. F. (2001). Mutant GABA$_A$ receptor gamma2-subunit in childhood absence epilepsy and febrile seizures. *Nat. Genet.* **28**, 49–52.

Wang, J. M., Zhang, L., Yao, Y., Viroonchatapan, N., Rothe, E., and Wang, Z. Z. (2002). A transmembrane motif governs the surface trafficking of nicotinic acetylcholine receptors. *Nat. Neurosci.* **5**, 963–970.

**Stephen L. Boehm II*, Igor Ponomarev[†], Yuri A. Blednov[†], and R. Adron Harris[†]**

*Department of Psychology, State University of New York at Binghamton, New York 13902

[†]Waggoner Center for Alcohol and Addiction Research University of Texas at Austin, Texas 78712

# From Gene to Behavior and Back Again: New Perspectives on GABA$_A$ Receptor Subunit Selectivity of Alcohol Actions[1]

## I. Abstract

$\gamma$-Aminobutyric acid A (GABA$_A$) receptors are believed to mediate a number of alcohol's behavioral actions. Because the subunit composition of GABA$_A$ receptors determines receptor pharmacology, behavioral sensitivity to alcohol (ethanol) may depend on which subunits are present (or absent). A number of knockout and/or transgenic mouse models have been developed ($\alpha$1, $\alpha$2, $\alpha$5, $\alpha$6, $\beta$2, $\beta$3, $\gamma$2S, $\gamma$2L, $\delta$) and tested for behavioral sensitivity to ethanol. Here we review the current GABA$_A$ receptor subunit knockout and transgenic literature for ethanol sensitivity, and integrate these results into those obtained using quantitative trait loci (QTL) analysis and gene

[1] This is a revised and updated version of an article entitled "$\gamma$-Aminobutyric Acid A Receptor Subunit Mutant Mice: New Perspectives on Alcohol Actions" that appeared in *Biochem. Pharmacol.* **68**, 1581–1602 (2004).

*Advances in Pharmacology, Volume 54*

1054-3589/06 $35.00
DOI: 10.1016/S1054-3589(06)54008-6

expression assays. Converging evidence from these three approaches support the notion that different behavioral actions of ethanol are mediated by specific subunits, and suggest that new drugs that target specific $GABA_A$ subunits may selectively alter some behavioral actions of ethanol without altering others. Current data sets provide strongest evidence for a role of $\alpha1$ subunits in ethanol-induced loss of righting reflex and $\alpha5$ subunits in ethanol-stimulated locomotion. Nevertheless, three-way validation is hampered by the incomplete behavioral characterization of many of the mutant mice, and additional subunits are likely to be linked to alcohol actions as behavioral testing progresses.

## II. Chapter Overview

$GABA_A$ receptors represent the major inhibitory class of neurotransmitter receptors in the mammalian brain. $GABA_A$ receptors have a pentameric structure with five subunits forming an ion pore. Agonist binding promotes the passage of chloride ions through the pore and into the cell. The net result is an influx of negatively charged ions and hyperpolarization of the neuron.

$GABA_A$ receptors mediate a number of drug effects, including sedation/hypnosis, anxiolysis, and anesthesia. Ethanol as well as barbiturates, benzodiazepines, neuroactive steroids, and volatile and intravenous anesthetics enhance $GABA_A$ receptor function in the presence of agonist resulting in the induction of the above behavioral drug effects. Most native $GABA_A$ receptors are thought to consist of two $\alpha$, two $\beta$, and a $\gamma$ subunit. However, seven classes of $GABA_A$ receptor subunits have been described to date ($\alpha1$–6, $\beta1$–3, $\gamma1$–3, $\delta$, $\varepsilon$, $\theta1$–3, $\pi$, $\rho1$–3) allowing for extensive heterogeneity in receptor subunit composition across neuronal cell types and brain regions. Moreover, the subunit composition of $GABA_A$ receptors has profound effects on receptor pharmacology (Ebert *et al.*, 1997) suggesting the possibility that behavioral sensitivity to ethanol (and other drugs that alter $GABA_A$ receptor function) may depend on which subunits are present (or absent) within specific brain circuits.

The present chapter reviews the actions of alcohol in $GABA_A$ receptor knockout (null mutant) mice. A number of genetic knockout models have been developed and tested, including the $\alpha1$, $\alpha2$, $\alpha5$, and $\alpha6$, the $\beta2$ and $\beta3$, the $\gamma$2L, and the $\delta$ knockout mice. Transgenic mice that overexpress either the $\gamma$2S (short) or $\gamma$2L (long) splice variants of the $GABA_A$ receptor $\gamma$ subunit have also been developed and tested. These studies have revealed a complicated picture of subunit specific behavioral pharmacology. Together, they support the notion that specific $GABA_A$ receptor subunits may indeed mediate specific ethanol- or drug-related behavioral phenotypes. Such results have important implications for studies aimed at developing drugs with fewer side effects; compounds could be engineered to target GABA$_A$ receptors possessing specific subunits thereby altering very specific ethanol-related behaviors. Comparison of the null mutant data with behavioral and gene expression data from the recombinant inbred strains will provide an interesting and powerful new way of examining the link between genes, brain, and behavioral sensitivity to ethanol. Future work will include the production of knock-in mice in which GABA$_A$ receptor subunit function remains largely intact except for a specific loss in ethanol sensitivity.

## III. $\alpha$-Subunit Knockout Mice

### A. $\alpha 1$ Subunit

The $\alpha 1$-receptor subunit of the GABA$_A$ receptor is the most widely expressed $\alpha$ subunit, having expression in the olfactory bulb, cortex, thalamus, hypothalamus, hippocampus, amygdala, midbrain, and cerebellum (Pirker *et al.*, 2000). Two different $\alpha 1$-subunit knockout mouse models have been developed (Sur *et al.*, 2001; Vicini *et al.*, 2001). Whereas the knockouts developed by Sur and colleagues (2001) displayed strong body tremor, those developed by Vicini and colleagues (2001) exhibited spontaneous body tremor and increased sensitivity to bicuculline-induced seizures (Kralic *et al.*, 2002). Indeed, Vicini's $\alpha 1$ knockouts exhibit phenotypic similarities to patients with human essential tremor, suggesting a role for $\alpha 1$-containing GABA$_A$ receptors in the etiology of this disease (Kralic *et al.*, 2005). Nevertheless, both mutant mouse models bred and developed normally, although the number of mutant births observed by both groups was somewhat lower than that predicted by Mendelian genetics.

Binding studies suggest that both populations of $\alpha 1$-subunit knockout mice lost about 50% of all GABA$_A$ receptors (Sur *et al.*, 2001), consistent with this subunit's wide distribution throughout the brain. Genetic deletion of the $\alpha 1$ subunit also resulted in a relative upregulation of $\alpha 2$- (37%) and $\alpha 3$- (39%) receptor subunits (Kralic *et al.*, 2002; Sur *et al.*, 2001) and downregulation of $\beta 2/3$- (65%) and $\gamma 2$- (47%) receptor subunits (Kralic *et al.*, 2002). There was also a selective downregulation of $\alpha 6$ receptor subunits in the cerebellum (Sur *et al.*, 2001). These alterations likely represent some of the compensatory changes that can occur following genetic deletion of specific genes and must be considered when interpreting data from knockout mice.

In addition to the changes in GABA$_A$ receptor subunit expression, a number of other notable phenotypic changes were observed in $\alpha 1$-null mutant mice. Both $\alpha 1$-subunit knockout mouse populations had lower body weights that normalized by 3 months of age and displayed handling-induced tremors (Kralic *et al.*, 2002; Sur *et al.*, 2001). Moreover, *in vitro* work demonstrated that the changes in cerebellar inhibitory synaptic currents that are associated with normal development were absent in the null mutants (Vicini *et al.*, 2001), and that hippocampal miniature inhibitory postsynaptic currents (IPSCs) were less frequent, smaller in amplitude, and longer in duration in $\alpha$1-subunit knockout mice (Goldstein *et al.*, 2002). Longer IPSC durations were also observed in neurons from the supraoptic nucleus of the hypothalamus (Koksma *et al.*, 2003) and layers II–III of the visual cortex (Bosman *et al.*, 2002), and at least in the visual cortex (layers II–III), these changes were associated with a decreased density of mushroom-shaped dendridic spines (Heinen *et al.*, 2003). Despite these observations, the genotypes displayed similar motor abilities and levels of spontaneous locomotion (Sur *et al.*, 2001).

Table I summarizes the results of studies examining the effects of $\alpha$1-subunit gene deletion on ethanol behavioral sensitivity. Sensitivity to other GABAergic compounds was also examined in $\alpha$1 and other $GABA_A$ subunit knockout mouse models. However, a summary of this literature is beyond the scope of this chapter. The interested reader is referred to Boehm II *et al.* (2004).

The Sur *et al.* (2001) and Vicini *et al.* (2001) $\alpha$1 mutant mouse models were both tested for behavioral sensitivity to ethanol. These studies indicated that loss of this subunit increased sensitivity to the locomotor stimulant effects of ethanol (Blednov *et al.*, 2003b; Kralic *et al.*, 2003). Using the female mutants developed by Sur *et al.* (2001), Blednov *et al.* (2003b) showed that the mutation decreased ethanol preference drinking and enhanced the aversive effects of ethanol without altering ethanol conditioned place preference (ethanol's reinforcing properties) or chronic ethanol withdrawal. Moreover, although not yet published, Blednov *et al.* has also observed reduced acute ethanol withdrawal severity in male $\alpha$1-subunit knockout mice. Using the Vicini mice, Kralic *et al.* (2003) showed that $\alpha$1 mutant and wild-type mice did not differ in sensitivity to ethanol's anxiolytic, motor incoordinating, or anticonvulsant actions, nor did the null mutation alter acute tolerance to ethanol's motor incoordinating effects. Finally, whereas the male mutants tested by Blednov and colleagues (2003a) displayed reduced sensitivity to ethanol's hypnotic actions as assessed by the loss of righting reflex assay, the mutants tested by Kralic *et al.* (2003) did not differ. Thus, despite the negative finding in the place-conditioning assay, the collective data suggest that $\alpha$1-containing $GABA_A$ receptors may have some role in modulating ethanol's reinforcing and/or motivational properties. In support of this contention, a recent report suggests that intraventral pallidal injections of an $\alpha$1-selective benzodiazepine antagonist reduce ethanol maintained responding in alcohol-preferring P rats (Harvey *et al.*, 2002).

## B. $\alpha$2 Subunit

The $\alpha$2-receptor subunit is expressed at low levels in a number of structures throughout the brain, including the cortex, hypothalamus, hippocampus,

**TABLE I** Change in Behavioral Sensitivity to Ethanol in $GABA_A$ Subunit Knockout and Transgenic Mice: A Summary of the Data

| *Subunit* | *Drink* | *CTA* | *CPP* | *Stim* | *LORR* | *Hypotherm* | *Ataxia* | *Anxiolysis* | *Anticonv* | *Acute tolerance* | *Chronic tolerance* | *Acute withdrawal* | *Chronic withdrawal* | *Discrim* |
|---|---|---|---|---|---|---|---|---|---|---|---|---|---|---|
| α1 | ↓ | ↑ | = | ↑ | ↓, = | | = | = | = | = | | ↓ | = | |
| α2 | = | | | | ↓ | | | = | | | | = | | |
| α5 | ↓ | | | ↑ | = | | | = | | = | | ↓ | | |
| α6 | | | | | = | | | | | = | = | | = | |
| β2 | = | = | = | = | ↓ | | | | | | | ↑ | = | |
| β3 | | | | | = | | | | | | | | | |
| γ2S | | | | | | | | | | ↓ (Tg) | | | | |
| γ2L | | | | = | =(Tg), = | | | = | | ↓ (Tg), = | | =(Tg) | = | |
| δ | ↓ | | | | = | = | | = | ↓ | = | = | | ↓ | = |

Results are from null mutant mice unless otherwise indicated. Results from transgenic mice are designated by Tg. Drinking, preference and/or consumption; CTA, conditioned taste aversion, aversion; CPP, conditioned place preference, reinforcement; Stimulation, locomotor stimulation; LORR, loss of righting reflex, hypnotic actions; Ataxia, motor incoordination—rotarod; Anxiolysis, anxiolytic actions—elevated plus maze; Anticonv, anticonvulsant actions; Acute Tolerance, acute tolerance to motor incoordinating actions—dowel rod; chronic tolerance, chronic tolerance to hypnotic actions—LORR; Discrim, ethanol discriminative stimulus effects.

and amygdala (Pirker *et al.*, 2000). α2-Subunit knockout mice were recently generated by Paul Whiting, Elisabeth Garrett, and Thomas Rosahl at Merck Sharp and Dohme (Harlow, United Kingdom). Although early on there was about a 30% decrease in the number of mutants surviving to weaning, α2-subunit knockouts now appear to breed and develop normally. It is currently unknown whether genetic deletion of this subunit has altered the expression of other $GABA_A$ receptor subunits. When tested for locomotor response to novelty, nonhabituated α2 knockout mice were less active compared to their wild-type counterparts (Boehm II *et al.*, 2004).

We recently assessed a number of ethanol behavioral phenotypes in α2 knockout mice (Boehm II *et al.*, 2004; Table I). α2 knockout mice displayed shorter durations of ethanol-induced loss of righting reflex and reduced ethanol-induced time and entries into the open arms of an elevated plus maze (although this result depended on how we analyzed the data), suggesting a role for the α2 subunit in the mediation of ethanol's hypnotic and anxiolytic actions. The genotypes did not significantly differ in sensitivity to acute ethanol withdrawal, although knockouts tended to experience less severe withdrawal. Female mutants preferred and consumed significantly less ethanol than did their wild-type counterparts. However, the null mutants also trended toward lower preference for the bitter tasting quinine, suggesting that the female α2 knockouts may have preferred and consumed less ethanol because of an enhanced aversion to bitter tastants. Male α2-subunit knockout mice did not differ in preference or consumption of ethanol.

## C. α5 Subunit

The α5-receptor subunit is not widely expressed in brain. Expression is restricted to structures like the hippocampus, olfactory bulb, areas of cortex, and the hypothalamus (Pirker *et al.*, 2000). Moreover, whereas α1, α2, and α3 receptor subunits are localized to the synapse, studies examining subunit expression in olfactory bulb and hippocampal pyramidal cells suggest that α5 receptor subunits are largely localized to extrasynaptic sites (Brünig *et al.*, 2002; Fritschy *et al.*, 1998), where they likely modulate tonic GABAergic inhibition (Caraiscos *et al.*, 2004). Interestingly studies suggest that the molecular sites of at least some of ethanol's actions are extrasynaptic, although α5-receptor subunits were not directly studied (Liang *et al.*, 2004; Wallner *et al.*, 2003).

Only two published reports have examined the role of α5-receptor subunits in ethanol sensitivity. One study showed that intra-hippocampal (CA1 and CA3) injection of a selective α5-receptor subunit benzodiazepine inverse agonist attenuated ethanol self-administration in rats (June *et al.*, 2001), suggesting that null mutation of the α5-receptor subunit may attenuate alcohol's reinforcing properties. More recently the same group demonstrated that this receptor subunit regulates the reinforcing (ethanol-maintained responding), motor incoordinating (oscillating bar task), and sedative (open field activity) actions of ethanol using a novel benzodiazepine inverse agonist with high affinity for $\alpha$5-containing GABA$_A$ receptors (McKay *et al.*, 2004).

$\alpha$5-Receptor subunit null mutant mice were recently developed, and although hippocampal benzodiazepine binding sites were reduced by 16%, there were no apparent alterations in the expression levels of other GABA$_A$ receptor subunits (Collinson *et al.*, 2002). Compared to their wild-type counterparts, $\alpha$5-subunit knockout mice exhibited improved performance in a water maze of spatial learning, but not in a non-hippocampal learning or anxiety task (Collinson *et al.*, 2002). However, the genotypes did not differ in locomotor response to novelty (Boehm II *et al.*, 2004). $\alpha$5-Subunit knockout mice also displayed lower IPSC amplitudes, and greater facilitation of paired-pulse facilitation of field excitatory postsynaptic potential amplitudes in hippocampal brain slices (Collinson *et al.*, 2002). Taken together, these results suggest that $\alpha$5-receptor subunits have an important role in mediating hippocampal-dependent learning processes.

We established a colony of $\alpha$5-receptor subunit knockout mice and assessed them for ethanol behavioral sensitivity (Boehm II *et al.*, 2004; Table I). $\alpha$5-Subunit knockout mice did not differ in sensitivity to ethanol-induced loss of righting reflex or ethanol's anxiolytic effects. However, the knockouts displayed lower handling-induced convulsion scores, suggesting a blunted acute withdrawal syndrome. Moreover, male null mutants preferred and consumed less ethanol than did their male wild-type counterparts in the absence of any differences in preference for the sweet tasting saccharine or the bitter tasting quinine, suggesting that deletion of the $\alpha$5-subunit gene may have also altered ethanol's reinforcing properties. Interestingly the null mutation also blunted sensitivity to ethanol's locomotor stimulant properties, as assessed using the elevated plus maze. Thus, deletion of the $\alpha$5-subunit gene may have altered the motivational effects of ethanol. However, this result should be interpreted with some caution as sensitivity to ethanol's locomotor stimulant effects has not been directly assessed.

## D. $\alpha$6-Subunit

Expression of GABA$_A$ $\alpha$6-receptor subunits is restricted to the postmigratory granule cells of the cerebellum and cochlear nuclei (Laurie *et al.*, 1992; Varecka *et al.*, 1994; Zheng *et al.*, 1993). Some 40–60% of cerebellar GABA$_A$ receptors contain the $\alpha$6 subunit (Khan *et al.*, 1996; Quirk *et al.*, 1995). Given the role of the cerebellum in motor control (Miall, 1998), the above-mentioned pattern of expression makes $\alpha$6-receptor subunits attractive candidates for modulation of ethanol's motor impairing actions. In support of this notion, an investigation reported that GABA$_A$ receptors composed of $\alpha6\beta3\delta$ or $\alpha4\beta3\delta$ are 10 times more sensitive to ethanol concentrations known to have intoxicating actions in humans (Wallner *et al.*, 2003).

Mutant mice lacking the $\alpha$6-receptor subunit were developed by two different research groups (Homanics *et al.*, 1997b; Jones *et al.*, 1997). Deletion of the $\alpha$6 subunit resulted in a reduction in cerebellar $\beta$2, $\beta$3, and $\gamma$2 subunits (Nusser *et al.*, 1999). $\delta$-Subunit expression was also reduced, despite the presence of a normal messenger ribonucleic acid (mRNA) level (Jones *et al.*, 1997). These results suggest that $\delta$ may associate with $\alpha$6 *in vivo* (Jones *et al.*, 1997). However, this interpretation should be made with some caution as $\alpha$1 and $\beta$2 subunit expression levels were also reduced in the forebrain, a structure that does not posses $\alpha$6-receptor subunits (Uusi-Oukari *et al.*, 2000). Nevertheless, these results indicate that insertion of the neomycin resistance cassette into the $\alpha$6-subunit gene had the unexpected effect of downregulating expression of other subunits clustered very near the $\alpha$6 subunit on mouse chromosome 11 (Uusi-Oukari *et al.*, 2000). Finally, binding affinity for muscimol was reduced in the cerebellum of the mutant mice (Homanics *et al.*, 1997b), as was tonic conductance in cerebellar granule cells (Brickley *et al.*, 2001).

Despite the above-mentioned changes in subunit expression, the $\alpha$6 deficient and wild-type mice developed by Jones *et al.* (1997) appeared to breed and develop normally. Moreover, when tested for the mutation's effects on naïve behavior, the genotypes displayed similar levels of open field activity, and did not differ in performance on the horizontal wire task (Jones *et al.*, 1997). The $\alpha$6-subunit knockout mice developed by Homanics *et al.* (1997b) were also viable and fertile, and had grossly normal cerebellar cytoarchitecture. However, no basal behavioral data were published on these animals.

Given the fairly strong expression of $\alpha$6 subunits in the cerebellum, one would predict that mice lacking this subunit would display altered behavioral responses to ethanol. Several ethanol-related behaviors were examined in $\alpha$6-subunit knockout and wild-type mice. However, the knockouts did not differ in sensitivity to ethanol's hypnotic effects as measured using the loss of righting reflex test (Homanics *et al.*, 1997b), nor did they develop different acute or chronic tolerance to ethanol, or chronic ethanol withdrawal (Homanics *et al.*, 1998). These results are summarized in Table I. Thus, despite the strong cerebellar expression, deletion of the $\alpha$6-subunit gene did not alter behavioral sensitivity to ethanol. However, one report suggests that neuronal adaptations may have countered the loss of this subunit, allowing for normal sensitivity to ethanol's motor impairing actions. Brickley *et al.* (2001) showed that normal cerebellar granule cell excitability was maintained by an adaptive enhancement in voltage-independent $K^+$ leak conductance in $\alpha$6-subunit knockout mice.

One of the benefits of summarizing all the $GABA_A$ receptor knockout data in one place is that it allows for identification of gaps in our knowledge. Several studies have demonstrated that a naturally occurring point mutation in the $\alpha$6-subunit gene is responsible for ethanol's impairment of postural reflexes in rat lines genetically selected to differ in ethanol sensitivity (Korpi *et al.*, 1993). Consequently, it may be that α6-subunit gene deletion altered sensitivity to ethanol's motor incoordinating effects, but that the appropriate behavioral tasks were not employed. Finally, as the available evidence suggests that this same mutation may also alter ethanol preference (Carr *et al.*, 2003; Saba *et al.*, 2001), α6-subunit knockout and wild-type mice should also be tested in a two-bottle choice-drinking paradigm, or in other paradigms that assess ethanol's reinforcing and/or motivational properties.

## IV. β-Subunit Knockout Mice

### A. β2 Subunit

β2 subunits are the most abundant of the β subunits, and GABA$_A$ receptors containing them are found in virtually all brain structures, including olfactory bulb, cortex, hippocampus, thalamus, hypothalamus, amygdala, cerebellum, and midbrain (Pirker *et al.*, 2000). Given this wide distribution, one would predict that β2 subunits are important for normal GABAergic functioning, and that they may also be important mediators of ethanol's behavioral effects.

Consistent with its widespread distribution, deletion of the β2-subunit gene reduced the total number of brain GABA$_A$ receptors (O'Meara *et al.*, 2004). Moreover, although β3-subunit expression was not altered, the expression of all six α subunits was reduced (40–70% reduction). These results suggest that β2 subunits can co-assemble with any α subunit, and that other β subunits do not substitute for β2.

Despite the widespread distribution of β2 subunits, these mutants bred and developed normally, and did not display any spontaneous seizures (Sur *et al.*, 2001). The knockouts also did not show any major deficits in motor function as measured by the rotarod, balance beam, or swimming ability tasks. However, the knockouts did display greater spontaneous locomotor activity (Sur *et al.*, 2001). When ethanol sensitivity was assessed knockouts were less sensitive to ethanol's hypnotic actions as determined by the loss of righting reflex test (Blednov *et al.*, 2003a), although this differential action of ethanol was only seen among male mice. Although it is not immediately clear why female knockouts did not display a similar reduction in hypnotic sensitivity, it is notable that the dose–response curves for the male knockouts overlapped the curves for the female knockouts and wild-types. Thus, it is possible that a floor effect masked any further reduction in hypnotic sensitivity in the female β2-subunit knockout mice. Gender specific effects were also seen when β2-subunit knockout mice were assessed for acute ethanol withdrawal severity; male knockouts experienced more severe acute ethanol withdrawal (Blednov *et al.*, unpublished). The genotypes did not differ in sensitivity to ethanol's locomotor stimulant effects, nor did they differ in ethanol preference drinking, ethanol conditioned taste aversion, or ethanol conditioned place preference (Blednov *et al.*, 2003b). $\beta 2$-Subunit knockout mice exhibited more robust chronic ethanol withdrawal following exposure to a chronic ethanol liquid diet. However, they also consumed more of the ethanol liquid diet (Blednov *et al.*, 2003b), making interpretation of these results difficult. These data are summarized in Table I.

## B. $\beta 3$ Subunit

$\beta 3$-Receptor subunits are strongly expressed in the olfactory bulb, cortex, hypothalamus, and amygdala, but can be found in many other cell types throughout the brain (Pirker *et al.*, 2000) and spinal cord (Persohn *et al.*, 1991). Its strong expression in cerebellar granule cells (Pirker *et al.*, 2000) makes it an attractive candidate for mediating behavioral sensitivity to ethanol. Indeed, a recent study suggests that $GABA_A$ receptors composed of $\alpha 6$, $\beta 3$, and $\delta$ receptors are particularly sensitive to ethanol (Wallner *et al.*, 2003).

$\beta 3$-Receptor knockout mice were developed by Homanics and colleagues (1997a). Knockout of the $\beta 3$-subunit gene reduced the total number of brain $GABA_A$ receptors containing $\alpha 2$ and $\alpha 3$ subunits (Ramadan *et al.*, 2003), and severely impaired $GABA_A$ receptor function as assessed by recordings from hippocampal (Krasowski *et al.*, 1998), dorsal root ganglion (Homanics *et al.*, 1997a; Krasowski *et al.*, 1998), and cortical (Ramadan *et al.*, 2003) neurons. However, brain morphology was grossly normal. Most $\beta 3$ null mutants died shortly after birth, and most (but not all) of these deaths were associated with cleft palate. The development of cleft palate is consistent with work suggesting a link between $\beta 3$ subunits and development of this condition (Culiat *et al.*, 1995). The surviving knockouts were initially smaller than their wildtype counterparts, but achieved normal body weight after weaning. Moreover, they bred normally but exhibited a shortened life span.

Consistent with the widespread distribution of the subunit, $\beta 3$-subunit knockout mice displayed a number of abnormal behaviors (Homanics *et al.*, 1997a). $\beta 3$-Subunit knockout mice were hyperactive and hyperresponsive to sensory stimuli. When lifted by the tail, the mutants showed signs of neurological impairment, and experienced difficulty walking on grids, platforms, and rotarods. $\beta 3$-Deficient mice also displayed occasional epileptic seizures, confirmed by electroencephalographic recordings. These phenotypes are consistent with Angelman syndrome, a severe human neurodevelopmental disorder resulting from deletion and/or mutation of maternal chromosome 15q11-13 (DeLorey *et al.*, 1998). The $\beta 3$-subunit gene is contained within this chromosomal region. Finally, $\beta 3$ knockout mice display impaired REM sleep and altered EEG spectral phenomena associated with non-REM sleep (Wisor *et al.*, 2002).

Although $\beta 3$-receptor subunit knockout mice were found to differ in sensitivity to a number of different $GABA_A$ acting compounds (Boehm II *et al.*, 2004), only one ethanol-related behavior has been assessed to date. This may be, in part, due to the severe behavioral consequences of $\beta$3-subunit knockout that are detailed above. Compared to their wild-type counterparts, $\beta$3-subunit knockout mice did not differ in sensitivity to ethanol's hypnotic actions as measured by the loss of righting reflex task (Quinlan *et al.*, 1998).

## V. $\gamma$2-Subunit Knockout and Transgenic Mice

### A. $\gamma$2 Subunit

$\gamma$2 subunits are widely expressed in brain (Pirker *et al.*, 2000). They are found in an estimated 60% of GABA$_A$ receptors (Whiting, 2003), and are believed to have a role in their synaptic clustering (Essrich *et al.*, 1998). The $\gamma$2 subunit can be alternatively spliced, creating two different splice variants, the $\gamma$2S and $\gamma$2L. The $\gamma$2L splice variant differs from its shorter relative because it possesses eight additional amino acids in the third intracellular loop. These additional amino acids contain a protein kinase C phosphorylation site, and work by Wafford and collegues (Wafford *et al.*, 1991) suggested that these eight amino acids are required for ethanol-enhancement of GABA$_A$ receptors possessing the $\gamma$2 subunit. However, another study did not support this finding (Sigel *et al.*, 1993).

$\gamma$2-Subunit knockout mice were first developed by Günther *et al.* (1995). The knockouts appeared normal at birth. However, the majority died shortly after birth with few surviving to postnatal day 18. Moreover, those that survived to postnatal day 18 displayed abnormal gait, impaired grasping and righting reflex, and were hyperactive. More recently conditional $\gamma$2 knockout mice (Schweizer *et al.*, 2003), as well as $\gamma$2 knockdown mice (Chandra *et al.*, 2005) have been generated. However, none of these mutant mouse models have been tested for ethanol sensitivity.

### B. $\gamma$2S Subunit

As mentioned previously, the $\gamma$2 subunit can be alternatively spliced, creating a short ($\gamma$2S) and a long ($\gamma$2L) splice variant. The distribution of $\gamma$2S and $\gamma$2L are fairly similar throughout the brain. However, the relative expression intensity varies depending on brain region and neuronal cell type. For example, whereas $\gamma$2S subunits are more abundant in the olfactory bulb, cortex, and hippocampus, $\gamma$2L subunits exhibit stronger expression in cerebellar Purkinje cells (Gutiérrez *et al.*, 1994).

Mice lacking the $\gamma$2S subunit have not been generated. However, transgenic mice that overexpress the $\gamma$2S subunit have been developed by Wick and colleagues (2000). There are no available data on basal behaviors in these mutant mice. However, when ethanol sensitivity was studied, it was determined that $\gamma$2S-subunit transgenic mice developed less acute tolerance to ethanol's motor incoordinating effects. Thus, it appears that the $\gamma$2S subunit may indeed have a role in mediating behavioral sensitivity to ethanol. However, more work will be necessary to more fully elucidate the role of $\gamma$2S in the mediation of ethanol's behavioral actions.

### C. $\gamma$2L Subunit

Knockout mice lacking the $\gamma$2L subunit were developed by Homanics *et al.* (1999). These mice were viable, and indistinguishable from wild-type mice. However, despite some *in vitro* evidence suggesting that this $GABA_A$ receptor subunit is important for ethanol's actions (Wafford *et al.*, 1991), $\gamma$2L-subunit deficient mice displayed similar sensitivities to ethanol's hypnotic (loss of righting reflex), anxiolytic (elevated plus maze), and locomotor stimulant actions (Homanics *et al.*, 1999). Moreover, the genotypes developed similar chronic ethanol withdrawal and acute tolerance to ethanol's motor incoordinating actions. Electrophysiological recordings in dorsal root ganglion neurons also did not reveal any differences between $\gamma$2L-subunit knockout and wild-type mice. A caveat was that total $\gamma$2-subunit protein levels were unchanged in the knockouts, suggesting that the $\gamma$2S-subunit may have substituted for the $\gamma$2L subunit in these mutant mice.

The same group that developed the $\gamma$2S-subunit transgenic mice also developed transgenic mice that overexpress the $\gamma$2L subunit (Wick *et al.*, 2000). These mice were also impaired in their ability to develop acute tolerance to ethanol's motor incoordinating actions. Thus, whereas the $\gamma$2L subunit appears to alter acute tolerance in transgenic mice, it has no such effect in knockout mice. These results are contrary to the prediction that the effects of transgenic overexpression would be phenotypically opposite those of gene knockout, and provide a mixed support, at best, for a role of the $\gamma$2L subunit in mediating ethanol sensitivity. Furthermore, it should also be noted that both $\gamma$2S- and $\gamma$2L-subunit transgenic mice displayed similar ethanol phenotypes (i.e., impaired acute tolerance), arguing against the importance of the eight amino acid segment in mitigating ethanol sensitivity in $\gamma$2-containing $GABA_A$ receptors. Nevertheless, given the normal $\gamma$2-subunit protein levels and lack of ethanol phenotype in the $\gamma$2L-subunit knockouts, it might be prudent to assess ethanol sensitivity in the heterozygous, global $\gamma$2-subunit knockout mice developed by Günther *et al.* (1995).

## VI. $\delta$-Subunit Knockout Mice

$\delta$-Receptor subunits are found in most brain structures, although with limited abundance (Pirker *et al.*, 2000). The $\delta$ subunit is more prevalant in cerebellar granule cells where its localization is almost exclusively extrasynaptic (Nusser *et al.*, 1998). Electrophysiological evidence also suggests an extrasynaptic localization of $\delta$-containing receptors on thalamic relay neurons (Porcello *et al.*, 2003) and granule cells of the mouse dentate gyrus (Wei *et al.*, 2003). Evidence suggests that extrasynaptic $\delta$-containing GABA$_A$ receptors are particularly sensitive to ethanol (Sundstrom-Poromaa *et al.*, 2002; Wallner *et al.*, 2003). Furthermore, recent work indicates that $\delta$-containing GABA$_A$ receptors, especially those also composed of $\alpha$4 and $\beta$, may be upregulated during hormonal states (i.e., premenstrual syndrome) associated with enhanced sensitivity to ethanol (Sundstrom-Poromaa *et al.*, 2002). Thus, $\delta$-subunit knockout mice would be expected to display altered behavioral sensitivity to ethanol.

$\delta$-Subunit knockout mice were developed by Mihalek *et al.* (1999). Immunoaffinity chromatography of cerebellar extracts indicated an increased co-assembly of $\alpha$6 and $\gamma$2 subunits in the $\delta$-subunit knockouts (Tretter *et al.*, 2001). Because 97% of all $\delta$ subunits were co-assembled with $\alpha$6 subunits in the cerebellum of wild-type mice, the above results suggest that $\alpha 6\beta\gamma 2$ and $\alpha\beta$ replaced $\delta$-containing GABA$_A$ receptors in the cerebellum of $\delta$-subunit deficient mice. Thus, it appears that the availability of the $\delta$ subunit influences the assembly of $\gamma$2 with other subunits, even though $\delta$ and $\gamma$2 subunits do not co-assemble in the same receptor. Similar results were seen in forebrain where $\delta$ subunits normally co-assemble with $\alpha$4 subunits; $\gamma$2-subunit expression and co-assembly with $\alpha$4 was increased in $\delta$-subunit knockout mice (Korpi *et al.*, 2002b; Peng *et al.*, 2002). $\delta$-Subunit gene deletion also reduced $\alpha$4-subunit expression in forebrain (Peng *et al.*, 2002) and hippocampus (Spigelman *et al.*, 2003).

Hippocampal slices from $\delta$-subunit knockout mice displayed a faster decay of mIPSC, but no change in mIPSC amplitude or frequency (Mihalek *et al.*, 1999). However, the mutants bred and developed normally (Mihalek *et al.*, 1999). Moreover, basal behaviors were not altered by the $\delta$-subunit null mutation. Mutants and wild-types displayed similar anxiety levels, and normal fear conditioning, exploratory activity, and pain sensitivity (Mihalek *et al.*, 1999), although a report suggests that female $\delta$-knockout mice exhibit enhanced acquisition of tone and context fear in a hippocampal-dependent trace fear conditioning paradigm (Wiltgen *et al.*, 2005).

Evidence suggests that extrasynaptic $\delta$-containing GABA$_A$ receptors are particularly sensitive to ethanol (Sundstrom-Poromaa *et al.*, 2002; Wallner *et al.*, 2003). Thus, deletion of the $\delta$ subunit should have profound effects on ethanol behavioral sensitvity. $\delta$-Subunit knockout mice preferred and consumed less ethanol, exhibited reduced chronic ethanol withdrawal severity, and displayed reduced sensitivity to the anticonvulsant actions of ethanol (Mihalek *et al.*, 2001). However, the hypnotic (loss of righting reflex), anxiolytic (elevated plus maze), and hypothermic actions of ethanol were not changed, nor was chronic tolerance to the hypnotic actions, or acute tolerance to the motor incoordinating actions of ethanol. Deletion of the $\delta$ subunit also did not alter the acquisition of ethanol/saline discrimination or the substitution patterns of $GABA_A$-positive modulators (Shannon *et al.*, 2004). These data are summarized in Table I. Consequently, at least some of the behavioral data appears to support *in vitro* studies suggesting a role for this $GABA_A$ receptor subunit in the mediation of ethanol sensitivity. Based on work suggesting a role neurosteroids in the modulation of ethanol's actions at $\delta$-containing receptors (Sundstrom-Poromaa *et al.*, 2002), future studies should assess the combined actions of ethanol and various neuroactive steroids in $\delta$-subunit knockout mice.

## VII. $GABA_A$ Receptor Subunit Knock-in Mice

A more elegant strategy for associating different $GABA_A$ receptor subunit genes with specific ethanol-related behaviors is the creation of knock-in mice. Knock-in mice possess a point mutation that alters some aspect of protein function, leaving all other aspects of protein function in tact. Perhaps the greatest advantage to this approach is that the protein is not entirely eliminated (as it is in knockout mice), but is present, and in large part functional. This approach has been successfully used to investigate the $\alpha$-subunit selectivity of diazepam's behavioral actions.

Two different groups have developed mutant mice possessing genetically altered $\alpha1$-receptor subunits. Rudolph *et al.* (1999) were the first to report knock-in mice possessing a point mutation (H101R) that eliminated diazepam-potentiation of $GABA_A$ currents *in vitro*, and a second group duplicated the feat with the same point mutation (McKernan *et al.*, 2000). Both knock-in mouse models were less sensitive to the sedative actions of diazepam. Moreover, Rudolph *et al.* (1999) provided additional evidence that sensitivity to the amnestic and anticonvulsant actions of diazepam were selectively attenuated in the knock-ins. Although the groups were in disagreement on whether the point mutation attenuated sensitivity to the motor impairing effects of diazepam, the combined data sets provide the evidence that certain $GABA_A$ receptor subunits mediate specific diazepam-induced behaviors, presumably without the possible confound of developmental compensation.

Since this initial work, a number of other $GABA_A$ receptor subunit knock-in mouse models have been developed, including the $\alpha1$ S270H (Homanics *et al.*, 2005), $\alpha2$ H101R (Low *et al.*, 2000; Reynolds *et al.*, 2001), $\alpha5$ H101R (Crestani *et al.*, 2002), $\beta2$ N265S (Reynolds *et al.*, 2003b), $\beta3$ N265M (Jurd *et al.*, 2003), and $\gamma2$ F77I (Cope *et al.*, 2004) knock-in mouse models. Mutagenesis studies continue to identify ethanol sensitive sites on $GABA_A$ receptor subunits (Harris, 1999; Jung *et al.*, 2005; Ueno *et al.*, 1999). Given continued progress along these lines, it will not be long before a mutation is identified that eliminates ethanol sensitivity while maintaining the actions of GABA *in vitro*. Such a mutation would make a good candidate for the production of GABA$_A$ subunit knock-in mice, and subsequent studies aimed at identifying which GABA$_A$ receptor subunits modulate which ethanol-related behaviors. The hope is that such animal models will bypass many of the developmental compensatory changes observed in the GABA$_A$ subunit knockout mice (i.e., up/down-regulation of other subunits) because the mutated subunits will remain intact and functional. If achieved, such mutant mouse models would be powerful new tools in the association between certain GABA$_A$ receptor subunits and specific ethanol-related behaviors.

## VIII. Functional Compensation in Genetically Altered Mice: Gene–Behavior Associations Put into Context

Despite some marked effects of genetic mutations at the cellular and molecular level, the behavioral profiles of some GABA$_A$ receptor mutants do not severely deviate from the norm. The lack of salient behavioral abnormalities is often attributed to developmental compensation for the disruption of function produced by the mutation. However, mechanisms of such compensation are largely unknown. One general assumption is that other subunits could substitute for the lost one. Indeed, this hypothesis received some support when Kralic and colleagues (2002) discovered up-regulation of $\alpha$2- and $\alpha$3-subunit proteins in their $\alpha$1 null mutants. However, subunit substitution does not appear to play a central role in other GABA$_A$ receptor subunit mutants with largely normal behavioral phenotypes, such as $\beta$2 or $\alpha$6 knockouts.

To understand the mechanisms of functional compensation in GABA$_A$ receptor mutant mice, it is important to understand what is compensated for. GABA$_A$ receptors mediate the majority of fast inhibitory neurotransmission in the CNS. Changes in receptor function produced by a genetic mutation of one of the subunits may result in an overall change in inhibitory tone, thus shifting the balance between excitation and inhibition in brain. Studies suggest that it is this shift in neuronal activity that triggers neuroplasticity mechanisms directed at restoring the balance. Research shows that such plasticity can occur at both inhibitory and excitatory synapses and can also affect intrinsic neuronal excitability (Ozaki, 2002; Turrigiano, 1999; Turrigiano and Nelson, 2004). One example of the latter mechanism comes from an elegant study by Brickley and colleagues (2001) showing that loss of tonic inhibition in GABA$_A$ receptor $\alpha$6-subunit null mutant mice triggers a change in the magnitude of a voltage-independent potassium conductance that maintains neuronal excitability within a physiologically relevant range.

The concept of plasticity driven by patterns of neuronal activity implies that functional compensation in $GABA_A$ mutants is not limited to changes at the GABA synapse. This notion is, in part, supported by a number of pharmacological studies in $\alpha 1$ knockout mice showing differential sensitivity to glutamatergic and dopaminergic drugs (Kralic *et al.*, 2003; Reynolds *et al.*, 2003a). A study used gene expression profiles and electrophysiological techniques to provide additional support for compensatory modulation in these mutants. In addition to pre- and post-synaptic changes in GABA transmission, the $\alpha 1$ knockouts showed an altered expression of several genes involved in regulation of glutamate signaling. Transcripts implicated in the regulation of neurotransmitter release, such as vesicular glutamate transporter VGLUT2, metabotropic glutamate receptors mGluR7 and mGluR8, and postsynaptic signaling, such as AMPA receptor $\alpha 3$ subunit and RACK1 protein, were differentially expressed between mutant and wild-type mice (Ponomarev *et al.*, 2006).

It is important to realize that while some forms of neuronal plasticity result in normalization of behavior, as may be the case for the $\alpha 6$ null mutants, other plasticity mechanisms may contribute to expression of the altered behavioral phenotype, thus complicating interpretation of the relationships between gene mutation and behavior. Creation of knock-in mice (discussed in Section VII) attempts to avoid this compensatory response by maintaining an intact GABA binding site on an otherwise mutated subunit. However, even knock-ins may display neuronal adaptive responses triggered by subtle changes in $GABA_A$ receptor properties. Thus, caution should be exercised when interpreting phenotypic data from genetically modified animals. Nevertheless, linking genetic mutations and altered behaviors through studying single neurons and neuronal networks should help our understanding of a gene–behavior relationship and its modulation by neuronal plasticity.

## IX. $GABA_A$ Receptor Subunit-Associated Quantitative Trait Loci

Another way to determine whether different $GABA_A$ receptor subunits modulate specific ethanol-related behavioral phenotypes is to examine the available QTL literature. Ethanol-related behaviors are complex traits. This means that many different genes influence genetic vulnerability to ethanol's behavioral actions. Over the past decade QTL analysis has emerged as a strategy for mapping the many chromosomal regions that contain genes influencing sensitivity to a number of ethanol-related behaviors.

The basic premise of QTL analysis is simple (Phillips and Belknap, 2002). First, one must measure a specific phenotype within a population. Next, the population must be genotyped at a hundred or more marker loci distributed across the genome, and the genotype (at each marker locus) of each individual animal compared with its phenotypic score. The idea is to identify animals of one genotype that score differently on the phenotypic trait than animals of another genotype. If such animals are found, a QTL is detected and mapped to the chromosomal region containing the associated marker.

To date a number of significant QTLs for different alcohol-related traits in mice have been identified. Most of these have been reviewed by Crabbe *et al.* (1999) and Crabbe (2002), and include QTLs for acute alcohol withdrawal severity, alcohol reinforcement/motivational effects (alcohol preference drinking, conditioned taste aversion, conditioned place preference, locomotor stimulation, and locomotor sensitzation), hypnosis (loss of righting reflex), hypothermia, and motor incoordination. Moreover, a number of candidate genes are known to reside within the regions spanned by these QTLs. However, confirmation of these candidate genes is difficult as the initial mapping of a QTL usually occurs with a resolution of 10–30 cM (Crabbe *et al.*, 1999), a region containing hundreds of possible candidate genes. Thus, it is essential to proceed from QTL to gene by both narrowing the region spanned by the QTL and by testing any suggested candidate genes lying within the region spanned by the QTL.

A number of QTLs span chromosomal regions known to contain GABA$_A$ receptor subunit genes. These genes are clustered on five different chromosomes, including 4, 5, 7, 11, and the X chromosome (Korpi *et al.*, 2002a; Table II). For example, a gene cluster containing the $\alpha1$, $\alpha6$, $\beta2$, and $\gamma2$ subunits can be found on chromosome 11, at about 23 cM. A QTL for acute ethanol withdrawal spans this region (Buck *et al.*, 1997). Other notable gene clusters include the $\alpha2$-, $\alpha4$-, $\beta1$-, and $\gamma1$-subunit cluster on chromosome 5 (40 cM), the $\alpha5$-, $\beta3$-, and $\gamma3$-subunit cluster on chromosome 7 (28 cM), the $\rho1$- and $\rho2$-subunit cluster on chromosome 4 (11 cM), and the $\alpha3$-, $\theta$-, and $\varepsilon$-subunit cluster on the X chromosome (29 cM). The $\delta$ subunit is located by itself on chromosome 4 (79 cM).

**TABLE II** Chromosomal Localization of Known GABA$_A$ Receptor Gene Clusters in Mice

| *Chromosome* | *Location (cM)* | *GABA$_A$ gene* |
|---|---|---|
| 4 | 10.5 | $\rho1$, $\rho2$ |
| 4 | 79 | $\delta$ |
| 5 | 40 | $\alpha2$, $\alpha4$, $\beta1$, $\gamma1$ |
| 7 | 28 | $\alpha5$, $\beta3$, $\gamma3$ |
| 11 | 23 | $\alpha l$, $\alpha6$, $\beta2$, $\gamma2$ |
| X | 29 | $\alpha3$, $\theta$, $\epsilon$ |

As mentioned above, the region spanned by a QTL can harbor hundreds of genes, any of which may influence the trait of interest. Besides narrowing the region spanned by the QTL, another strategy has been to turn to mutant mice for confirmation or exclusion of candidate genes. QTLs overlapping the locations of known $GABA_A$ receptor subunit genes are listed in Table III. Not all of the listed QTLs are among the most highly significant in the studies in which they were detected. However, all span regions that overlap or are in close proximity to the locations of known $GABA_A$ receptor genes. For example, inspection of Table III reveals that a number of significant QTLs for such phenotypes as acute ethanol withdrawal, chronic ethanol withdrawal, loss of righting reflex, ethanol-induced motor incoordination, ethanol conditioned taste aversion, ethanol-induced hypothermia, and chronic tolerance to ethanol were detected, which span a region of mouse chromosome 11 (Bergeson *et al.*, 2003; Browman and Crabbe, 2000; Buck *et al.*, 1997; Crabbe *et al.*, 1994; Kirstein *et al.*, 2002; Phillips *et al.*, 1996; Risinger and Cunningham, 1998). This particular region contains a cluster of $GABA_A$ receptor genes that includes the $\alpha1$-, $\alpha6$-, $\beta2$-, and $\gamma2$-subunit genes. Because it is known that ethanol modulates $GABA_A$ receptor function, it is reasonable to include these subunits among a list of potential candidate genes responsible for the significant QTLs.

Comparison of the QTL results in Table III with the data obtained from $GABA_A$ subunit knockout and transgenic mouse models summarized in Table I reveals some interesting trends. For example, a significant QTL for ethanol's hypnotic actions as assessed by the loss of righting reflex test was detected on chromosome 11 in a region containing the $\alpha1$-, $\alpha6$-, $\beta2$-, and $\gamma2$-subunit genes (Browman and Crabbe, 2000). Genetic deletion of the $\alpha1$ and $\beta2$ subunits also reduced sensitivity to ethanol's hypnotic actions as assessed by the same behavioral assay (Blednov *et al.*, 2003a). Thus, the knockout data provide strong evidence that at least one of these two receptor subunits likely account for the QTL. Moreover, that genetic deletion of the $\alpha6$ (Homanics *et al.*, 1997b) and $\gamma2L$ (Homanics *et al.*, 1999) subunits, or overexpression of the $\gamma2L$ (Gutiérrez *et al.*, 1994) subunit had no such effect provides evidence against these subunits as possible candidate genes for this QTL. Similar convergence was seen regarding a significant QTL for ethanol conditioned taste aversion also detected on chromosome 11 (Risinger and Cunnningham, 1998). The QTL spanned the same $GABA_A$ receptor gene cluster, and $\alpha1$-subunit knockout mice developed greater ethanol conditioned taste aversion (Blednov *et al.*, 2003b).

Of the remaining QTLs, several others overlapping $GABA_A$ receptor gene clusters were also supported by results from knockout mice. QTLs for ethanol-induced loss of righting reflex were detected on mouse chromosome 5 that spanned a region containing a cluster of genes coding for the $\alpha2$, $\alpha4$, $\beta1$, and $\gamma1$ subunits (Radcliffe *et al.*, 2000; Rodriguez *et al.*, 1995). Whereas knockouts for the $\alpha4$, $\beta1$, and $\gamma1$ subunits are not currently available, we

**TABLE III** GABA$_A$ Receptor Subunit Gene Expression Patterns Are Associated with Ethanol Behavioral QTLs That Map to Chromosomal Regions Harboring These Subunits

| *Chromosome: cM* | *Ethanol phenotype* | *Mouse population* | *Reference* | *Maps near (chromosome:cM)* | *Correlated with subunit expression [p value]*[a] |
|---|---|---|---|---|---|
| 11:16–19 | Acute withdrawal | BXD | Buck *et al.*, 1997 | $\alpha$1, $\alpha$6, $\beta$2, $\gamma$2 (11:23) | |
| 11:46 | Chronic tolerance—hypothermia | BXD | Crabbe *et al.*, 1994 | $\alpha$1, $\alpha$6, $\beta$2, $\gamma$2 (11:23) | $\alpha$1*, CB (0.002), $\beta$2*, CB (0.001), $\gamma$2*, CB (0.052) |
| 11:15–36 | Chronic withdrawal | IP2 X IR1 F2 | Bergeson *et al.*, 2003 | $\alpha$1, $\alpha$6, $\beta$2, $\gamma$2 (11:23) | |
| 11:40–45 | CTA | BXD | Risinger and Cunningham, 1998 | $\alpha$1, $\alpha$6, $\beta$2, $\gamma$2 (11:23) | |
| 11:12 | Hypothermia | BXD | Crabbe *et al.*, 1994 | $\alpha$1, $\alpha$6, $\beta$2, $\gamma$2 (11:23) | $\alpha$1*, WB (0.014), $\beta$2*, CB (0.028), $\gamma$2*, WB (0.004) |
| 11:26 | LORR | BXD | Browman and Crabbe, 2000 | $\alpha$1, $\alpha$6, $\beta$2, $\gamma$2 (11:23) | $\alpha$1**, WB (0.059) |
| 11:29–43 | Motor incoordination—dowel | BXD | Kirstein *et al.*, 2002 | $\alpha$1, $\alpha$6, $\beta$2, $\gamma$2 (11:23) | $\alpha$1*, CB (0 051), $\gamma$2*, CB (0.028) |
| 11:35–40 | Motor incoordination—grid | BXD | Phillips *et al.*, 1996 | $\alpha$1, $\alpha$6, $\beta$2, $\gamma$2 (11:23) | $\beta$2*, WB (0.011) |
| 11:26–32 | Motor incoordination—screen | BXD | Browman and Crabbe, 2000 | $\alpha$1, $\alpha$6, $\beta$2, $\gamma$2 (11:23) | $\alpha$1*, CB (0.041) |
| 5:58 | Chronic tolerance—grid | BXD | Phillips *et al.*, 1996 | $\alpha$2, $\alpha$4, $\beta$1, $\gamma$1 (5:40) | |
| 5:25–63 | Chronic tolerance—hypothermia | BXD | Crabbe *et al.*, 1994 | $\alpha$2, $\alpha$4, $\beta$1, $\gamma$1 (5:40) | |
| 5:47 | Hypothermia | BXD | Crabbe *et al.*, 1994 | $\alpha$2, $\alpha$4, $\beta$1, $\gamma$1 (5:40) | $\alpha$2*, WB (0.057) |
| 5:20 | LORR | B6 X D2 F2 | Radcliffe *et al.*, 2000 | $\alpha$2, $\alpha$4, $\beta$1, $\gamma$1 (5:40) | |
| 5:17 | LORR | BXD | Rodriguez *et al.*, 1995 | $\alpha$2, $\alpha$4, $\beta$1, $\gamma$1 (5:40) | |

(continues)

**TABLE III** (continued)

| *Chromosome: cM* | *Ethanol phenotype* | *Mouse population* | *Reference* | *Maps near (chromosome:cM)* | *Correlated with subunit expression [p value]*[a] |
|---|---|---|---|---|---|
| 5:26 | LORR-female | B6 X D2 F2 | Radcliffe *et al.*, 2000 | $\alpha$2, $\alpha$4, $\beta$1, $\gamma$1 (5:40) | |
| 7:7 | Acute tolerance—dowel | BXD | Gallaher *et al.*, 1996 | $\alpha$5, $\beta$3, $\gamma$3 (7:28) | |
| 7:50 | Chronic tolerance—grid | BXD | Phillips *et al.*, 1996 | $\alpha$5, $\beta$3, $\gamma$3 (7:28) | |
| 7:10–15 | Chronic tolerance—hypothermia | BXD | Crabbe *et al.*, 1994 | $\alpha$5, $\beta$3, $\gamma$3 (7:28) | $\beta$3*, WB (0.044), $\beta$3*, CB (0.026) |
| 7:36 | Hypothermia | BXD | Crabbe *et al.*, 1994 | $\alpha$5, $\beta$3, $\gamma$3 (7:28) | $\beta$3*, CB (0.026) |
| 7:6–20 | Locomotor stimulation | BXD | Phillips *et al.*, 1996 | $\alpha$5, $\beta$3, $\gamma$3 (7:28) | |
| 7:10–16 | Locomotor stimulation | BXD | Cunningham, 1995 | $\alpha$5, $\beta$3, $\gamma$3 (7:28) | $\alpha$5**, CB (0.053), $\beta$3*, WB (0.035) |
| 7:13 | LORR | BXD | Rodriguez *et al.*, 1995 | $\alpha$5, $\beta$3, $\gamma$3 (7:28) | |
| 7:27 | Preference | BXD | Phillips *et al.*, 1998 | $\alpha$5, $\beta$3, $\gamma$3 (7:28) | |
| 7:13 | Preference | B6 X D2 F2 | Tarantino *et al.*, 1998 | $\alpha$5, $\beta$3, $\gamma$3 (7:28) | $\beta$3*, CB (0.013) |
| 7:11 | Preference | BXD | Phillips *et al.*, 1994 | $\alpha$5, $\beta$3, $\gamma$3 (7:28) | |
| 7:22 | Preference | BXD | Rodriguez *et al.*, 1995 | $\alpha$5, $\beta$3, $\gamma$3 (7:28) | $\beta$3*, CB (0.038) |
| 4:81 | Acute tolerance—dowel | BXD | Gallaher *et al.*, 1996 | $\delta$ (4:79) | $\delta$*, WB (0.016) |
| 4:70–? | Chronic tolerance—grid | BXD | Phillips *et al.*, 1996 | $\delta$ (4:79) | $\delta$*, WB (0.056) |
| 4:46–79 | CPP | BXD | Cunningham, 1995 | $\delta$ (4:79) | |
| 4:75–94 | CTA | BXD | Risinger and Cunningham, 1998 | $\delta$ (4: 79) | |
| 4:60–69 | Hypothermia | BXD | Crabbe *et al.*, 1994 | $\delta$ (4:79) | $\delta$*, WB (0.014) |
| 4:66–78 | Locomotor stimulation | BXD | Demarest *et al.*, 1999 | $\delta$ (4:79) | $\delta$*, WB (0.054) |
| 4:81 | Preference | BXD | Phillips *et al.*, 1998 | $\delta$ (4:79) | |

| | | | | | |
|---|---|---|---|---|---|
| 4:65 | Preference | B6 X D2 F2 | Tarantino *et al.*, 1998 | $\delta$ (4:79) | |
| 4:57–61 | Preference | BXD | Phillips *et al.*, 1994 | $\delta$ (4:79) | |
| 4:0–22 | Acute tolerance—dowel | BXD | Gallaher *et al.*, 1996 | $\rho1$, $\rho2$ (4:11) | $\rho2$*, WB (0.005), $\rho2$, CB (0.008) |
| 4:14 | Acute withdrawal | BXD | Buck *et al.*, 1997 | $\rho1$, $\rho2$ (4:11) | $\rho1$*, WB (0.009) |
| 4:0–16 | Chronic tolerance—grid | BXD | Phillips *et al.*, 1996 | $\rho1$, $\rho2$ (4:11) | |
| 4:25 | Chronic tolerance—hypothermia | BXD | Crabbe *et al.*, 1994 | $\rho1$, $\rho2$ (4:11) | $\rho2$*, CB (0.042) |
| 4:2 | LORR | BXD | Rodriguez *et al.*, 1995 | $\rho1$, $\rho2$ (4:11) | |
| 4:0–26 | Motor incoordination—dowel | BXD | Gallaher *et al.*, 1996 | $\rho1$, $\rho2$ (4:11) | $\rho2$*, CB (0.037) |
| 4:35–36 | Motor incoordination—screen | BXD | Browman and Crabbe, 2000 | $\rho1$, $\rho2$ (4:11) | |

[a] WebQTL (www.genenetwork.org) provides access to behavioral and gene expression data from the BXD recombinant inbred strains. These data can then be accessed for data mining purposes. We used WebQTL to perform correlational analyses between the ethanol behavioral parameters above and $GABA_A$ receptor subunit gene expression in the BXD recombinant inbred strains.

* Change in subunit expression is consistent with a significant QTL.

** Change in subunit expression is consistent with a significant QTL and data from knockout mice.

CB, cerebellum; WB, whole brain.

showed that α2-subunit knockout mice exhibit reduced sensitivity to ethanol's hypnotic actions as assessed by the loss of righting reflex test (Boehm II *et al.*, 2004), supporting the α2 subunit as a viable candidate gene underlying the QTL. QTLs for ethanol preference drinking (Phillips *et al.*, 1994; Rodriguez *et al.*, 1995; Tarantino *et al.*, 1998), and ethanol-induced locomotor stimulation (Crabbe *et al.*, 1994; Cunningham, 1995) were detected on chromosome 7 that span the same region as the α5-, β3-, and γ3-subunit genes. Although β3-subunit knockout mice have not been tested and γ3-subunit knockouts have yet to be developed, we have shown that α5-subunit knockout mice prefer and consume less ethanol, and that these same mutants may also be more sensitive to ethanol's locomotor stimulant properties. Thus, these results provide additional support for the α5 subunit as a possible candidate gene for both ethanol-related QTLs. Finally, three QTLs for ethanol preference drinking were detected on chromosome 4 in a region harboring the δ-subunit gene (Phillips *et al.*, 1994, 1998), and δ-subunit knockout mice exhibited reduced ethanol preference drinking (Mihalek *et al.*, 2001). Thus, the mutant mouse literature can be used to confirm the possibility that suspected candidate genes contained within a region spanned by a QTL may indeed underlie the QTL.

As can also be seen by comparison of Tables I and III, there are also a number of QTLs for which $GABA_A$ receptor subunits are viable candidate genes, but the corresponding knockout and/or transgenic mouse models were not assessed using the appropriate behavioral assays. For example, whereas three different groups identified QTLs for sensitivity to ethanol's motor incoordinating actions in a region of mouse chromosome 11 that contains the α1-, α6-, β2-, and γ2-subunit genes (Browman and Crabbe, 2000; Kirstein *et al.*, 2002; Phillips *et al.*, 1996), only α1-subunit knockout mice were tested for sensitivity to this ethanol-related trait (Kralic *et al.*, 2003), and these mice did not differ. Moreover, whereas a number of QTLs were detected that span the α5-, β3-, and γ3-subunit gene cluster on mouse chromosome 7 (Crabbe *et al.*, 1994; Gallaher *et al.*, 1996; Phillips *et al.*, 1994; Rodriguez *et al.*, 1995; Tarantino *et al.*, 1998), only the α5-subunit knockouts were tested in more than one behavioral assay. β3-Subunit knockout mice were only tested for sensitivity to ethanol's hypnotic actions using the loss of righting reflex test (Quinlan *et al.*, 1998), and γ3-subunit knockout mice have yet to even be developed. Finally, a number of QTLs were detected that overlap a cluster of genes coding for the ρ1 and ρ2 subunits on mouse chromosome 4 (Buck *et al.*, 1997; Crabbe *et al.*, 1994; Gallaher *et al.*, 1996; Risinger and Cunningham, 1998; Rodriguez *et al.*, 1995). Although ρ2-subunit knockout mice do not currently exist, two different groups have developed ρ1-subunit knockout and wild-type mice (McCall *et al.*, 2002; Zheng *et al.*, 2003). Given that behaviors such as acute tolerance to ethanol, acute ethanol withdrawal, chronic tolerance to ethanol, ethanol-induced loss of righting reflex, and ethanol-induced motor incoordination have each been mapped to this region, it will be interesting to assess ethanol sensitivity in these new mutant mice.

## X. GABA$_A$ Receptor Subunit-Associated Gene Expression Patterns

A genetic difference in DNA sequence at the coding region of an underlying gene is one mechanism by which significant QTLs might influence their associated traits. Such a mechanism might alter the amino acid sequence of the subunit, thereby altering GABA$_A$ receptor function and changing behavioral sensitivity to ethanol. For example, a report identified a polymorphism in $\gamma 2$-subunit gene that predicts a difference in amino acid sequence between the C57BL6/J (B6) and DBA/2J (D2) inbred strains, the progenitors of the BXD recombinant inbred strains (Buck and Hood, 1998). This polymorphism was shown to associate with acute ethanol withdrawal severity, likely explaining the earlier detection of a QTL that spanned a region of chromosome 11 harboring the $\gamma 2$-subunit gene.

Despite the story for the $\gamma 2$-subunit gene and acute ethanol withdrawal, all to often detection of significant QTLs are not always followed by the identification of sequence variants. The B6 and D2 strains exhibited identical polypeptide sequences for the $\alpha 1$- (Wang *et al.*, 1992) and $\beta 2$- (Kamatchi *et al.*, 1995) subunit genes, also contained within the spanned region of the acute ethanol withdrawal QTL on chromosome 11 (Buck and Hood, 1998). Although it is possible that these two GABA$_A$ receptor subunits do not contribute to acute ethanol withdrawal severity, it may be that they actually do contribute by virtue of differing genotypic expression patterns of the $\alpha 1$- and $\beta 2$-subunit genes. In other words, differences in subunit expression patterns may also regulate GABA$_A$ receptor function, altering behavioral sensitivity to ethanol.

WebQTL (www.genenetwork.org) is a web-based resource for the analysis of complex traits (Chesler *et al.*, 2003; Wang *et al.*, 2003) containing more than 600 published phenotypes tested in a panel of mouse strains. These strains include the B6 and D2 inbred strains, their F1 hybrids, and their 32 derived BXD recombinant inbred strains (Taylor *et al.*, 1999; Williams *et al.*, 2001). WebQTL also contains estimates of gene expression patterns across these 35 strains. mRNA expression patterns in whole brain (excluding cerebellum) and cerebellum were determined in naïve mice using Affymetrix (whole brain, UTHSC Brain mRNA U74Av2 [Dec03] MAS5 database; cerebellum, SJUT mRNA M430 [Oct03] MAS5 database) micorarrays (Taylor *et al.*, 1999) (see www.genenetwork.org for animal, sample, and preparation details). In sum, WebQTL allows for the comparisons of gene expression patterns with various ethanol-related phenotypes. More specifically, WebQTL allows for calculating genetic correlations between mRNA expression and behavioral variables, which provide yet another way to verify potential candidate genes that might underlie significant QTLs.

Using WebQTL, we calculated Pearson's correlations between various ethanol-related behavioral traits and $GABA_A$ receptor subunit mRNA abundance values in the BXD recombinant inbred strains. Our goal was to relate these findings to ethanol behavior QTLs that overlap the known locations of subunit gene clusters, and ultimately to data from $GABA_A$ receptor subunit knockout mice. Thus, with a few exceptions, we restricted the number of correlations to only those that involved subunits for which knockout mice are currently available. This approach yielded about 125 significant correlations.

Of the ethanol related-traits that correlated with $GABA_A$ receptor subunit gene expression, only a handful overlapped previously mapped ethanol behavior QTLs. Correlated differences in gene expression were observed for traits like ethanol preference drinking, ethanol-induced locomotor stimulation, ethanol-induced loss of righting reflex, ethanol-induced hypothermia and motor incoordination, as well as tolerance to these effects, and acute ethanol withdrawal. For example, QTL analysis suggests that each of the $GABA_A$ receptor gene clusters (except for the one on mouse chromosome 4 that codes for the $\rho$ subunits) may contain viable candidate genes influencing sensitivity to ethanol's hypothermic actions (Crabbe *et al.*, 1994). Whereas any number of the genes contained within these clusters may actually underlie the QTLs, correlational analysis reveals strong associations between this ethanol behavioral phenotype and expression of $\alpha1$, $\alpha2$, $\beta2$, $\beta3$, $\gamma2$, and $\delta$ subunits. These results support a role for these $GABA_A$ receptor subunits in the mediation of ethanol's hypothermic actions, and effectively eliminate $\alpha5$ and $\alpha6$ subunits (at least in the brain regions for which mRNA expression data are available) as viable candidate genes.

Perhaps the most intriguing of the significant correlations are those that overlap both a previously mapped ethanol behavior QTL and the $GABA_A$ receptor subunit knockout mouse literature. This was not the case for the above ethanol hypothermia correlations. In fact, except for $\delta$, none of the subunits whose expression correlated with the behavior were even tested using mutant mouse models, and the $\delta$-subunit knockout and wild-type mice did not differ in sensitivity to this action of ethanol (Table I). Inspection of Table III reveals just two cases where a significant correlation consistent with both QTL and knockout data was found. Sensitivity to loss of righting reflex correlated with $\alpha1$-subunit mRNA expression in whole brain, confirming a significant QTL for this behavior detected on mouse chromosome 11 (Browman and Crabbe, 2000), and coinciding with data showing the $\alpha1$-subunit knockout mice are less sensitive to this action of ethanol (Blednov *et al.*, 2003b). Moreover, three-way convergence was also found for a correlation between ethanol's locomotor stimulant actions and $\alpha5$-subunit expression in cerebellum. This result is consistent with a significant QTL on mouse chromosome 7 (Cunningham, 1995; Phillips *et al.*, 1996) as well as our data suggesting that α5-subunit knockout mice are more sensitive to this ethanol effect (Boehm II *et al.*, 2004). Thus, comparison of phenotypic data from these very different behavioral genetic approaches can yield powerful evidence for or against suspected candidate genes, in this case $GABA_A$ receptor subunits.

Finally, we earlier discussed a very interesting series of ethanol behavioral QTLs that mapped to the proximal portion of mouse chromosome 4. These QTLs spanned or were very close to a cluster of genes coding for the ρ1- and ρ2-subunit genes (Buck *et al.*, 1997; Crabbe *et al.*, 1994; Gallaher *et al.*, 1996; Phillips *et al.*, 1996; Risinger and Cunningham, 1998). We pointed out that although ρ2-subunit knockout mice are not currently available, ρ1-subunit knockouts were recently developed (McCall *et al.*, 2002; Zheng *et al.*, 2003) and have yet to be tested for sensitivity to ethanol's behavioral actions. Several highly significant correlations were detected between ρ1- and ρ2-subunit expression and several different ethanol-related traits. Of particular interest is highly significant correlation between ρ1-subunit expression in whole brain and acute ethanol withdrawal severity. Buck and colleagues (1997) detected an acute ethanol withdrawal QTL very near the ρ-gene cluster. These results may suggest a role for ρ1 subunits in mediating acute ethanol withdrawal severity, and that future work should examine this ethanol-related behavior in the new knockout mice.

## XI. Conclusions

$GABA_A$ receptors are known to have a role in the modulation of a number of ethanol's behavioral actions. Evidence suggests that the subunit composition of individual $GABA_A$ receptors may determine behavioral sensitivity to ethanol (Ebert *et al.*, 1997). Indeed, studies of subunit knockout mice have yielded considerable insights into the subunit specificity of ethanol's behavioral actions. These studies complement experiments aimed at mapping chromosomal regions (QTLs) underlying behavioral sensitivity to ethanol. A number of ethanol behavioral QTLs span regions harboring $GABA_A$ receptor subunit gene clusters, and examination of the knockout literature provides a means by which to investigate the potential that these subunit genes might underlie these QTLs.

Subunit gene expression data has also been generated for many of the inbred strains used in the above QTL analyses. These data sets have been uploaded to an online database (WebQTL) allowing for the correlation of $GABA_A$ receptor subunit gene expression with various ethanol-related traits. The results of these correlational analyses may also be compared to the results of QTL studies to more precisely determine the role of certain $GABA_A$ receptor subunits in behavioral sensitivity to ethanol.

Convergence of results between knockout, QTL, and gene expression studies offer the strongest evidence supporting the role of any particular $GABA_A$ receptor subunit in mediating sensitivity to a specific ethanol-related behavior. Although future studies will undoubtedly refine the above techniques (such as by the development of knock-in mouse models), the converging results of these studies will undoubtedly aid in the development of subunit specific drugs for the treatment of alcohol abuse and dependence. These studies indicate that it may be possible to engineer drugs that selectively alter certain behavioral actions of ethanol. As just one example, convergent evidence from knockout, QTL, and gene expression data suggest that drugs that target $\alpha 5$-containing $GABA_A$ receptors may be particularly useful in altering ethanol's reinforcing/motivational properties. Such drugs are currently being developed and tested in animal models (June *et al.*, 2001).

## References

Bergeson, S. E., Warren, R. K., Crabbe, J. C., Metten, P., Erwin, V. G., and Belknap, J. K. (2003). Chromosome loci influencing chronic alcohol withdrawal severity. *Mamm. Genome* **14**, 454–463.

Blednov, Y. A., Jung, S., Alva, H., Wallace, D., Rosahl, T., Whiting, P.-J., and Harris, R. A. (2003a). Deletion of the $\alpha 1$ or $\beta 2$ subunit of $GABA_A$ receptors reduces actions of alcohol and other drugs. *J. Pharmacol. Exp. Ther.* **304**, 30–36.

Blednov, Y. A., Walker, D., Alva, H., Creech, K., Findlay, G., and Harris, R. A. (2003b). $GABA_A$ receptor $\alpha 1$ and $\beta 2$ subunit null mutant mice: Behavioral responses to ethanol. *J. Pharmacol. Exp. Ther.* **305**, 854–863.

Boehm, S. L., II, Ponomarev, I., Jennings, A. W., Whiting, P. J., Rosahl, T. W., Garrett, E. M., Blednov, Y. A., and Harris, R. A. (2004). $\gamma$-Aminobutyric acid A receptor subunit mutant mice: New perspectives on alcohol actions. *Biochem. Pharmacol.* **68**, 1581–1602.

Bosman, L. W. J., Rosahl, T. W., and Brussaard, A. B. (2002). Neonatal development of the rat visual cortex: Synaptic function of $GABA_A$ receptor $\alpha$ subunits. *J. Physiol.* **541**(1), 169–181.

Browman, K. E., and Crabbe, J. C. (2000). Quantitative trait loci affecting ethanol sensitivity in BXD recombinant inbred mice. *Alcohol. Clin. Exp. Res.* **24**, 17–23.

Brickley, S. G., Revilla, V., Cull-Candy, S. G., Wisden, W., and Farrant, M. (2001). Adaptive regulation of neuronal excitability by a voltage-independent potassium conductance. *Nature* **409**, 88–92.

Brünig, I., Scotti, E., Sidler, C., and Fritschy, J.-M. (2002). Intact sorting, targeting, and clustering of $\gamma$-aminobutyric acid A receptor subtypes in hippocampal neurons *in vitro*. *J. Comp. Neurol.* **443**, 43–55.

Buck, K. J., and Hood, H. M. (1998). Genetic association of a $GABA_A$ receptor $\gamma 2$ subunit variant with acute physiological dependence on alcohol. *Mamm. Genome* **9**, 975–978.

Buck, K. J., Metten, P., Belknap, J. K., and Crabbe, J. C. (1997). Quantitative trait loci involved in genetic predisposition to acute alcohol withdrawal in mice. *J. Neurosci.* **17**, 3946–3955.

Caraiscos, V. B., Elliot, E. M., You-Ten, K. E., Cheng, V. Y., Belelli, D., Newell, J. G., Jackson, M. F., Lambert, J. J., Rosahl, T. W., Wafford, K. A., MacDonald, J. F., and Orser, B. A. (2004). Tonic inhibition in mouse hippocampal CA1 pyramidal neurons is mediated by $\alpha 5$

subunit-containing $\gamma$-aminobutyric acid type A receptors. *Proc. Natl. Acad. Sci. USA* **101**, 3662–3667.

Carr, L. G., Spence, J. P., Eriksson, P., Lumeng, C. J., and Li, T. K. (2003). AA and ANA rats exhibit the R100Q mutation in the $GABA_A$ receptor $\alpha6$ subunit. *Alcohol* **31**, 93–97.

Chandra, D., Korpi, E. R., Miralles, C. P., DeBlas, A. L., and Homanics, G. E. (2005). $GABA_A$ receptor $\gamma2$ subunit knockdown mice have enhanced anxiety-like behavior but unaltered hypnotic response to benzodiazepines. *BMC Neurosci.* **6**, 30.

Chesler, E. J., Wang, J., Lu, L., Qu, Y., Manly, K. F., and Williams, R. W. (2003). Genetic correlates of gene expression in recombinant inbred strains: A relational model system to explore neurobehavioral phenotypes. *Neuroinformatics* **1**, 343–357.

Collinson, N., Kuenzi, F. M., Jarolimek, W., Maubach, K. A., Cothliff, R., Sur, C., Smith, A., Out, F. M., Howell, O., Atack, J. R., McKernan, R. M., Seabrook, G. R., *et al.* (2002). Enhanced learning and memory and altered GABAergic synaptic transmission in mice lacking the $\alpha5$ subunit of the $GABA_A$ receptor. *J. Neurosci.* **22**, 5572–5580.

Cope, D. W., Wulff, P., Oberto, A., Aller, M. I., Capogna, M., Ferraguti, F., Halbsguth, C., Hoeger, H., Jolin, H. E., Jones, A., Mckenzie, A. N. J., Ogris, W., *et al.* (2004). Abolition of zolpidem sensitivity in mice with a point mutation in the $GABA_A$ receptor $\gamma2$ subunit. *Neuropharmacology* **47**, 17–34.

Crabbe, J. C. (2002). Alcohol and genetics: New Models. *Am. J. Med. Genet.* **114**, 969–974.

Crabbe, J. C., Belknap, J. K., Mitchell, S. R., and Crawshaw, L. I. (1994). Quantitative trait loci mapping of genes that influence the sensitivity and tolerance to ethanol-induced hypothermia in BXD recombinant inbred mice. *J. Pharmacol. Exp. Ther.* **269**, 184–192.

Crabbe, J. C., Phillips, T. J., Buck, K. J., Cunningham, C. L., and Belknap, J. K. (1999). Identifying genes for alcohol and drug sensitivity: Recent progress and future directions. *Trends Neurosci.* **22**, 173–179.

Crestani, F., Keist, R., Fritschy, J.-M., Benke, D., Vogt, K., Prut, L., Blüthmann, H., Möhler, H., and Rudolph, U. (2002). Trace fear conditioning involves hippocampal $\alpha5$ $GABA_A$ receptors. *Proc. Natl. Acad. Sci. USA* **99**, 8980–8985.

Culiat, C. T., Stubbs, L. J., Woychik, R. P., Russell, L. B., Johnson, D. K., and Rinchik, E. M. (1995). Deficiency of the $\beta3$ subunit of the type A $\gamma$-aminobutyric acid receptor causes cleft palate in mice. *Nat. Genet.* **11**, 344–346.

Cunningham, C. L. (1995). Localization of genes influencing ethanol-induced conditioned place preference and locomotor activity in BXD recombinant inbred mice. *Psychopharmacology* **120**, 28–41.

DeLorey, T. M., Handforth, A., Anagnostaras, S. G., Homanics, G. E., Minassian, B. A., Asatourian, A., Fanselow, M. S., Delgado-Escueta, A., Ellison, G. D., and Olsen, R. W. (1998). Mice lacking the $\beta3$ subunit of the $GABA_A$ receptor have the epilepsy phenotype and many of the behavioral characteristics of Angelman syndrome. *J. Neurosci.* **18**, 8505–8514.

Demarest, K., McCaughran, J., Jr., Mahjubi, E., Cipp, L., and Hitzemann, R. (1999). Identification of an acute ethanol response quantitative trait locus on chromosome 2. *J. Neurosci.* **19**, 549–561.

Ebert, B., Thompson, S. A., Saounatsou, K., McKernan, R., Krogsgaard-Larsen, P., and Wafford, K. A. (1997). Differences in agonist/antagonist binding affinity and receptor transduction using recombinant human $\gamma$-aminobutyric acid type A receptors. *Mol. Pharmacol.* **52**, 1150–1156.

Essrich, C., Lorez, M., Benson, J. A., Fritschy, J. M., and Luscher, B. (1998). Postsynaptic clustering of major $GABA_A$ receptor subtypes requires the $\gamma2$ subunit and gephyrin. *Nat. Neurosci.* **1**, 563–571.

Fritschy, J.-M., Johnson, D. K., Möhler, H., and Rudolph, U. (1998). Independent assembly and subcellular targeting of $GABA_A$-receptor subtypes demonstrated in mouse hippocampal and olfactory neurons *in vivo*. *Neurosci. Lett.* **249**, 99–102.

Gallaher, E. J., Jones, G. E., Belknap, J. K., and Crabbe, J. C. (1996). Identification of genetic markers for initial sensitivity and rapid tolerance to ethanol-induced ataxia using quantitative trait locus analysis in BXD recombinant inbred mice. *J. Pharmacol. Exp. Ther.* **277**, 604–612.

Goldstein, P. A., Elsen, F. P., Ying, S.-W., Ferguson, C., Homanics, G. E., and Harrison, N. L. (2002). Prolongation of hippocampal inhibitory postsynaptic currents in mice lacking the $GABA_A$ receptor $\alpha1$ subunit. *J. Neurophysiol.* **88**, 3208–3217.

Günther, U., Benson, J., Benke, D., Firtschy, J.-M., Reyes, G., Knoflach, F., Crestani, F., Aguzzi, A., Arigoni, M., Lang, Y., Bluethmann, H., Möhler, H., *et al.* (1995). Benzodiazepine-insensitive mice generated by targeted disruption of the $\gamma2$ subunit gene of $\gamma$-aminobutyric acid type A receptors. *Proc. Natl. Acad. Sci. USA* **92**, 7749–7753.

Gutiérrez, A., Khan, Z. U., and De Blas, A. L. (1994). Immunocytochemical localization of $\gamma2$ short and long subunits of the $GABA_A$ receptor in the rat brain. *J. Neurosci.* **14**, 7168–7179.

Harris, R. A. (1999). Ethanol actions on multiple ion channels: Which are important? *Alcohol. Clin. Exp. Res.* **23**, 1563–1570.

Harvey, S. C., Foster, K. L., McKay, P. F., Carroll, M. R., Seyoum, R., Woods, J. E., II, Grey, C., Jones, C. M., McCane, S., Cummings, R., Mason, D., Ma, C., *et al.* (2002). The $GABA_A$ $\alpha1$ subtype in the ventral pallidum regulates alcohol-seeking behaviors. *J. Neurosci.* **22**, 3765–3775.

Heinen, K., Baker, R. E., Spijker, S., Rosahl, T., Van Pelt, J., and Brussaard, A. B. (2003). Impaired dendritic spine maturation in $GABA_A$ receptor $\alpha1$ subunit knock out mice. *Neuroscience* **122**, 699–705.

Homanics, G. E., DeLorey, T. M., Firestone, L. L., Quinlan, J. J., Handforth, A., Harrison, N. L., Drasowski, M. D., Rick, C. E. M., Korpi, E. R., Mäkelä, R., Brilliant, M. H., Hagiwara, N., *et al.* (1997a). Mice devoid of $\gamma$-aminobutyrate type A receptor $\beta3$ subunit have epilepsy, cleft palate, and hypersensitive behavior. *Proc. Natl. Acad. Sci. USA* **94**, 4143–4148.

Homanics, G. E., Ferguson, C., Quinlan, J. J., Daggett, J., Snyder, K., Lagenaur, C., Mi, A.-P., Wang, X.-H., Grayson, D. R., and Firestone, L. L. (1997b). Gene knockout of the $\alpha6$ subunit of the $\gamma$-aminobutyric acid type A receptor: Lack of effect on responses to ethanol, pentobarbital, and general anesthetics. *Mol. Pharmacol.* **51**, 588–596.

Homanics, G. E., Le, N. Q., Mihalek, R., Hart, A. R., and Quinlan, J. J. (1998). Ethanol tolerance and withdrawal responses in $GABA_A$ receptor alpha 6 subunit null allele mice and in inbred C57BL/6J and strain 129/SvJ mice. *Alcohol. Clin. Exp. Res.* **22**, 259–265.

Homanics, G. E., Harrison, N. L., Quinlan, J. J., Krasowski, M. D., Rick, C. E. M., de Blas, A. L., Mehta, A. K., Kist, F., Mihalek, R. M., Aul, J. J., and Firestone, L. L. (1999). Normal electrophysiological and behavioral responses to ethanol in mice lacking the long splice variant of the $\gamma2$ subunit of the $\gamma$-aminobutyrate type A receptor. *Neuropharmacology* **38**, 253–265.

Homanics, G. E., Elsen, F. P., Ying, S.-W., Jenkins, A., Ferguson, C., Sloat, B., Yuditskaya, S., Goldstein, P. A., Kralic, J. E., Morrow, A. L., and Harrison, N. L. (2005). A gain-of-function mutation in the $GABA_A$ receptor produces synaptic and behavioral abnormalities in the mouse. *Gene Brain Behav.* **4**, 10–19.

Jones, A., Korpi, E. R., McKernan, R. M., Pelz, R., Nusser, Z., Mäkelä, R., Mellor, J. R., Pollard, S., Bahn, S., Stephenson, F. A., Randall, A. D., Sieghart, W., *et al.* (1997). Ligand-gated ion channel subunit partnerships: $GABA_A$ receptor $\alpha6$ subunit gene inactivation inhibits $\delta$ subunit expression. *J. Neurosci.* **17**, 1350–1362.

June, H. L., Harvey, S. C., Foster, K. L., Mckay, P. F., Cummings, R., Garcia, M., Mason, D., Grey, C., McCane, S., Williams, L. S., Johnson, T. B., He, X., *et al.* (2001). $GABA_A$ receptors containing $\alpha5$ subunits in the CA1 and CA3 hippocampal fields regulate ethanol-motivated behaviors: An extended ethanol reward circuitry. *J. Neurosci.* **21**, 2166–2177.

Jung, S., Akabas, M. H., and Harris, R. A. (2005). Functional and structural analysis of the GABAA receptor $\alpha$1 subunit during channel gating and alcohol modulation. *J. Biol. Chem.* **280**, 308–316.

Jurd, R., Arras, M., Lambert, S., Drexler, B., Siegwart, R., Crestani, F., Zaugg, M., Vogt, K. E., Ledermann, B., Antkowiak, B., and Rudolph, U. (2003). General anesthetic actions *in vivo* strongly attenuated by a point mutation in the GABA$_A$ receptor $\beta$3 subunit. *FASEB J.* **17**, 250–252.

Kamatchi, G. L., Kofuji, P., Wang, J. B., Fernando, J. C., Liu, Z., Mathura, J. R., and Burt, D. R. (1995). GABA$_A$ receptor $\beta$1, $\beta$2, and $\beta$3 subunits: Comparisons in DBA/2J and C57BL/6J mice. *Biochim. Biophys. Acta* **1261**, 134–142.

Khan, Z. U., Gutierrez, A., and De Blas, A. L. (1996). The $\alpha$1 and $\alpha$6 subunits can coexist in the same cerebellar GABA$_A$ receptor maintaining their individual benzodiazepine-binding specificities. *J. Neurochem.* **66**, 685–691.

Kirstein, S. L., Davidson, K. L., Ehringer, M. A., and Sikela, J. M. (2002). Quantitative trait loci affecting initial sensitivity and acute functional tolerance to ethanol-induced ataxia and brain cAMP signaling in BXD recombinant inbred mice. *J. Pharmacol. Exp. Ther.* **302**, 1238–1245.

Koksma, J.-J., van Kesteren, R. E., Rosahl, T. W., Zwart, R., Smit, A. B., Lüddens, H., and Brussaard, A. B. (2003). Oxytocin regulates neurosteroid modulation of GABA$_A$ receptors in supraoptic nuecleus around parturition. *J. Neurosci.* **23**, 788–797.

Korpi, E. R., Kleingoor, C., Kettenmann, H., and Seeburg, P. H. (1993). Benzodiazepine-induced motor impairment in cerebellar GABA$_A$ receptor. *Nature* **361**, 356–359.

Korpi, E. R., Gründer, G., and Lüddens, H. (2002a). Drug interactions at GABA$_A$ receptors. *Prog. Neurobiol.* **67**, 113–159.

Korpi, E. R., Mihalek, R. M., Sinkkonen, S. T., Hauer, B., Hevers, W., Homanics, G. E., Sieghart, W., and Lüddens, H. (2002b). Altered receptor subtypes in the forebrain of GABA$_A$ receptor $\delta$ subunit-deficient mice: Recruitment of $\gamma$2 subunits. *Neuroscience* **109**, 733–743.

Kralic, J. E., Korpi, E. R., O'Buckley, T. K., Homanics, G. E., and Morrow, A. L. (2002). Molecular and pharmacological characterization of GABA$_A$ receptor $\alpha$1 subunit knockout mice. *J. Pharmacol. Exp. Ther.* **302**, 1037–1045.

Kralic, J. E., Wheeler, M., Renzi, K., Ferguson, C., O'Buckley, T. K., Grobin, A. C., Morrow, A. L., and Homanics, G. E. (2003). Deletion of GABA$_A$ receptor $\alpha$1 subunit-contianing receptors alters responses to ethanol and other anesthetics. *J. Pharmacol. Exp. Ther.* **305**, 600–607.

Kralic, J. E., Criswell, H. E., Osterman, J. L., O'Buckley, T. K., Wilkie, M. E., Matthews, D. B., Hamre, K., Breese, G. R., Homanics, G. E., and Morrow, A. L. (2005). Genetic essential tremor in $\gamma$-aminobutyric acid$_A$ receptor $\alpha$1 subunit knockout mice. *J. Clin. Invest.* **115**, 774–779.

Krasowski, M. D., Rick, C. E., Harrison, N. L., Firestone, L. L., and Homanics, G. E. (1998). A deficit of functional GABA$_A$ receptors in neurons of $\beta$3 subunit knockout mice. *Neurosci. Lett.* **240**, 81–84.

Laurie, B. J., Wisden, W., and Seeburg, P. H. (1992). The distribution of thirteen GABA$_A$ receptor subunit mRNAs in the rat brain. III. Embryonic and postnatal development. *J. Neurosci.* **12**, 4151–4172.

Liang, J., Cagetti, E., Olsen, R. W., and Spigelman, I. (2004). Altered pharmacology of synaptic and extrasynaptic GABA$_A$ receptors on CA1 hippocampal neurons is consistent with subunit changes in a model of alcohol withdrawal and dependence. *J. Pharmacol. Exp. Ther.* **310**, 1234–1245.

Low, K., Crestani, F., Keist, R., Benke, D., Brunig, I., Benson, J. A., Fritschy, J.-M., Rulicke, T., Bluethmann, H., Mohler, H., and Rudolph, U. (2000). Molecular and neuronal substrate for selective attenuation of anxiety. *Science* **290**, 131–134.

McCall, M., Lukasiewicz, P. D., Gregg, R. G., and Peachey, N. S. (2002). Elimination of the $\rho 1$ subunit abolishes $GABA_C$ receptor expression and alters visual processing in the mouse retina. *J. Neurosci.* **22**, 4163–4174.

McKay, P. F., Foster, K. L., Mason, D., Cummings, R., Garcia, M., Williams, L. S., Grey, C., McCane, S., He, X., Cook, J. M., and June, H. L. (2004). A high affinity ligand for $GABA_A$-receptor containing $\alpha 5$ subunit antagonizes ethanol's neurobehavioral effects in Long-Evans rats. *Psychopharmacology* **172**, 455–462.

McKernan, R. M., Rosahl, T. W., Reynolds, D. S., Sur, C., Wafford, K. A., Atack, J. R., Farrar, S., Myers, J., Cook, G., Ferris, P., Garrett, L., Bristow, L., *et al.* (2000). Sedative but not anxiolytic properties of benzodiazepines are mediated by the $GABA_A$ receptor $\alpha 1$ subtype. *Nat. Neurosci.* **3**, 587–592.

Miall, R. C. (1998). The cerebellum, predictive control and motor coordination. *Novartis. Found. Symp.* **218**, 272–284.

Mihalek, R. M., Banerjee, P. K., Korpi, E. R., Quinlan, J. J., Firestone, L. L., Mi, Z.-P., Lagenaur, C., Tretter, V., Sieghart, W., Anagnostaras, S. G., Sage, J. R., Fanselow, M. S., *et al.* (1999). Attenuated sensitivity to neuroactive steroids in $\gamma$-aminobutyrate type A receptor delta subunit knockout mice. *Proc. Nat. Acad. Sci. USA* **96**, 12905–12910.

Mihalek, R. M., Bowers, B. J., Wehner, J. M., Kralic, J. E., VanDoren, M. J., Morrow, A. L., and Homanics, G. E. (2001). $GABA_A$-receptor $\delta$ subunit knockout mice have multiple defects in behavioral responses to ethanol. *Alcohol. Clin. Exp. Res.* **25**, 1708–1718.

Nusser, Z., Sieghart, W., and Somogy, P. (1998). Segregation of different $GABA_A$ receptors to synaptic and extrasynaptic membranes of cerebellar granule cells. *J. Neurosci.* **18**, 1693–1703.

Nusser, Z., Ahmad, Z., Tretter, V., Fuchs, K., Wisden, W., Sieghart, W., and Somogy, P. (1999). Alterations in the expression of $GABA_A$ receptor subunits in cerebellar granule cells after the disruption of the $\alpha 6$ subunit gene. *Eur. J. Neurosci.* **11**, 1685–1697.

O'Meara, G. F., Newman, R. J., Fradley, R. L., Dawson, G. R., and Reynolds, D. S. (2004). The GABA-A $\beta 3$ subunit mediates anaesthesia induced by etomidate. *Neuroreport* **15**, 1653–1656.

Ozaki, M. (2002). Analysis of patterned neuronal impulses and function of neuregulin. *Neurosignals* **11**, 191–196.

Peng, Z., Hauer, B., Mihalek, R. M., Homanics, G. E., Sieghart, W., Olsen, R. W., and Houser, C. R. (2002). $GABA_A$ receptor changes in $\delta$ subunit-deficient mice: Altered expression of $\alpha 4$ and $\gamma 2$ subunits in the forebrain. *J. Comp. Neurol.* **446**, 179–197.

Persohn, E., Malherbe, P., and Richards, J. G. (1991). *In situ* hybridization reveals a diversity of $GABA_A$ receptor subunit mRNAs in neurons of the rat spinal cord and dorsal root ganglia. *Neuroscience* **42**, 497–507.

Phillips, T. J., Crabbe, J. C., Metten, P., and Belknap, J. K. (1994). Localization of genes affecting alcohol drinking in mice. *Alcohol. Clin. Exp. Res.* **18**, 931–941.

Phillips, T. J., Lessov, C. N., Harland, R. D., and Mitchell, S. R. (1996). Evaluation of potential genetic associations between ethanol tolerance and sensitization in BXD/Ty recombinant inbred mice. *J. Pharmacol. Exp. Ther.* **277**, 613–623.

Phillips, T. J., Belknap, J. K., Buck, K. J., and Cunningham, C. L. (1998). Genes on mouse chromosome 2 and 9 determine variation in ethanol consumption. *Mamm. Genome* **9**, 936–941.

Phillips, T. J., and Belknap, J. K. (2002). Complex-trait genetics: Emergence of multivariate strategies. *Nat. Rev.* **3**, 478–485.

Pirker, S., Schwarzer, C., Wieselthaler, A., Sieghart, W., and Sperk, G. (2000). $GABA_A$ receptors: Immunocytochemical distribution of 13 subunits in the adult brain. *Neuroscience* **4**, 815–850.

Ponomarev, I., Maiya, R., Harnett, M. T., Schafer, G. L., Ryabinin, A. E., Blednov, Y. A., Morikawa, H., Boehm, II, S. L., Homanics, G. E., Berman, A., Lodowski, K. H., Bergeson, S. E., *et al.* (2006). Transcriptional signatures of cellular plasticity in mice lacking the alpha1 subunit of GABA$_A$ receptors. *J. Neurosci.* (In Press).

Porcello, D. M., Huntsman, M. M., Mihalek, R. M., Homanics, G. E., and Huguenard, J. R. (2003). Intact synaptic GABAergic inhibition and altered neurosteroid modulation of thalamic relay neurons in mice lacking $\delta$ subunit. *J. Neurophysiol.* **89**, 1378–1386.

Quinlan, J. J., Homanics, G. E., and Firestone, L. L. (1998). Anesthesia sensitivity in mice that lack the $\beta 3$ subunit of the $\gamma$-aminobutyric acid type A receptor. *Anesthesiology* **88**, 775–780.

Quirk, K., Gillar, N. P., Ragan, C. I., Whiting, P. J., and McKernan, R. M. (1995). Model of subunit composition of $\gamma$-aminobutyric acid A receptor subtypes expressed in rat cerebellum with respect to their $\alpha$ and $\gamma/\delta$ subunits. *J. Biol. Chem.* **269**, 16020–16028.

Radcliffe, R. A., Bohl, M. L., Lowe, M. V., Cycowski, C. S., and Wehner, J. M. (2000). Mapping of quantitative trait loci for hypnotic sensitivity to ethanol in crosses derived form the C57BL/6 and DBA/2 mouse strains. *Alcohol. Clin. Exp. Res.* **24**, 1335–1342.

Ramadan, E., Fu, Z., Losi, G., Homanics, G. E., Neale, J. H., and Vicini, S. (2003). GABA$_A$ receptor $\beta 3$ subunit deletion decreases $\alpha 2/3$ subunits and IPSC duration. *J. Neurophysiol.* **89**, 128–134.

Reynolds, D. S., McKernan, R. M., and Dawson, G. R. (2001). Anxiolytic-like action of diazepam: Which GABA$_A$ receptor subtype is involved? *Trends Pharmacol. Sci.* **22**, 402–403.

Reynolds, D. S., O'Meara, G. F., Newman, R. J., Bromidge, F. A., Atack, J. R., Whiting, P. J., Rosahl, T. W., and Dawson, G. R. (2003a). GABA$_A$ alpha 1 subunit knock-out mice do not show a hyperlocomotor response following amphetamine or cocaine treatment. *Neuropharmacology* **44**, 190–198.

Reynolds, D. S., Rosahl, T. W., Cirone, J., O'Meara, G. F., Haythornthwaite, A., Newman, R. J., Myers, J., Sur, C., Howell, O., Rutter, A. R., Atack, J., Macaulay, A. J., *et al.* (2003b). Sedation and anesthesia mediated by distinct GABA$_A$ receptor isoforms. *J. Neurosci.* **23**, 8608–8617.

Risinger, F. O., and Cunningham, C. L. (1998). Ethanol-induced conditioned taste aversion in BXD recombinant inbred mice. *Alcohol. Clin. Exp. Res.* **22**, 1234–1244.

Rodriguez, L. A., Plomin, R., Blizard, D. A., Jones, B. C., and McClearn, G. E. (1995). Alcohol acceptance, preference, and sensitivity in mice. II. Quantitative trait loci mapping analysis using BXD recombinant inbred strains. *Alcohol. Clin. Exp. Res.* **19**, 367–373.

Rudolph, U., Crestani, F., Benke, D., Brunig, I., Benson, J. A., Fritschy, J.-M., Martin, J. R., Bluethmann, H., and Möhler, H. (1999). Benzodiazepine actions mediated by specific $\gamma$-aminobutyric acid$_A$ receptor subtypes. *Nature* **401**, 796–800.

Saba, L., Porcella, A., Congeddu, E., Colombo, G., Peis, M., Pistis, M., Gessa, G. L., and Pani, L. (2001). The R100Q mutation of the GABA$_A$ $\alpha 6$ receptor subunit may contribute to voluntary aversion to ethanol in the sNP rat line. *Mol. Brain Res.* **87**, 263–270.

Schweizer, C., Balsiger, S., Bluethmann, H., Mansuy, I. M., Fritschy, J.-M., Mohler, H., and Lüscher, B. (2003). The $\gamma 2$ subunit of GABA$_A$ receptors is required for maintenance of receptors at mature synapses. *Mol. Cell. Neurosci.* **24**, 442–450.

Shannon, E. E., Shelton, K. L., Vivian, J. A., Yount, I., Morgan, A. R., Homanics, G. E., and Grant, K. E. (2004). Discriminative stimulus effects of ethanol in mice lacking the $\gamma$-aminobutyric acid type A receptor $\delta$ subunit. *Alcohol. Clin. Exp. Res.* **28**, 906–913.

Sigel, E., Baur, R., and Malherbe, P. (1993). Recombinant GABA$_A$ receptor function and ethanol. *FEBS J.* **324**, 140–142.

Spigelman, I., Li, Z., Liang, J., Gagetti, E., Samzadeh, S., Mihalek, R. M., Homanics, G. E., and Olsen, R. W. (2003). Reduced inhibition and sensitivity to neurosteroids in hippocampus of mice lacking the GABA$_A$ receptor $\delta$ subunit. *J. Neurophysiol.* **90**, 903–910.

Sundstrom-Poromaa, I., Smith, D. H., Gong, Q. H., Sabado, T. N., Li, X., Light, A., Wiedmann, M., Williams, K., and Smith, S. S. (2002). Hormonally regulated $\alpha 4\beta 2\delta$ $GABA_A$ receptors are a target for alcohol. *Nat. Neurosci.* **5**, 721–722.

Sur, C., Wafford, K. A., Reynolds, D. S., Hadingham, K. L., Bromidge, F., Macaulay, A., Collinson, N., O'Meara, G., Howell, O., Newman, R., Myers, J., Atack, J. R., *et al.* (2001). Loss of the major $GABA_A$ receptor subtype in the brain is not lethal in mice. *J. Neurosci.* **21**, 3409–3418.

Tarantino, L. M., McClearn, G. E., Rodriguez, L. A., and Plomin, R. (1998). Confirmation of quantitative trait loci for alcohol preference in mice. *Alcohol. Clin. Exp. Res.* **22**, 1099–1105.

Taylor, B. A., Wnek, C., Kotlus, B. S., Roemer, N., MacTaggart, T., and Phillips, S. J. (1999). Genotyping new BXD recombinant inbred mouse strains and comparison of BXD and consensus maps. *Mamm. Genome* **10**, 335–348.

Tretter, V., Hauer, B., Nusser, Z., Mihalek, R. M., Höger, H., Homanics, G. E., Somogy, P., and Sieghart, W. (2001). Targeted disruption of the $GABA_A$ receptor $\delta$ subunit gene leads to an up-regulation of $\gamma 2$ subunit-containing receptors in cerebellar granule cells. *J. Biol. Chem.* **276**, 10532–10538.

Turrigiano, G. G. (1999). Homeostatic plasticity in neuronal networks: The more things change, the more they stay the same. *Trends Neurosci.* **22**, 221–227.

Turrigiano, G. G., and Nelson, S. B. (2004). Homeostatic plasticity in the developing nervous system. *Nat. Rev. Neurosci.* **5**, 97–107.

Ueno, S., Wick, M. J., Ye, Q., Harrison, N. L., and Harris, R. A. (1999). Subunit mutations affect ethanol actions on $GABA_A$ receptors expressed in Xenopus oocytes. *Br. J. Pharmacol.* **127**, 377–382.

Uusi-Oukari, M., Heikkila, J., Sinkkonen, S. T., Mäkelä, R., Hauer, B., Homanics, G. E., Sieghart, W., Wisden, W., and Korpi, E. R. (2000). Long-range interactions in neuronal gene expression: Evidence from gene targeting in the $GABA_A$ receptor $\beta 2$–a6–$\alpha 1$–$\gamma 2$ subunit gene cluster. *Mol. Cell. Neurosci.* **16**, 34–41.

Varecka, L., Wu, C.-H., Rotter, A., and Frostholm, A. (1994). $GABA_A$/benzodiazepine receptor $\alpha 6$ subunit mRNA in granule cells of the cerebellar cortex and cochlear nuclei: Expression in developing and mutant mice. *J. Comp. Neurol.* **339**, 341–352.

Vicini, S., Ferguson, C., Prybylowski, K., Kralic, J., Morrow, A. L., and Homanics, G. E. (2001). $GABA_A$ receptor $\alpha 1$ subunit deletion prevents developmental changes of inhibitory synaptic currents in cerebellar neurons. *J. Neurosci.* **21**, 3009–3016.

Wafford, K. A., Burnett, D. M., Leidenheimer, N. J., Burt, D. R., Wang, J. B., Kofuji, P., Dunwiddie, T. V., Harris, R. A., and Sikela, J. M. (1991). Ethanol sensitivity of the $GABA_A$ receptor expressed in Xenopus oocyte requires 8 amino acids contained in the $\gamma$2L subunit. *Neuron* **7**, 27–33.

Wallner, M., Hanchar, H. J., and Olsen, R. W. (2003). Ethanol enhances $\alpha 4\beta 3\delta$ and $\alpha 6\beta 3\delta$ $\gamma$-aminobutyric acid type A receptors at low concentrations known to affect humans. *Proc. Natl. Acad. Sci. USA* **100**, 15218–15223.

Wang, J., Williams, R. W., and Manly, K. F. (2003). WebQTL: Web-based complex trait analysis. *Neuroinformatics* **1**, 299–308.

Wang, J. B., Kofuji, P., Fernando, J. C., Moss, S. J., Huganir, R. L., and Burt, D. R. (1992). The $\alpha 1$, $\alpha 2$, and $\alpha 3$ subunits of $GABA_A$ receptors: Comparison in seizure-prone and resistant mice and during development. *J. Mol. Neurosci.* **3**, 177–184.

Wei, W., Zhang, N., Peng, Z., Houser, C. R., and Mody, I. (2003). Perisynaptic localization of $\delta$ subunit-contianing $GABA_A$ receptors and their activation by GABA spillover in the mouse dentate gyrus. *J. Neurosci.* **23**, 10650–10661.

Whiting, P. J. (2003). The $GABA_A$ receptor gene family: New opportunities for drug development. *Curr. Opin. Drug Discov. Develop.* **6**, 648–657.

Wick, M. J., Radcliffe, R. A., Bowers, B. J., Mascia, M. P., Lüscher, B., Harris, R. A., and Wehner, J. M. (2000). Behavioural changes produced by transgenic overexpression of $\gamma$2L and $\gamma$2S subunits of the $GABA_A$ receptor. *Eur. J. Neurosci.* **12**, 2634–2638.

Williams, R. W., Gu, J., Qi, S., and Lu, L. (2001). The genetic structure of recombinant inbrerd mice: High-resolution consensus maps for complex trait analysis. *Gen. Biol.* **2**, research 0046.1–0046.18.

Wiltgen, B. J., Sanders, M. J., Ferguson, C., Homanics, G. E., and Fanselow, M. S. (2005). Trace fear conditioning is enhanced in mice lacking the $\delta$ subunit of the $GABA_A$ receptor. *Learn Mem.* **12**, 327–333.

Wisor, J. P., DeLorey, T. M., Homanics, G. E., and Edgar, D. M. (2002). Sleep states and sleep electroencephalographic spectral power in mice lacking the $\beta$3 subunit of the $GABA_A$ receptor. *Brain Res.* **955**, 221–228.

Zheng, T., Santi, M. R., Bovolin, P., Marlier, L. N., and Grayson, D. R. (1993). Developmental expression of the $\alpha$6 $GABA_A$ receptor subunit mRNA occurs only after cerebellar granule cell migration. *Dev. Brain Res.* **75**, 91–103.

Zheng, W., Xie, W., Zhang, J., Strong, J., Wang, L., and Xu, M. (2003). Function of $\gamma$-aminobutyric acid receptor/channel $\rho$1 subunits in spinal cord. *J. Bio. Chem.* **278**, 48321–48329.

**George F. Koob**
Molecular and Integrative
Neurosciences Department
The Scripps Research Institute
La Jolla, California

# A Role for GABA in Alcohol Dependence[1]

## I. Chapter Overview

Low doses of alcohol have been hypothesized to act directly via proteins that form ligand-gated receptor channels, such as the $\gamma$-aminobutyric acid (GABA) receptor complex, to allosterically alter function, particularly in specific brain areas such as those hypothesized to be involved in alcohol reinforcement. Specific GABA subunits involving the $\alpha4$, $\alpha6$, $\beta3$, and $\delta$ subunits have been found to be particularly sensitive to alcohol. At the pharmacological level, one can antagonize the effects of alcohol with GABA antagonists and $GABA_B$ agonists, particularly its sedative, anxiolytic-like, and acute reinforcing actions. Brain sites involved in the GABAergic component of alcohol

[1] This is a revised and updated version of an article entitled "A role for GABA mechanisms in the motivational effects of alcohol" that appeared in *Biochem. Pharmacol.* **68**, 1515–1525 (2004).

*Advances in Pharmacology, Volume 54*
1054-3589/06 $35.00
DOI: 10.1016/S1054-3589(06)54009-8

reinforcement include the ventral tegmental area, elements of the extended amygdala (including the central nucleus of the amygdala), and the globus pallidus. Chronic administration of alcohol sufficient to produce dependence and increased alcohol intake are associated with increased GABA release in the amygdala, and GABA agonists block alcohol withdrawal and reduce excessive alcohol intake in dependent animals during withdrawal. Human studies in alcoholics reveal, during dependence, reduced responses to benzodiazepines and higher GABA receptor function during acute withdrawal. Significant associations between $\alpha 6$ $GABA_A$ subunit gene *Gabra6* polymorphisms are observed in certain human alcoholic populations. A hypothesis is proposed that GABAergic interactions with the brain stress neurotransmitter corticotropin-releasing factor (CRF) in specific elements of the extended amygdala may be an important component for the motivation for excessive drinking associated with the transition from social drinking to addiction.

## II. Alcohol and GABA

Alcohol to date does not have an identified specific neurotransmitter-binding site in the brain, but alcohol-receptive elements within membranes—and a protein component of neuronal membranes in particular—may provide a sensitive site for alcohol actions (Deitrich and Erwin, 1996; Tabakoff and Hoffman, 1992). The question is how these alcohol-receptive elements convey specificity of action and how this translates into behavioral action.

Alcohol has been hypothesized to interact with a number of ligand-gated ion channels, and low doses of alcohol (10–50 mM) have been hypothesized to act directly on proteins that form ligand-gated receptor channels such as the GABA receptor complex, particularly in specific brain areas such as those hypothesized to be involved in alcohol reinforcement (Allan and Harris, 1986; Liljequist and Engel, 1982; Mihic and Harris, 1996; Ming *et al.*, 2001; Suzdak *et al.*, 1986; Ticku *et al.*, 1986). The *in vitro* actions of alcohol on the $GABA_A$ receptor are some of its most potent effects, with doses as low as 1–3 mM being effective at altering GABA-gated current measures (Sundstrom-Poromaa *et al.*, 2002). Alcohol appears to modulate the GABA receptor complex allosterically to basically open the chloride channel and hyperpolarize cells or at least potentiate the hyperpolarization produced by GABA. At the pharmacological level, one can antagonize the effects of alcohol with $GABA_A$ antagonists. Approach-avoidance behavior is reduced by alcohol (Masserman and Yum, 1946), and alcohol produces anticonflict actions in the social interaction test, elevated plus maze, and in operant procedures (Koob and Britton, 1996). These anticonflict effects are blocked by drugs that interact with the GABA receptor complex to decrease functional activity. The anticonflict effect of alcohol is blocked by the GABA antagonist picrotoxin (Liljequist and Engel, 1984) but not by the benzodiazepine antagonist flumazenil (Koob *et al.*, 1986). Isopropylbicyclophosphate, a compound that binds near or at the chloride ionophore regulated by GABA, blocks the anticonflict effects of alcohol at low doses (Koob *et al.*, 1989) (Fig. 1). Low doses of benzodiazepine inverse agonists also block the anticonflict effects of alcohol but can have anxiogenic-like effects on their own at these doses (Britton *et al.*, 1988; Koob *et al.*, 1986).

Systemic injections of $GABA_A$ antagonists also reverse the motor-impairing effects of alcohol (Frye and Breese, 1982; Liljequist and Engel, 1982). The GABA agonist muscimol potentiated the sedative effects of alcohol, and the noncompetitive $GABA_A$ antagonist picrotoxin reduced alcohol-induced sedation (Liljequist and Engel, 1982). Both direct and

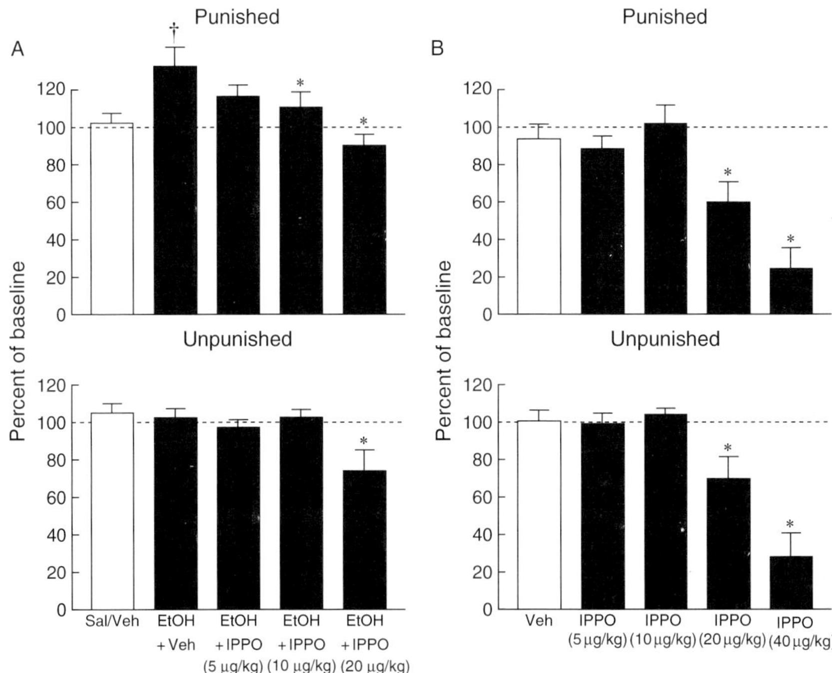


**FIGURE 1** (A) The effects of ethanol and three doses of isopropylbicyclophosphate (IPPO) + ethanol on responding during an operant conflict test. Ethanol produced a significant increase in responding during the conflict component (top) that was dose-dependently reversed by IPPO. Ethanol and IPPO + ethanol had no effect on reinforcers earned during the unpunished fixed-interval component (bottom) except at the highest dose of IPPO. The dagger (†) indicates significant difference from saline/vehicle group ($p < 0.05$; Newman-Keuls); *, Significant difference from ethanol vehicle ($p < 0.05$; Newman-Keuls). Ethanol + 5 μg/kg IPPO was not significantly different from Ethanol + 10 μg/kg IPPO ($p > 0.05$; Newman-Keuls). (B) Effects of IPPO alone on responding during the operant conflict test. IPPO produced a dose-dependent reduction in responding in the punished and unpunished fixed-interval components. Asterisks (*) indicate significant difference from the vehicle group ($p < 0.05$; Newman-Keuls). Taken from Koob *et al.* (1989) with permission.

indirect GABA agonists potentiated alcohol-induced increases in the aerial righting reflex, while the competitive $GABA_A$ antagonist bicuculline reversed the effects of alcohol on the righting response (Frye *et al.*, 1983).

Other modulators of the GABA system may act not only through modulation of the $GABA_A$ receptor but also may modulate GABA release by interactions with the $GABA_B$ receptor. The selective $GABA_B$ receptor agonist baclofen decreased alcohol self-administration in nondependent rats (Janak and Gill, 2003) and decreased the alcohol deprivation effect in alcohol-preferring rats (Colombo *et al.*, 2003a,b). Several clinical studies also have shown potential efficacy of the $GABA_B$ agonist baclofen in reducing alcohol craving and alcohol withdrawal (Addolorato *et al.*, 2002a,b).

An important question is whether there is subunit dependence for the actions of alcohol on the GABA/benzodiazepine ionophore complex. Molecular studies have revealed multiple $GABA_A$ subunits that can be divided by homology into subunit classes with several members: $\alpha$1–6, $\beta$1–4, $\gamma$1–3, $\delta$, $\varepsilon$, and $\tau$ (Sieghart and Sperk, 2002). A number of subunits and mechanisms have been implicated in alcohol's enhancement of $GABA_A$ currents at reasonable doses (10–50 mM). The presence of the $\gamma_2$ long subunit of the $\alpha1\beta2\gamma2$ GABA receptor (Wafford *et al.*, 1991), the $\alpha4\beta1\delta$ subunit (Sundstrom-Poromaa *et al.*, 2002), and the $\alpha4\beta3\delta$ and $\alpha6\beta3\delta$ subunits (Wallner *et al.*, 2003) have all been implicated in sensitivity to alcohol.

Studies have suggested a direct, highly sensitive action of alcohol on $GABA_A$ receptors at specific $\alpha$4, $\alpha$6, $\beta$3, and $\delta$ subunits. Recombinant $\alpha4\beta3\delta$ and $\alpha6\beta3\delta$ subunits expressed in *Xenopus* oocytes are particularly sensitive to alcohol with thresholds as low as 0.1 mM (Wallner *et al.*, 2003). Alcohol also was much more effective at $\beta$3 subunits than at $\beta$2 subunits with a tenfold increase when the $\beta$2 subunit was replaced by the $\beta$3 (Wallner *et al.*, 2003). The authors hypothesized as a result of this increased sensitivity that extrasynaptic receptors in some cells are composed of $\alpha4\beta3\delta$ and $\alpha6\beta3\delta$ subunits and may be the primary targets for alcohol in the GABA receptor system, including such functions as intoxication, sleep, anxiety, memory, and cognition (Hanchar *et al.*, 2004, 2005; Olsen *et al.*, 2004). Mice with a *Gabra6* gene product polymorphism of one allele showed increased sensitivity to alcohol and increased alcohol-induced motor impairment (Hanchar *et al.*, 2005). However, total knockout of the $\alpha6\beta3$ and $\delta$ GABA receptor subunits did not show dramatic changes in alcohol sensitivity (Homanics *et al.*, 1997; Mihalek *et al.*, 2001; Quinlan *et al.*, 1998; Shannon *et al.*, 2004), although $\delta$ knockout mice did drink less alcohol (Mihalek *et al.*, 2001). Nevertheless, it has been argued that point mutations can show more pronounced phenotypes than total knockouts, so the hypothesis of a critical role for the $\beta$3 and $\delta$ subunits awaits further study (Hanchar *et al.*, 2004; Jurd *et al.*, 2003). Deletion of the $\alpha$1 subunit and the $\alpha$5 subunit in knockout studies decreased alcohol drinking and increased the locomotor stimulant effects of alcohol (Blednov *et al.*, 2003; Boehm *et al.*, 2004; see also Boehm *et al.*, this volume).

## III. Targets Within the Addiction Cycle Relevant for Actions of GABA

The purpose of this review is to address the hypothesis that the neurotransmitter GABA in specific neurocircuits forms an important component of reinforcement mechanisms that drive substance dependence on alcohol or alcoholism. Alcoholism can be defined as a complex behavioral disorder characterized by preoccupation with obtaining alcohol and a narrowing of the behavioral repertoire toward excessive consumption (loss of control over consumption). Alcoholism also is usually accompanied by the development of tolerance and dependence and impairment in social and occupational functioning. The *Diagnostic and Statistical Manual of Mental Disorders* (DSM-IV) (American Psychiatric Association, 1994) defines substance dependence on alcohol as a cluster of cognitive, behavioral, and physiological symptoms, indicating that an individual continues use of alcohol despite significant alcohol-related problems and lists seven criteria that incorporate the symptoms mentioned previously. For the purposes of this discussion, *Substance Dependence on Alcohol*, as defined by the DSM-IV, will be considered to be operationally equivalent to the syndrome of *alcoholism*. It is recognized that animal models of a complete syndrome as complex as alcoholism are difficult to achieve, but validated animal models exist for many of the different components of the syndrome, providing a heuristic means by which to pursue the underlying neurobiological basis for the disorder (Table I).

In this context of substance dependence, there are two major sources for the reinforcing actions of alcohol. The first is that there are obviously positive reinforcing effects of alcohol, and this psychological construct often is linked to the positive hedonic or pleasurable effects of alcohol. However, a second motivational aspect of alcoholism or substance dependence on alcohol is the negative reinforcing properties associated with relief of a negative affective state associated with alcohol dependence. The construct of negative reinforcement refers to the increase in the probability of a response by removal of a stimulus (usually aversive). Negative reinforcement in alcoholism can involve a genetic vulnerability for pathology, such as anxiety, which is relieved by alcohol self-administration such as drinking to reduce the anxiety associated with a comorbid anxiety disorder. Alternatively, drinking excessively can engage the brain stress systems, and drinking may produce negative reinforcement by reducing stress responses. The combination of positive reinforcement, genetic vulnerability, psychosocial stressors, and drug-reduced stress may constitute a powerful substrate for alcohol reinforcement that may involve changes in GABAergic function that provide a key component of the motivation to seek alcohol in alcohol dependence. Although less explored to date, some of the changes in GABAergic function may persist into protracted abstinence to contribute to vulnerability to relapse.

**TABLE I** Animal Models for the DSM-IV Criteria for Alcoholism

| *DSM-IV criteria* | *Animal models* |
|---|---|
| A maladaptive pattern of alcohol use, leading to clinically significant impairment or distress occurring at any time in the same 12-month period: | |
| 1. Need for markedly increased amounts of alcohol to achieve intoxication or desired effect; or markedly diminished effect with continued use of the same amount of alcohol | Increased ethanol intake with dependence induction |
| 2. The characteristic withdrawal syndrome for alcohol; or alcohol is taken to relieve or avoid withdrawal symptoms | Increased reward thresholds and increased anxiety-like responses |
| 3. Persistent desire or one or more unsuccessful attempts to cut down or control alcohol use | Conditioned positive reinforcing effects |
| 4. Alcohol used in larger amounts or over a longer period that the person intended | Alcohol intake in dependent animals<br>Alcohol deprivation effect |
| 5. Important social, occupational, or recreational activities given up or reduced because of alcohol use | Choice paradigms behavioral economics—loss of plasticity |
| 6. A great deal of time spent in activities necessary to obtain alcohol, to use alcohol, or to recover from its effects | Alcohol self-administration during withdrawal |
| 7. Continued alcohol use despite knowledge of having a persistent problem that is likely to be caused or exacerbated by alcohol use | Binge alcohol intake in selectively bred animal lines following alcohol deprivation |

## IV. Extended Amygdala: A Basal Forebrain Macrostructure as a Focal Point for GABAergic Actions on Alcohol Reinforcement

The anatomical construct termed the *extended amygdala* represents a macrostructure that shares similarities in morphology, neurochemistry, and connectivity and is composed of several basal forebrain structures: the lateral and medial bed nucleus of the stria terminalis (BNST), the central and medial amygdala, the area termed the sublenticular substantia innominata, and a transition zone in the posterior medial part of the nucleus accumbens (e.g., shell) (Heimer and Alheid, 1991). This system receives limbic and olfactory afferents and projects heavily to the hypothalamus and midbrain. As such, the extended amygdala links the basal forebrain to the classical reward systems of the lateral hypothalamus via the medial forebrain bundle reward system. A guiding hypothesis is that many of the neuropharmacological effects of alcohol on GABAergic function, including its rewarding and "anxiolytic" effects, may be mediated by this circuitry and that neuroadaptive changes in this reward circuit also may provide the motivation for excessive drinking characterized by dependence and relapse (Koob *et al.*, 1998) (see the next section).

## V. Role for GABA in Acute Alcohol Reinforcement

Animal models for the acute reinforcing effects of alcohol were greatly facilitated by advances in animal models for drinking. Whereas early paradigms which assessed the reinforcing effects of alcohol typically used an oral preference paradigm where animals were allowed to drink alcohol or water, a validated operant procedure for limited access to alcohol subsequently provided a reliable procedure for measuring the motivation for drinking pharmacologically relevant doses of alcohol (Samson, 1986; Samson *et al.*, 1988). A major breakthrough in this domain was the development of a training procedure involving access to a sweetened solution and a subsequent fading in of alcohol to avoid the aversiveness of the alcohol taste. As a result, this procedure is a reliable means of measuring the reinforcing effects of alcohol and a reliable means for exploring the neuropharmacological basis for alcohol reinforcement (Samson *et al.*, 1993).

## VI. Effects of GABAergic Agents on Self-Administration of Alcohol in Nondependent Rats

$GABA_A$ antagonists decreased operant alcohol self-administration (Samson *et al.*, 1987) and blocked the alcohol stimulus effects in drug discrimination (Grant *et al.*, 2000). Using an operant model of alcohol self-administration, pretreatment with RO 15-4513, a benzodiazepine inverse agonist, at low doses selectively decreased responding for alcohol but not for water. RO 15-4513 did not affect responding for a saccharin solution, suggesting a specific action (Rassnick *et al.*, 1993a) (Fig. 2). Isopropylbicyclophosphate, a picrotoxinin site ligand, selectively decreased responding for alcohol at very low doses in alcohol-preferring, alcohol-nonpreferring, and Wistar rats (Rassnick *et al.*, 1993a) (Fig. 3). Chlordiazepoxide, a benzodiazepine, had no effect on responding for alcohol under these conditions. These results suggest that acute blockade of $GABA_A$ receptor function can block the motivation for responding for alcohol, supporting the hypothesis that activation of GABA is an important component of the acute reinforcing effects of alcohol.

$GABA_B$ receptors are metabotropic receptors that regulate potassium and calcium channels through a G-protein–mediated mechanism and exert an inhibitory cellular action in the central nervous system (CNS). A selective $GABA_B$ agonist decreased alcohol self-administration in

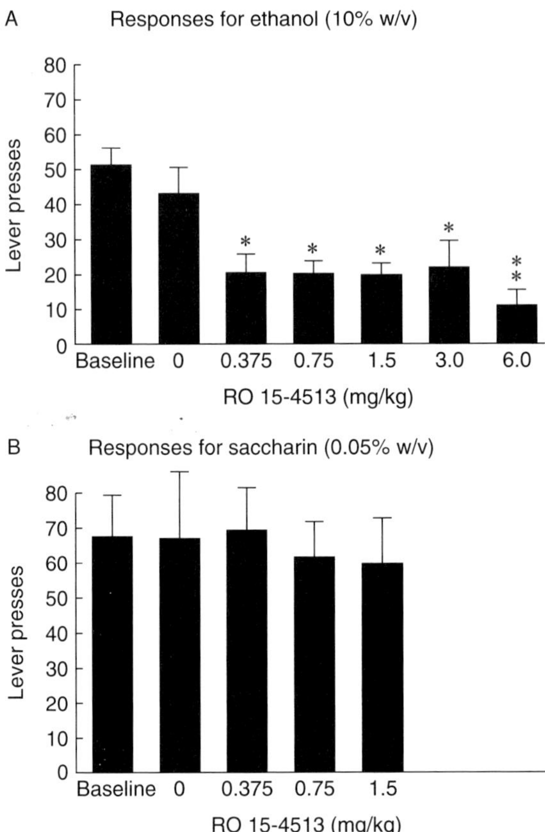


**FIGURE 2** (A) Effects of RO 15-4513 on responding for ethanol in a free-choice task. Responses on a fixed-ratio 1 schedule resulted in the delivery of response-contingent ethanol (10%) reinforcement. Values shown here represent the mean ± SEM number of lever presses for ethanol during 30 min sessions. Asterisks (*) indicate significant differences compared to vehicle (*$p < 0.05$; **$p < 0.01$; Newman-Keuls test). (B) Effects of RO 15-4513 on responding for saccharin in a free-choice saccharin self-administration task. Responses on a fixed-ratio 1 schedule resulted in the delivery of response-contingent saccharin (0.05%) reinforcement. Values shown here represent the mean ± SEM number of lever presses for saccharin during 30-min sessions. Taken from Rassnick *et al.* (1993a) with permission.

nondependent rats (Janak and Gill, 2003) and the alcohol deprivation effect in alcohol-preferring rats (Colombo *et al.*, 2003a,b). Several clinical studies also have shown potential efficacy of baclofen in reducing alcohol craving and alcohol withdrawal (Addolorato *et al.*, 2002a,b). These studies and evidence that $GABA_B$ receptor agonists may modulate mesolimbic dopamine neurons have provided a rationale for the hypothesis that activation of $GABA_B$ receptors may decrease the reinforcing actions of alcohol (Cousins *et al.*, 2002).

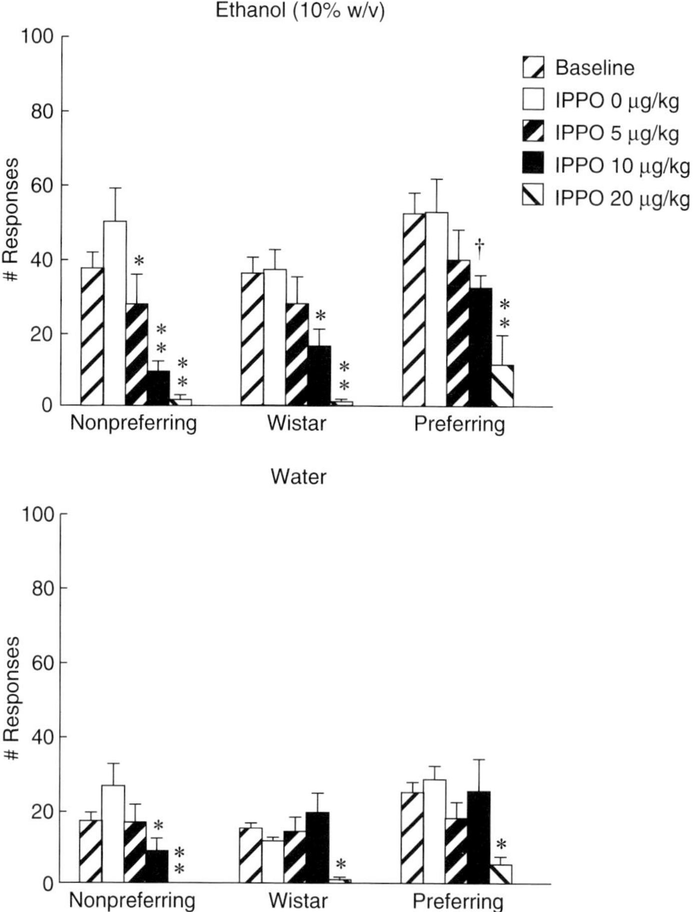


**FIGURE 3** Effects of isopropylbicyclophosphate (IPPO) on responding for ethanol or water in a free-choice operant task. Responses on a fixed-ratio 1 schedule resulted in the delivery of response-contingent ethanol (10% w/v) or water reinforcement. Values shown here represent the mean ± SEM number of lever presses for ethanol and water during 30-min sessions. Asterisks (*) indicate significant differences compared to vehicle (*$p < 0.05$; **$p < 0.01$; Newman-Keuls test). The dagger (†) indicates a significant difference from baseline (†$p < 0.05$; paired t-test). Taken from Rassnick *et al.* (1993a) with permission.

In addition, a very potent GABA antagonist, SR 95531, when microinjected into the basal forebrain, significantly decreased alcohol consumption (Hyytia and Koob, 1995). The GABA antagonist was injected bilaterally into the nucleus accumbens, BNST, and central nucleus of the amygdala in rats trained to self-administer alcohol in a limited access procedure. The most sensitive site was the central nucleus of the amygdala; doses as low as 2 and 4 ng of SR 95531, when injected into the central

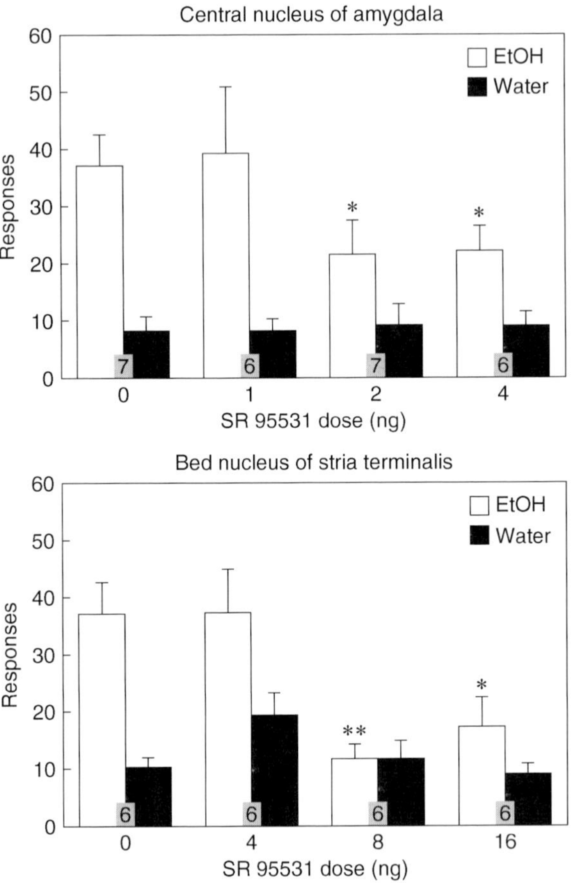


**FIGURE 4** The effect of SR 95531 injections into the central nucleus of the amygdala and the BNST on responding for ethanol (EtOH) and water. Data are expressed as the mean ± SEM numbers of responses for ethanol and water during 30-min sessions for each injection site. Asterisks (*) indicate significant differences from the corresponding saline control values (*$p < 0.05$, **$p < 0.01$ for ethanol responses). Taken from Hyytia and Koob (1995) with permission.

nucleus of the amygdala, decreased alcohol self-administration (Hyytia and Koob, 1995) (Fig. 4). Using alcohol as the cue for drug discrimination, the direct GABA agonist muscimol substituted for alcohol when injected into the nucleus accumbens core or central nucleus of the amygdala (Hodge and Cox, 1998). Others have observed that a mixed agonist/antagonist at the benzodiazepine site of the $GABA_A$ receptor that interacts with the $\alpha_1$ subunit of the $GABA_A$ receptor significantly decreased alcohol self-administration when injected into the central nucleus of the amygdala (Foster *et al.*, 2004) and the ventral pallidum—an important projection of the extended amygdala (Harvey *et al.*, 2002; June *et al.*, 2003).

## VII. Effects of GABAergic Agents on Self-Administration of Alcohol in Dependent Rats

The question of what circuits in the brain are involved in negative reinforcement associated with alcohol withdrawal has been focused on two dependent variables: motivational measures of withdrawal and animal models of excessive drinking during dependence. GABAergic mechanisms have been implicated in both domains and suggest a role for GABA in the neuroadaptations associated with the transition in humans from limited access to alcohol to chronic binging or chronic drinking on a daily basis.

Alcohol withdrawal in humans and animals is characterized by a CNS hyperexcitability that results in both physical and "affective" signs of dependence. In humans, early stages (up to 36 h) are characterized by tremor and elevated sympathetic responses including increased heart rate, blood pressure, and body temperature. Such physical signs are accompanied by insomnia, anxiety, anorexia, and dysphoria. Late stages of withdrawal, if untreated, which is now rare, can include more severe tremor, sympathetic responses, anxiety, and delirium tremens. In animals, physical signs include tremor, loss of the ventromedial distal flexion reflex, weight loss, and audiogenic- or stress-induced seizures. More "affective" signs have included increased responsiveness of acoustic startle (Rassnick *et al.*, 1992), disruption of operant behavior (Baldwin *et al.*, 1991), stimulus generalization to an anxiogenic drug (Lal *et al.*, 1988), and increased sensitivity in behavioral tests of anxiety and stress such as the elevated plus maze (Baldwin *et al.*, 1991). The time course of alcohol withdrawal in the rat ranges up to 7 days, with peak effects manifesting at 8–24 h (Hunter *et al.*, 1975). The severity of withdrawal is related to the blood alcohol levels attained, the duration of the treatment, and an individual's prior history of alcohol withdrawal (Baker and Cannon, 1979; Branchey *et al.*, 1971; Hunter *et al.*, 1975).

While physical or somatic signs of alcohol withdrawal are useful markers for the general hyperexcitability of the alcohol-dependent state, the more "motivational" signs have more relevance to the negative reinforcement construct described previously. Startle amplitude was enhanced during alcohol withdrawal (Edmonds *et al.*, 1982; Rassnick *et al.*, 1992) with maximal effects observed during the first 4–8 h. Alcohol withdrawal decreased prepulse inhibition (Rassnick *et al.*, 1992), a measure that may reflect increases in distractibility and that has been shown to be impaired in psychosis (Braff *et al.*, 1978). Alcohol withdrawal also disrupted ongoing behavior, decreasing operant responding on a mixed fixed-ratio/fixed-interval schedule of food reinforcement (Denoble and Begleiter, 1976). Alcohol withdrawal produced a pronounced anxiogenic-like response in animal models of anxiety. Rats exposed to a liquid diet of alcohol for 2–3 weeks and tested 8 h after withdrawal showed an "anxiogenic-like" response on the elevated plus maze (Baldwin *et al.*, 1991), including reductions in both the percentage of time spent on and the percentage number of entries onto the open arms of the elevated plus maze.

Finally, rats can be trained to discriminate CNS stimulants/convulsants from saline, and the stimulus properties of the stimulant/convulsant have been generalized to the stimulus properties of alcohol withdrawal (Lal *et al.*, 1988). When alcohol is administered by gavage or by liquid diet, the animals selected a pentylenetetrazol lever before the onset of overt physical signs of alcohol withdrawal.

Studies with pharmacological agonists and antagonists have implicated GABA systems in both the physical/somatic and the "affective" or more specifically the anxiogenic-like effects, of alcohol withdrawal. GABA agonists decreased CNS hyperexcitability during alcohol withdrawal and decreased alcohol withdrawal-induced convulsions (Cooper *et al.*, 1979; Frye *et al.*, 1983). GABA antagonists exacerbated many of the symptoms of alcohol withdrawal (Goldstein, 1973), and the partial inverse benzodiazepine agonist RO 15-4513 has been shown to increase the incidence of seizures during alcohol withdrawal (Lister and Karanian, 1987).

GABA also has been implicated in more "affective" measures of alcohol withdrawal. As described previously, using a drug discrimination procedure, alcohol withdrawal as a stimulus produced stimulus characteristics similar to injection of pentylenetetrazol—an anxiogenic drug (Lal *et al.*, 1988). This pentylenetetrazol-like interoceptive stimulus produced by alcohol withdrawal was potentiated by bicuculline and picrotoxin, suggesting that the anxiogenic-like response produced by alcohol withdrawal may be related to an alcohol-induced alteration in the function of the GABA/benzodiazepine ionophore complex (Idemudia *et al.*, 1989). Also, the benzodiazepine antagonist flumazenil (RO 15-1788) reversed the anxiogenic effects of alcohol withdrawal using the social interaction test in rats (File *et al.*, 1989). The flumazenil effect appeared to be very long lasting, suggesting some possible long-term interaction with the benzodiazepine ionophore complex or an endogenous ligand acting on this complex.

Another neurotransmitter system hypothesized to be involved in the "affective" aspects of alcohol withdrawal is the brain stress neurotransmitter corticotrophin-releasing factor (CRF). CRF itself has anxiogenic-like actions, and CRF antagonists have the opposite effects, reversing many behavioral responses to stress (Heinrichs and Koob, 2004). CRF antagonists also reverse the anxiogenic-like response of rats during alcohol withdrawal (Baldwin *et al.*, 1991). These actions of CRF antagonists have been linked to elements of the extended amygdala in that microinjection of the CRF antagonist into the central nucleus of the amygdala also reversed the anxiogenic-like responses of alcohol withdrawal at a dose which is ineffective when administered intraventricularly (Rassnick *et al.*, 1993b) (Fig. 5). There also is evidence that chronic alcohol increased the sensitivity of rats to the locomotor-activating effects of CRF (Ehlers *et al.*, 1987). Also, hypothalamic CRF was increased in rats that

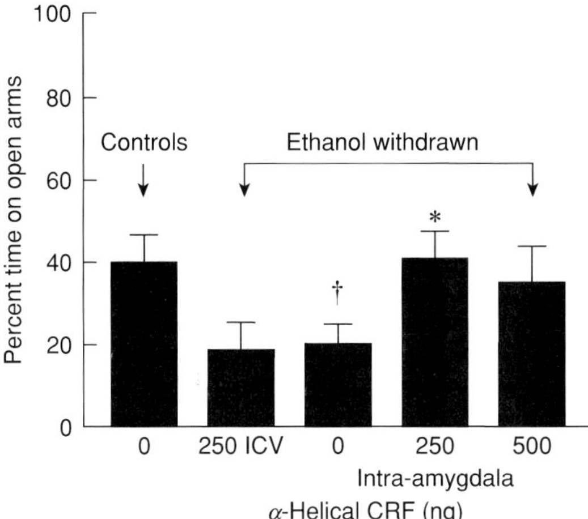


**FIGURE 5** Effects of microinfusion of $\alpha$-helical-CRF$_{9\text{–}41}$ into the central nucleus of the amygdala and i.c.v. administered $\alpha$-helical-CRF$_{9\text{–}41}$ in the elevated plus maze during ethanol withdrawal. Data are expressed as mean ± SEM of percent time exploring the open arms. The asterisk (*) indicates a significant difference compared to vehicle treatment ($^{*}p < 0.05$). The dagger (†) indicates a significant difference compared to pair-fed controls ($^{\dagger}p < 0.05$). Taken from Rassnick *et al.* (1993b) with permission.

showed a high preference for alcohol in a free-choice situation (George *et al.*, 1990). Extracellular levels of CRF were increased in the central nucleus of the amygdala during acute alcohol withdrawal (Merlo-Pich *et al.*, 1995), and even more compelling, a competitive CRF antagonist injected intracerebroventricularly reversed the excessive drinking of alcohol associated with alcohol withdrawal and protracted abstinence (Valdez *et al.*, 2003). These results suggested that selective extrahypothalamic CRF systems, in addition to the classic hypothalamic–pituitary–adrenal axis, may be altered during the alcohol dependence cycle, and this could be reflected in an overactivity during withdrawal.

To address the question of changes in the reward system associated with drug dependence and alcohol dependence, measures of reward function following chronic drug exposure were performed using the technique of intracranial self-stimulation. Acute administration of many drugs of abuse lowers thresholds for brain stimulation reward (Schulteis *et al.*, 1995). However, following chronic drug administration, thresholds are augmented or increased, which means there is a decrease in reward during acute withdrawal (i.e., more electrical current is required to activate the neurons of the medial forebrain bundle). During acute alcohol withdrawal there is a prolonged increase in reward thresholds that lasts up to 72 h (Schulteis *et al.*, 1995) (Fig. 6). Thus, one can hypothesize that the function of the medial forebrain bundle has been compromised by chronic administration.

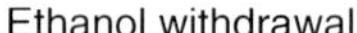


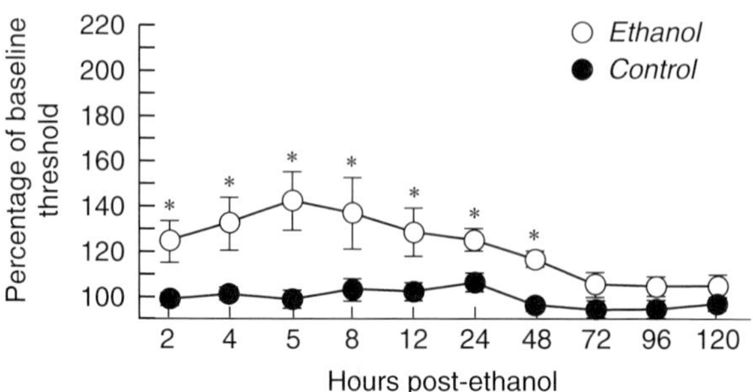


**FIGURE 6** Time-dependent elevation of intracranial self-stimulation thresholds during ethanol withdrawal. Mean blood alcohol levels achieved were 197.29 mg percent. Data are expressed as mean ± SEM percentage of baseline threshold. Asterisks (*) indicate thresholds that were significantly elevated above control levels at 2–48 h post-ethanol ($*p < 0.05$). Open circles indicate the control condition. Closed circles indicate the ethanol withdrawal condition. Taken from Schulteis *et al.* (1995) with permission.

GABAergic drugs can modify reward thresholds, suggesting that GABA mechanisms may modulate reward and may be involved in the changes in reward associated with acute withdrawal. Both $GABA_B$ agonists and antagonists can increase brain stimulation reward thresholds, suggesting a complex interaction with the reward system and GABA function, possibly reflecting differential effects at pre- and postsynaptic receptors (Macey *et al.*, 2001). These changes in reward function are accompanied by changes in neurochemical systems within the extended amygdala that include decreases in neurotransmitter function implicated in the acute reinforcing effects of alcohol (e.g., GABAergic systems). Using an animal model of alcohol self-administration in dependent rats, a GABA agonist was shown to selectively decrease alcohol self-administration in dependent but not nondependent rats (Roberts *et al.*, 1996).

Rats were trained to lever press for 10% alcohol using the saccharin fade-out procedure. Half of the rats were put into alcohol vapor chambers for dependence induction, and half of the rats were placed in control air chambers. After 2 weeks of vapor exposure, the rats were withdrawn every 4 days for a total of five tests. Immediately on removal from the vapor, the rats were placed in operant boxes and allowed to respond for alcohol and water across a 12-h period of withdrawal. Dependent rats responded to a greater degree than nondependent controls, and in fact, maintained blood alcohol levels above 100 mg percent over the 12-h period and as a result did not show the withdrawal signs present in dependent rats not allowed to respond for alcohol during the withdrawal phase (Roberts *et al.*, 1996) (Fig. 7).

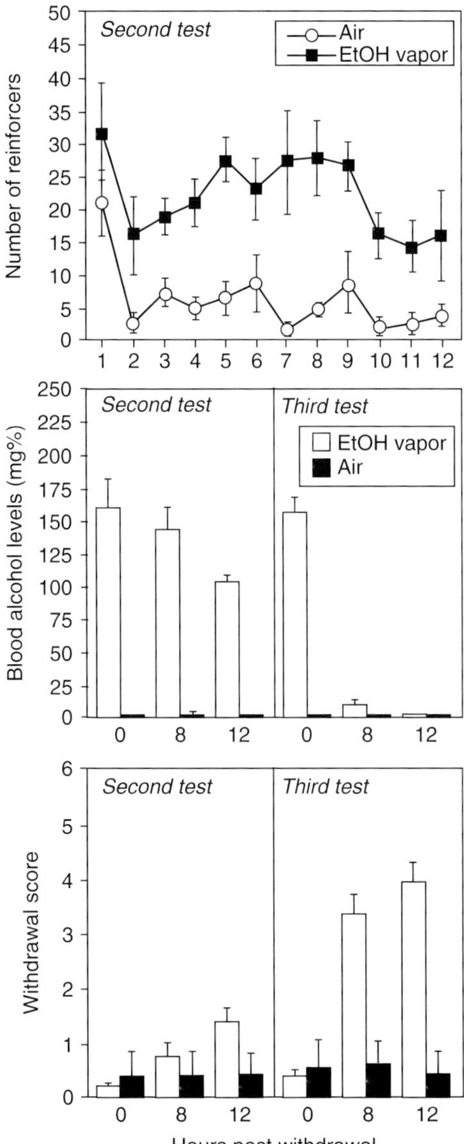


**FIGURE 7** Operant responding for ethanol (EtOH) across a 12-h test period by air-exposed and ethanol vapor-exposed rats (A). In addition, blood alcohol levels (B) and ethanol withdrawal severity (C) obtained during test 2 (while rats were allowed access to ethanol in the operant boxes) and test 3 (while in home cages) are shown. Data are expressed as means ± SEM. Taken from Roberts *et al.* (1996) with permission.

Subsequent work showed that responding across repeated withdrawal sessions increased, suggesting that the rats learned to respond in a manner that controlled their blood alcohol level and minimized or avoided withdrawal discomfort (Roberts *et al.*, 2000).

The enhanced alcohol self-administration during acute withdrawal was reduced dose dependently by intracerebral pretreatment of the GABA agonist muscimol into the central nucleus of the amygdala (Roberts *et al.*, 1996) (Fig. 8). Muscimol significantly decreased responding for alcohol in alcohol-dependent animals but had no effect in nondependent controls in either extended or limited access tests. These results suggest that increases in GABA activity in the amygdala selectively decrease alcohol consumption in dependent rats and suggests that GABAergic systems in the amygdala may change with the development of dependence.

Changes in GABAergic function in the amygdala during the development of dependence on alcohol are supported by biochemical, electrophysiological, and pharmacological studies. Pharmacological studies with GABA agonists show decreased sensitivity to GABA activation after chronic alcohol (Gonzalez and Czachura, 1989; Rassnick *et al.*, 1993c), and GABA agonists are well known to block acute withdrawal from alcohol (Cooper *et al.*, 1979; Frye *et al.*, 1983). In humans, alcohol dependence is associated with decreased responsiveness to the indirect GABA agonist midazolam (Lingford-Hughes *et al.*, 2005).

Chronic administration of alcohol decreased GABA-mediated responses in cerebral cortex (Morrow *et al.*, 1988; Sanna *et al.*, 1993), and nucleus

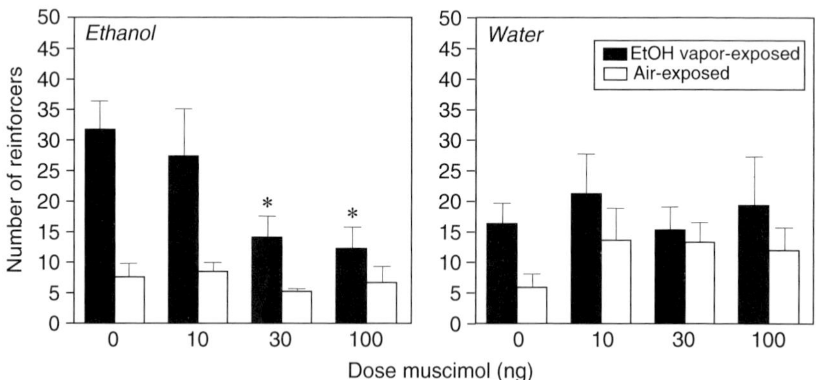


**FIGURE 8** Operant responding for ethanol and water in ethanol vapor-exposed and air-exposed rats after intra-amygdala administration of muscimol—a $GABA_A$ receptor agonist. Data are the means ± SEM of hours 7 and 8 postwithdrawal of 12-h withdrawal sessions in which animals had access to ethanol self-administration for all 12 h. Asterisks (*) indicate significant difference ($p < 0.05$). Modified from Roberts *et al.* (1996) with permission.

accumbens (Szmigielski *et al.*, 1992), and the functional activity of benzodiazepine inverse agonists are enhanced in chronic alcohol-exposed animals (Buck and Harris, 1990; Mehta and Ticku, 1989). Decreased muscimol-stimulated chloride uptake in the cortex of alcohol-exposed animals also suggests a decreased sensitivity of this system during the development of dependence (Allan and Harris, 1987; Morrow *et al.*, 1988, 1990).

Chronic alcohol also increased the release of GABA into the central nucleus of the amygdala and facilitated GABAergic neurotransmission (Roberto *et al.*, 2004). Using an *in vitro* slice preparation from the central nucleus of the amygdala, acute superfusion of alcohol (11–66 mM) enhanced $GABA_A$ inhibitory postsynaptic potential/current (IPSP/C), with recovery on washout. The alcohol effect on IPSP/Cs in chronically alcohol-exposed animals was quantitatively similar to that in neurons from naive rats, suggesting a lack of tolerance. In chronic alcohol-exposed rats, the overall amplitude of evoked IPSP/Cs was larger, spontaneous IPSP/C activity was increased, and baseline paired-pulse facilitation of IPSP/Cs was decreased compared to naive rats, suggesting that evoked GABA release was increased. *In vivo* administration of alcohol (0.1, 0.3, 1.0 M) via a microdialysis probe produced a dose-dependent increase of GABA release in central nucleus of the amygdala dialysates of both chronic alcohol treatment and naive rats. In the rat hippocampus, alcohol enhanced presynaptic $GABA_B$ autoreceptor function, possibly via an enhanced increase in spontaneous GABA release (Ariwodola and Weiner, 2004). A subthreshold dose of the $GABA_B$ agonist baclofen blocked alcohol potentiation of IPSCs. $GABA_B$ agonists also blocked the alcohol deprivation effect in Sardinian alcohol-preferring rats (Colombo *et al.*, 2004).

Such functional changes in the GABA system are accompanied by changes in the expression of specific subunits of the $GABA_A$ receptor with decreases in the $\alpha_1$ subunit and increases in the $\alpha_4$ and $\alpha_6$ subunit (Grobin *et al.*, 1998). These results suggest that changes in GABA neurotransmission and/or the GABA/benzodiazepine ionophore complex may contribute to the development of alcohol dependence. The neurocircuitry site of action for these changes remains unknown, but the differential distribution of the $\alpha_1$ and $\alpha_2$ subunits of the $GABA_A$ receptor within the extended amygdala with strong expression of the $\alpha_1$ in the medial amygdala, and strong expression of the $\alpha_2$ subunit in the central division of the extended amygdala, may have some relevance (Kaufmann *et al.*, 2003). Evidence for increased sensitivity of GABA receptors expressing the $\alpha 4$, $\alpha 6$, $\beta 3$, and $\delta$ subunits suggest that these subunits may be important targets for future study (Hanchar *et al.*, 2004, 2005; Olsen *et al.*, 2004). In addition, the specific brain sites critical for mediating these GABAergic effects on specific aspects of dependence, notably motivationally relevant aspects, remain to be determined. Human studies show significant associations between polymorphism of the $\alpha 6$ $GABA_A$ subunit gene *Gabra6* (Radel *et al.*, 2005), making the conceptual link between $GABA_A$ receptor subunits, the extended amygdala, and motivational aspects of alcohol dependence even more compelling.

CRF/GABA interactions have been shown in other brain areas and support a complex interaction that is dependent on the brain site. In the paraventricular nucleus of the hypothalamus, it appears that CRF neurons are under tonic inhibitory control of an intrinsic GABAergic circuit (Bartanusz *et al.*, 2004). GABAergic receptors are localized on CRF neurons in the paraventricular nucleus (Cullinan, 2000), and GABA may be co-localized in some CRF neurons of the parvocellular division of the paraventricular nucleus (Meister *et al.*, 1988). In contrast, in the frontal cortex, CRF may control GABAergic activity through an interaction with serotonin (Tan *et al.*, 2004), and such an interaction may be of relevance to pathological changes in the frontal cortex associated with CRF in suicide victims (Merali *et al.*, 2004). There is also evidence showing that CRF controls GABA release in the ventral pallidum (Sirinathsinghji and Heavens, 1989). Together these results suggest that GABA may control CRF activity within local circuits in the paraventricular nucleus of the hypothalamus, but in the basal forebrain, CRF activity may control GABAergic activity as seen in the amygdala.

The specific neural substrates for the anxiogenic effects of alcohol withdrawal are likely to involve the same neural elements of the extended amygdala that mediate the acute reinforcing effects of alcohol and may involve specific changes in both the GABA systems and other systems, such as CRF, classically associated with behavioral responses to stressors. Particularly intriguing are data suggesting that chronic alcohol exposure increased the release of GABA in the amygdala and that GABA may interact with the brain stress systems in the amygdala. Indeed, GABA and CRF are co-localized and co-synthesized in the central extended amygdala (Veinante *et al.*, 1997). In nondependent mice, alcohol (44 mM) in an amygdala slice preparation increased the activity of GABAergic neurotransmission as measured by GABA IPSPs (Nie *et al.*, 2004). Blockade of the $CRF_1$ receptor or molecular genetic knockout of the $CRF_1$ receptor blocked the GABAergic facilitation produce by alcohol or CRF in this model. Chronic alcohol increased both CRF and GABA release in the amygdala, suggesting that the two systems are intimately linked in the development of dependence. One possibility is that the stress-like aversive effects of CRF are modulated by the subsequent activation of GABA neurotransmission (Fig. 9).

Several pharmacological observations may support this conceptual framework. CRF antagonists are effective in blocking the excessive drinking associated with alcohol dependence (Valdez *et al.*, 2003), and as noted previously, a GABA agonist injected into the amygdala had the same effect. Neither treatment was effective in blocking alcohol self-administration in nondependent animals. Similarly, both GABA agonists and CRF antagonists blocked the anxiogenic-like effects of alcohol withdrawal (Rassnick

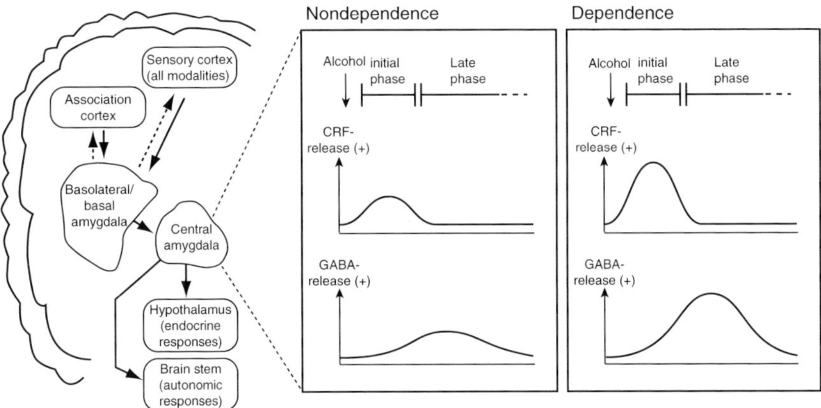


**FIGURE 9** Hypothetical interaction of CRF and GABA in the amygdala to contribute to the reinforcing effects of ethanol with a focus on the anxiolytic-like effects of acute alcohol administration and the anxiogenic-like effects of ethanol withdrawal. The amygdala has long been considered part of an integration of sensory and associative cortical information transduced to an output that activates endocrine, autonomic, and behavioral responses to stressors. Alcohol stimulates CRF release during the initial phase, which in turn activates GABA release. The increase in CRF release gets progressively greater as dependence develops and is followed by a concomitant increase in GABA release to help buffer the physiological effects of the CRF activation. Somewhat paradoxically, the increased CRF availability conveys an increased sensitivity to CRF antagonists but an increased sensitivity to GABA agonists, suggesting differential postsynaptic adaptations to functional activation of these systems. Regardless of the exact mechanism, CRF and GABA are hypothesized to interact to produce some of the motivation for the excessive drinking of alcohol in the dependent state. Derived from a conceptually similar figure involving neuropeptide Y from Heilig *et al.*, 1994.

*et al.*, 1993b) (see the preceding paragraph). Both GABA and CRF are co-synthesized in the same neurons in the central nucleus of the amygdala and the lateral BNST (Veinante *et al.*, 1997). Together these results suggest that there is an important alcohol/CRF/GABA interaction in the extended amygdala that may be of motivational significance for the transition from controlled, nondependent drinking to excessive drinking associated with the development of alcohol abuse and alcoholism in vulnerable individuals.

## Acknowledgments

This is publication number 17712-NP from The Scripps Research Institute. Research was supported by National Institutes of Health grants AA06420 and AA08459 from the National Institute on Alcohol Abuse and Alcoholism and by the Pearson Center for Alcoholism and Addiction Research at The Scripps Research Institute. The author would like to thank Mike Arends and Mellany Santos for their help with the preparation of this manuscript.

## References

Addolorato, G., Caputo, F., Capristo, E., Domenicali, M., Bernardi, M., Janiri, L., Agabio, R., Colombo, G., Gessa, G. L., and Gasbarrini, G. (2002a). Baclofen efficacy in reducing alcohol craving and intake: A preliminary double-blind randomized controlled study. *Alcohol Alcohol.* **37**, 504–508.

Addolorato, G., Caputo, F., Capristo, E., Janiri, L., Bernardi, M., Agabio, R., Colombo, G., Gessa, G. L., and Gasbarrini, G. (2002b). Rapid suppression of alcohol withdrawal syndrome by baclofen. *Am. J. Med.* **112**, 226–229.

Allan, A. M., and Harris, R. A. (1986). Gamma-aminobutyric acid and alcohol actions: Neurochemical studies of long sleep and short sleep mice. *Life Sci.* **39**, 2005–2015.

Allan, A. M., and Harris, R. A. (1987). Acute and chronic ethanol treatments alter GABA receptor-operated chloride channels. *Pharmacol. Biochem. Behav.* **27**, 665–670.

American Psychiatric Association (1994). "Diagnostic and Statistical Manual of Mental Disorders," 4th edition. American Psychiatric Press, Washington DC.

Ariwodola, O. J., and Weiner, J. L. (2004). Ethanol potentiation of GABAergic synaptic transmission may be self-limiting: Role of presynaptic GABAB receptors. *J. Neurosci.* **24**, 10679–10686.

Baker, T. B., and Cannon, D. S. (1979). Potentiation of ethanol withdrawal by prior dependence. *Psychopharmacology* **60**, 105–110.

Baldwin, H. A., Rassnick, S., Rivier, J., Koob, G. F., and Britton, K. T. (1991). CRF antagonist reverses the "anxiogenic" response to ethanol withdrawal in the rat. *Psychopharmacology* **103**, 227–232.

Bartanusz, V., Muller, D., Gaillard, R. C., Streit, P., Vutskits, L., and Kiss, J. Z. (2004). Local gamma-aminobutyric acid and glutamate circuit control of hypophyseotrophic corticotropin-releasing factor neuron activity in the paraventricular nucleus of the hypothalamus. *Eur. J. Neurosci.* **19**, 777–782.

Blednov, Y. A., Walker, D., Alva, H., Creech, K., Findlay, G., and Harris, R. A. (2003). GABAA receptor alpha 1 and beta 2 subunit null mutant mice: Behavioral responses to ethanol. *J. Pharmacol. Exp. Ther.* **305**, 854–863.

Boehm, S. L., II, Ponomarev, I., Jennings, A. W., Whiting, P. J., Rosahl, T. W., Garrett, E. M., Blednov, Y. A., and Harris, R. A. (2004). Gamma-aminobutyric acid A receptor subunit mutant mice: New perspectives on alcohol actions. *Biochem. Pharmacol.* **68**, 1581–1602.

Braff, D. L., Stone, C., Callaway, E., Geyer, M., Glick, I., and Bali, L. (1978). Prestimulus effects on human startle reflex in normals and schizophrenics. *Psychophysiology* **15**, 339–343.

Branchey, M., Rauscher, G., and Kissin, B. (1971). Modifications in the response to alcohol following the establishment of physical dependence. *Psychopharmacologia* **22**, 314–322.

Britton, K. T., Ehlers, C. L., and Koob, G. F. (1988). Is ethanol antagonist Ro 15-4513 selective for ethanol. *Science* **239**, 648–650.

Buck, K. J., and Harris, R. A. (1990). Benzodiazepine agonist and inverse agonist actions on GABAA receptor-operated chloride channels: II. Chronic effects of ethanol. *J. Pharmacol. Exp. Ther.* **253**, 713–719.

Colombo, G., Serra, S., Brunetti, G., Vacca, G., Carai, M. A., and Gessa, G. L. (2003a). Suppression by baclofen of alcohol deprivation effect in Sardinian alcohol-preferring (sP) rats. *Drug Alcohol Depend.* **70**, 105–108.

Colombo, G., Vacca, G., Serra, S., Brunetti, G., Carai, M. A., and Gessa, G. L. (2003b). Baclofen suppresses motivation to consume alcohol in rats. *Psychopharmacology* **167**, 221–224.

Colombo, G., Addolorato, G., Agabio, R., Carai, M. A., Pibiri, F., Serra, S., Vacca, G., and Gessa, G. L. (2004). Role of GABA(B) receptor in alcohol dependence: Reducing effect of baclofen on alcohol intake and alcohol motivational properties in rats and amelioration of alcohol withdrawal syndrome and alcohol craving in human alcoholics. *Neurotox. Res.* **6**, 403–414.

Cooper, B. R., Viik, K., Ferris, R. M., and White, H. L. (1979). Antagonism of the enhanced susceptibility to audiogenic seizures during alcohol withdrawal in the rat by gamma-aminobutyric acid (GABA) and "GABA-mimetic" agents. *J. Pharmacol. Exp. Ther.* **209**, 396–403.

Cousins, M. S., Roberts, D. C., and de Wit, H. (2002). GABA(B) receptor agonists for the treatment of drug addiction: A review of recent findings. *Drug Alcohol Depend.* **65**, 209–220.

Cullinan, W. E. (2000). GABA(A) receptor subunit expression within hypophysiotropic CRH neurons: A dual hybridization histochemical study. *J. Comp. Neurol.* **419**, 344–351.

Deitrich, R. A., and Erwin, V. G. E. (1996). "Pharmacological Effects of Ethanol on the Nervous System." CRC Press, Boca Raton.

Denoble, U., and Begleiter, H. (1976). Response suppression on a mixed schedule of reinforcement during alcohol withdrawal. *Pharmacol. Biochem. Behav.* **5**, 227–229.

Edmonds, H. L., Jr., Sytinsky, I. A., Sylvester, D. M., and Bellin, S. I. (1982). Neurochemical, electroencephalographic and behavioral correlates of ethanol withdrawal in the rat. *Neurobehav. Toxicol. Teratol.* **4**, 33–41.

Ehlers, C. L., Chaplin, R. I., and Koob, G. F. (1987). Antidepressants modulate the CNS effects of corticotropin releasing factor in rats. *Med. Sci. Res.* **15**, 719–720.

File, S. E., Baldwin, H. A., and Hitchcott, P. K. (1989). Flumazenil but not nitrendipine reverses the increased anxiety during ethanol withdrawal in the rat. *Psychopharmacology* **98**, 262–264.

Foster, K. L., McKay, P. F., Seyoum, R., Milbourne, D., Yin, W., Sarma, P. V., Cook, J. M., and June, H. L. (2004). GABA(A) and opioid receptors of the central nucleus of the amygdala selectively regulate ethanol-maintained behaviors. *Neuropsychopharmacology* **29**, 269–284.

Frye, G. D., and Breese, G. R. (1982). GABAergic modulation of ethanol-induced motor impairment. *J. Pharmacol. Exp. Ther.* **223**, 750–756.

Frye, G. D., McCown, T. J., and Breese, G. R. (1983). Differential sensitivity of ethanol withdrawal signs in the rat to gamma-aminobutyric acid (GABA)mimetics: Blockade of audiogenic seizures but not forelimb tremors. *J. Pharmacol. Exp. Ther.* **226**, 720–725.

George, S. R., Fan, T., Roldan, L., and Naranjo, C. A. (1990). Corticotropin-releasing factor is altered in brains of animals with high preference for ethanol. *Alcohol. Clin. Exp. Res.* **14**, 425–429.

Goldstein, D. B. (1973). Alcohol withdrawal reactions in mice: Effects of drugs that modify neurotransmission. *J. Pharmacol. Exp. Ther.* **186**, 1–9.

Gonzalez, L. P., and Czachura, J. F. (1989). Reduced behavioral responses to intranigral muscimol following chronic ethanol. *Physiol. Behav.* **46**, 473–477.

Grant, K. A., Waters, C. A., Green-Jordan, K., Azarov, A., and Szeliga, K. T. (2000). Characterization of the discriminative stimulus effects of GABA(A) receptor ligands in Macaca fascicularis monkeys under different ethanol training conditions. *Psychopharmacology* **152**, 181–188.

Grobin, A. C., Matthews, D. B., Devaud, L. L., and Morrow, A. L. (1998). The role of GABA (A) receptors in the acute and chronic effects of ethanol. *Psychopharmacology* **139**, 2–19.

Hanchar, H. J., Wallner, M., and Olsen, R. W. (2004). Alcohol effects on gamma-aminobutyric acid type A receptors: Are extrasynaptic receptors the answer? *Life Sci.* **76**, 1–8.

Hanchar, H. J., Dodson, P. D., Olsen, R. W., Otis, T. S., and Wallner, M. (2005). Alcohol-induced motor impairment caused by increased extrasynaptic GABA(A) receptor activity. *Nat. Neurosci.* **8**, 339–345.

Harvey, S. C., Foster, K. L., McKay, P. F., Carroll, M. R., Seyoum, R., Woods, J. E., II, Grey, C., Jones, C. M., McCane, S., Cummings, R., Mason, D., Ma, C., *et al.* (2002). The GABA

(A) receptor alpha1 subtype in the ventral pallidum regulates alcohol-seeking behaviors. *J. Neurosci.* **22**, 3765–3775.

Heilig, M., Koob, G. F., Ekman, R., and Britton, K. T. (1994). Corticotropin-releasing factor and neuropeptide Y: Role in emotional integration. *Trends Neurosci.* **17**, 80–85.

Heimer, L., and Alheid, G. (1991). Piecing together the puzzle of basal forebrain anatomy. *In* "The Basal Forebrain: Anatomy to Function" (T. C. Napier, P. W. Kalivas, and I. Hanin, Eds.), Vol. 295, pp. 1–42. Plenum Press, New York.

Heinrichs, S. C., and Koob, G. F. (2004). Corticotropin-releasing factor in brain: A role in activation, arousal, and affect regulation. *J. Pharmacol. Exp. Ther.* **311**, 427–440.

Hodge, C. W., and Cox, A. A. (1998). The discriminative stimulus effects of ethanol are mediated by NMDA and GABA(A) receptors in specific limbic brain regions. *Psychopharmacology* **139**, 95–107.

Homanics, G. E., Ferguson, C., Quinlan, J. J., Daggett, J., Snyder, K., Lagenaur, C., Mi, Z. P., Wang, X. H., Grayson, D. R., and Firestone, L. L. (1997). Gene knockout of the alpha6 subunit of the gamma-aminobutyric acid type A receptor: Lack of effect on responses to ethanol, pentobarbital, and general anesthetics. *Mol. Pharmacol.* **51**, 588–596.

Hunter, B. E., Riley, J. N., and Walker, D. W. (1975). Ethanol dependence in the rat: A parametric analysis. *Pharmacol. Biochem. Behav.* **3**, 619–629.

Hyytia, P., and Koob, G. F. (1995). GABA-A receptor antagonism in the extended amygdala decreases ethanol self-administration in rats. *Eur. J. Pharmacol.* **283**, 151–159.

Idemudia, S. O., Bhadra, S., and Lal, H. (1989). The pentylenetetrazol-like interoceptive stimulus produced by ethanol withdrawal is potentiated by bicuculline and picrotoxinin. *Neuropsychopharmacology* **2**, 115–122.

Janak, P. H., and Gill, M. T. (2003). Comparison of the effects of allopregnanolone with direct GABAergic agonists on ethanol self-administration with and without concurrently available sucrose. *Alcohol* **30**, 1–7.

June, H. L., Foster, K. L., McKay, P. F., Seyoum, R., Woods, J. E., Harvey, S. C., Eiler, W. J., Grey, C., Carroll, M. R., McCane, S., Jones, C. M., Yin, W., *et al.* (2003). The reinforcing properties of alcohol are mediated by GABA(A1) receptors in the ventral pallidum. *Neuropsychopharmacology* **28**, 2124–2137.

Jurd, R., Arras, M., Lambert, S., Drexler, B., Siegwart, R., Crestani, F., Zaugg, M., Vogt, K. E., Ledermann, B., Antkowiak, B., and Rudolph, U. (2003). General anesthetic actions *in vivo* strongly attenuated by a point mutation in the GABA(A) receptor beta3 subunit. *FASEB J.* **17**, 250–252.

Kaufmann, W. A., Humpel, C., Alheid, G. F., and Marksteiner, J. (2003). Compartmentation of alpha 1 and alpha 2 GABA(A) receptor subunits within rat extended amygdala: Implications for benzodiazepine action. *Brain Res.* **964**, 91–99.

Koob, G. F., and Britton, K. T. (1996). Neurobiological substrates for the anti-anxiety effects of ethanol. *In* "The Pharmacology of Alcohol and Alcohol Dependence" (series title: "Alcohol and Alcoholism") (H. Begleiter and B. Kissin, Eds.), Vol. 2, pp. 477–506. Oxford University Press, New York.

Koob, G. F., Braestrup, C., and Thatcher-Britton, K. (1986). The effects of FG 7142 and RO 15-1788 on the release of punished responding produced by chlordiazepoxide and ethanol in the rat. *Psychopharmacology* **90**, 173–178.

Koob, G. F., Mendelson, W. B., Schafer, J., Wall, T. L., Britton, K. T., and Bloom, F. E. (1989). Picrotoxinin receptor ligand blocks anti-punishment effects of alcohol. *Alcohol* **5**, 437–443.

Koob, G. F., Roberts, A. J., Schulteis, G., Parsons, L. H., Heyser, C. J., Hyytia, P., Merlo-Pich, E., and Weiss, F. (1998). Neurocircuitry targets in ethanol reward and dependence. *Alcohol. Clin. Exp. Res.* **22**, 3–9.

Lal, H., Harris, C. M., Benjamin, D., Springfield, A. C., Bhadra, S., and Emmett-Oglesby, M. W. (1988). Characterization of a pentylenetetrazol-like interoceptive stimulus produced by ethanol withdrawal. *J. Pharmacol. Exp. Ther.* **247**, 508–518.

Liljequist, S., and Engel, J. (1982). Effects of GABAergic agonists and antagonists on various ethanol-induced behavioral changes. *Psychopharmacology* **78**, 71–75.

Liljequist, S., and Engel, J. A. (1984). The effects of GABA and benzodiazepine receptor antagonists on the anti-conflict actions of diazepam or ethanol. *Pharmacol. Biochem. Behav.* **21**, 521–525.

Lingford-Hughes, A. R., Wilson, S. J., Cunningham, V. J., Feeney, A., Stevenson, B., Brooks, D. J., and Nutt, D. J. (2005). GABA-benzodiazepine receptor function in alcohol dependence: A combined 11C-flumazenil PET and pharmacodynamic study. *Psychopharmacology* **180**, 595–606.

Lister, R. G., and Karanian, J. W. (1987). RO 15-4513 induces seizures in DBA/2 mice undergoing alcohol withdrawal. *Alcohol* **4**, 409–411.

Macey, D. J., Froestl, W., Koob, G. F., and Markou, A. (2001). Both GABA-B receptor agonist and antagonists decreased brain stimulation reward in the rat. *Neuropharmacology* **40**, 676–685.

Masserman, J. H., and Yum, K. S. (1946). An analysis of the influence of alcohol on experimental neuroses in cats. *Psychosom. Med.* **8**, 36–52.

Mehta, A. K., and Ticku, M. K. (1989). Chronic ethanol treatment alters the behavioral effects of Ro 15-4513, a partially negative ligand for benzodiazepine binding sites. *Brain Res.* **489**, 93–100.

Meister, B., Hokfelt, T., Geffard, M., and Oertel, W. (1988). Glutamic acid decarboxylase- and gamma-aminobutyric acid-like immunoreactivities in corticotropin-releasing factor-containing parvocellular neurons of the hypothalamic paraventricular nucleus. *Neuroendocrinology* **48**, 516–526.

Merali, Z., Du, L., Hrdina, P., Palkovits, M., Faludi, G., Poulter, M. O., and Anisman, H. (2004). Dysregulation in the suicide brain: mRNA expression of corticotropin-releasing hormone receptors and GABA(A) receptor subunits in frontal cortical brain region. *J. Neurosci.* **24**, 1478–1485.

Merlo-Pich, E., Lorang, M., Yeganeh, M., Rodriguez de Fonseca, F., Raber, J., Koob, G. F., and Weiss, F. (1995). Increase of extracellular corticotropin-releasing factor-like immunoreactivity levels in the amygdala of awake rats during restraint stress and ethanol withdrawal as measured by microdialysis. *J. Neurosci.* **15**, 5439–5447.

Mihalek, R. M., Bowers, B. J., Wehner, J. M., Kralic, J. E., VanDoren, M. J., Morrow, A. L., and Homanics, G. E. (2001). GABA(A)-receptor delta subunit knockout mice have multiple defects in behavioral responses to ethanol. *Alcohol. Clin. Exp. Res.* **25**, 1708–1718.

Mihic, S. J., and Harris, R. A. (1996). Alcohol actions at the GABA-A receptor/chloride channel complex. *In* "Pharmacological Effects of Ethanol on the Nervous System" (R. A. Deitrich and V. G. Erwin, Eds.), pp. 51–72. CRC Press, Boca Raton.

Ming, Z., Knapp, D. J., Mueller, R. A., Breese, G. R., and Criswell, H. E. (2001). Differential modulation of GABA- and NMDA-gated currents by ethanol and isoflurane in cultured rat cerebral cortical neurons. *Brain Res.* **920**, 117–124.

Morrow, A. L., Suzdak, P. D., Karanian, J. W., and Paul, S. M. (1988). Chronic ethanol administration alters gamma-aminobutyric acid, pentobarbital and ethanol-mediated $^{36}Cl^-$ uptake in cerebral cortical synaptoneurosomes. *J. Pharmacol. Exp. Ther.* **246**, 158–164.

Morrow, A. L., Montpied, P., Lingford-Hughes, A., and Paul, S. M. (1990). Chronic ethanol and pentobarbital administration in the rat: Effects on GABAA receptor function and expression in brain. *Alcohol* **7**, 237–244.

Nie, Z., Schweitzer, P., Roberts, A. J., Madamba, S. G., Moore, S. D., and Siggins, G. R. (2004). Ethanol augments GABAergic transmission in the central amygdala via CRF1 receptors. *Science* **303**, 1512–1514.

Olsen, R. W., Chang, C. S., Li, G., Hanchar, H. J., and Wallner, M. (2004). Fishing for allosteric sites on GABA(A) receptors. *Biochem. Pharmacol.* **68**, 1675–1684.

Quinlan, J. J., Homanics, G. E., and Firestone, L. L. (1998). Anesthesia sensitivity in mice that lack the beta3 subunit of the gamma-aminobutyric acid type A receptor. *Anesthesiology* **88**, 775–780.

Radel, M., Vallejo, R. L., Iwata, N., Aragon, R., Long, J. C., Virkkunen, M., and Goldman, D. (2005). Haplotype-based localization of an alcohol dependence gene to the 5q34 $\gamma$-aminobutyric acid type A gene cluster. *Arch. Gen. Psychiatry* **62**, 47–55.

Rassnick, S., Koob, G. F., and Geyer, M. A. (1992). Responding to acoustic startle during chronic ethanol intoxication and withdrawal. *Psychopharmacology* **106**, 351–358.

Rassnick, S., D'Amico, E., Riley, E., and Koob, G. F. (1993a). GABA antagonist and benzodiazepine partial inverse agonist reduce motivated responding for ethanol. *Alcohol. Clin. Exp. Res.* **17**, 124–130.

Rassnick, S., Heinrichs, S. C., Britton, K. T., and Koob, G. F. (1993b). Microinjection of a corticotropin-releasing factor antagonist into the central nucleus of the amygdala reverses anxiogenic-like effects of ethanol withdrawal. *Brain Res.* **605**, 25–32.

Rassnick, S., Krechman, J., and Koob, G. F. (1993c). Chronic ethanol produces a decreased sensitivity to the response-disruptive effects of GABA receptor complex antagonists. *Pharmacol. Biochem. Behav.* **44**, 943–950.

Roberto, M., Schweitzer, P., Madamba, S. G., Stouffer, D. G., Parsons, L. H., and Siggins, G. R. (2004). Acute and chronic ethanol alter glutamatergic transmission in rat central amygdala: An *in vitro* and *in vivo* analysis. *J. Neurosci.* **24**, 1594–1603.

Roberts, A. J., Cole, M., and Koob, G. F. (1996). Intra-amygdala muscimol decreases operant ethanol self-administration in dependent rats. *Alcohol. Clin. Exp. Res.* **20**, 1289–1298.

Roberts, A. J., Heyser, C. J., Cole, M., Griffin, P., and Koob, G. F. (2000). Excessive ethanol drinking following a history of dependence: Animal model of allostasis. *Neuropsychopharmacology* **22**, 581–594.

Samson, H. H. (1986). Initiation of ethanol reinforcement using a sucrose-substitution procedure in food- and water-sated rats. *Alcohol. Clin. Exp. Res.* **10**, 436–442.

Samson, H. H., Tolliver, G. A., Pfeffer, A. O., Sadeghi, K. G., and Mills, F. G. (1987). Oral ethanol reinforcement in the rat: Effect of the partial inverse benzodiazepine agonist RO15-4513. *Pharmacol. Biochem. Behav.* **27**, 517–519.

Samson, H. H., Pfeffer, A. O., and Tolliver, G. A. (1988). Oral ethanol self-administration in rats: Models of alcohol-seeking behavior. *Alcohol. Clin. Exp. Res.* **12**, 591–598.

Samson, H. H., Hodge, C. W., Tolliver, G. A., and Haraguchi, M. (1993). Effect of dopamine agonists and antagonists on ethanol-reinforced behavior: The involvement of the nucleus accumbens. *Brain Res. Bull.* **30**, 133–141.

Sanna, E., Serra, M., Cossu, A., Colombo, G., Follesa, P., Cuccheddu, T., Concas, A., and Biggio, G. (1993). Chronic ethanol intoxication induces differential effects on GABAA and NMDA receptor function in the rat brain. *Alcohol. Clin. Exp. Res.* **17**, 115–123.

Schulteis, G., Markou, A., Cole, M., and Koob, G. (1995). Decreased brain reward produced by ethanol withdrawal. *Proc. Natl. Acad. Sci. USA* **92**, 5880–5884.

Shannon, E. E., Shelton, K. L., Vivian, J. A., Yount, I., Morgan, A. R., Homanics, G. E., and Grant, K. A. (2004). Discriminative stimulus effects of ethanol in mice lacking the gamma-aminobutyric acid type A receptor delta subunit. *Alcohol. Clin. Exp. Res.* **28**, 906–913.

Sieghart, W., and Sperk, G. (2002). Subunit composition, distribution and function of GABA (A) receptor subtypes. *Curr. Topics Med. Chem.* **2**, 795–816.

Sirinathsinghji, D. J., and Heavens, R. P. (1989). Stimulation of GABA release from the rat neostriatum and globus pallidus *in vivo* by corticotropin-releasing factor. *Neurosci. Lett.* **100**, 203–209.

Sundstrom-Poromaa, I., Smith, D. H., Gong, Q. H., Sabado, T. N., Li, X., Light, A., Wiedmann, M., Williams, K., and Smith, S. S. (2002). Hormonally regulated alpha-4-beta-2-delta GABA-A receptors are a target for alcohol. *Nat. Neurosci.* **5**, 721–722.

Suzdak, P. D., Glowa, J. R., Crawley, J. N., Schwartz, R. D., Skolnick, P., and Paul, S. M. (1986). A selective imidazobenzodiazepine antagonist of ethanol in the rat. *Science* **234**, 1243–1247.

Szmigielski, A., Szmigielska, H., and Wejman, I. (1992). The effect of single and prolonged ethanol administration on the sensitivity of central GABA-A and benzodiazepine receptors *in vivo*. *Pol. J. Pharmacol. Pharm.* **44**, 271–280.

Tabakoff, B., and Hoffman, P. L. (1992). Alcohol: Neurobiology. *In* "Substance Abuse: A Comprehensive Textbook," 2nd edition. (J. H. Lowinson, P. Ruiz, and R. B. Millman, Eds.), pp. 152–185. Williams and Wilkins, Baltimore.

Tan, H., Zhong, P., and Yan, Z. (2004). Corticotropin-releasing factor and acute stress prolongs serotonergic regulation of GABA transmission in prefrontal cortical pyramidal neurons. *J. Neurosci.* **24**, 5000–5008.

Ticku, M. K., Lowrimore, P., and Lehoullier, P. (1986). Ethanol enhances GABA-induced 36Cl-influx in primary spinal cord cultured neurons. *Brain Res. Bull.* **17**, 123–126.

Valdez, G. R., Zorrilla, E. P., Roberts, A. J., and Koob, G. F. (2003). Antagonism of corticotropin-releasing factor attenuates the enhanced responsiveness to stress observed during protracted ethanol abstinence. *Alcohol* **29**, 55–60.

Veinante, P., Stoeckel, M. E., and Freund-Mercier, M. J. (1997). GABA- and peptide-immunoreactivities co-localize in the rat central extended amygdala. *Neuroreport* 8, 2985–2989.

Wafford, K. A., Burnett, D. M., Leidenheimer, N. J., Burt, D. R., Wang, J. B., Kofuji, P., Dunwiddie, T. V., Harris, R. A., and Sikela, J. M. (1991). Ethanol sensitivity of the GABAA receptor expressed in Xenopus oocytes requires 8 amino acids contained in the gamma 2L subunit. *Neuron* 7, 27–33.

Wallner, M., Hanchar, H. J., and Olsen, R. W. (2003). Ethanol enhances alpha 4 beta 3 delta and alpha 6 beta 3 delta gamma-aminobutyric acid type A receptors at low concentrations known to affect humans. *Proc. Natl. Acad. Sci. USA* **100**, 15218–15223.

**Werner Sieghart**

Division of Biochemistry and Molecular Biology
Center for Brain Research, and Section of Biochemical Psychiatry
University Clinic for Psychiatry, Medical University Vienna, Austria

# Structure, Pharmacology, and Function of $GABA_A$ Receptor Subtypes

## I. Chapter Overview

Gamma-aminobutyric acid type A ($GABA_A$) receptors are the most important inhibitory transmitter receptors in the central nervous system (CNS). They are chloride channels that can be opened by GABA and modulated by a variety of different drugs such as benzodiazepines, barbiturates, neuroactive steroids, anesthetics, and convulsants. These receptors are composed of five subunits that can belong to different subunit classes, giving rise to a large variety of distinct receptor subtypes. Depending on their subunit composition, these receptor subtypes exhibit distinct pharmacological and electrophysiological properties. In this chapter, the pharmacology of $GABA_A$ receptors is reviewed, new compounds interacting with these receptors are described, and novel receptor subtype-selective compounds are discussed. In addition, evidence for the function of distinct $GABA_A$ receptor subtypes in the brain is summarized. Finally, information

*Advances in Pharmacology, Volume 54*

1054-3589/06 $35.00
DOI: 10.1016/S1054-3589(06)54010-4

on the molecular structure of the extracellular and transmembrane domain of $GABA_A$ receptors based on the X-ray crystallographic structure of the acetylcholine binding protein and on the cryo-electronmicroscopic structure of the nicotinic acetylcholine receptor is provided. This structure contains multiple solvent accessible cavities that possibly are used by a variety of allosteric modulators for their interaction with $GABA_A$ receptors, thus explaining the rich pharmacology of these important receptors.

## II. Introduction

GABA is the most abundant inhibitory neurotransmitter in the CNS. In the brain, 17–20% of all neurons are GABAergic (Somogyi *et al.*, 1998). Most of the physiological actions of GABA are generated via $GABA_A$ receptors. These receptors are chloride ion channels that can be opened by GABA and can be modulated by a variety of pharmacologically and clinically important drugs such as benzodiazepines, barbiturates, steroids, anesthetics, and convulsants (Sieghart, 1995). These drugs produce at least part of their clinically relevant effects by interacting with distinct allosteric binding sites on $GABA_A$ receptors (Sigel and Buhr, 1997; Smith and Olsen, 1995). Based on the pharmacological action of these drugs, it was concluded that $GABA_A$ receptors are involved in controlling the excitability of the brain (Fritschy *et al.*, 1999; Olsen and Avoli, 1997), in the modulation of anxiety (Nutt *et al.*, 1990; Pratt, 1992), of feeding and drinking behavior (Berridge and Pecina, 1995; Cooper, 1989), circadian rhythms (Turek and Van Reeth, 1988; Wagner *et al.*, 1997), cognition, vigilance, memory, and learning (Izquierdo and Medina, 1991; Paulsen and Moser, 1998; Sarter *et al.*, 1988).

## III. Heterogeneity of $GABA_A$ Receptors

$GABA_A$ receptors are composed of five subunits that consist of a large N-terminal extracellular domain, four transmembrane (TM) domains, and a large intracellular loop between TM3 and TM4 (Nayeem *et al.*, 1994; Schofield *et al.*, 1987; Tretter *et al.*, 1997). So far, a total of six $\alpha$, three $\beta$, three $\gamma$, one $\delta$, one $\epsilon$, one $\pi$, one $\theta$, and three $\rho$ subunits of $GABA_A$ receptors have been cloned and sequenced from the mammalian nervous system, and for several of these subunits splice variants have been identified (Barnard *et al.*, 1998; Sieghart and Sperk, 2002). This set of 19 different subunits is the largest of any among the mammalian ion channel receptors. At least for the human brain this subunit set seems to be final. By applying search algorithms designed to recognize sequences of all known $GABA_A$ receptor type subunits in species from man down to nematodes, in a study no new $GABA_A$ receptor subunits were detectable in the human genome (Simon *et al.*, 2004). In nonmammalian species, however, additional subunit homologs have been identified (Barnard *et al.*, 1998; Hosie *et al.*, 1997; Schuske *et al.*, 2004).

$GABA_A$ receptors are widely distributed all over the brain, and evidence has accumulated indicating an enormous heterogeneity of these receptors (Sieghart and Sperk, 2002). Thus, *in situ* hybridization studies (Laurie *et al.*, 1992; Persohn *et al.*, 1992; Wisden *et al.*, 1992) and immunohistochemical studies (Fritschy *et al.*, 1992; Pirker *et al.*, 2000; Sperk *et al.*, 1997) have demonstrated that each one of the subunits has a distinct regional and cellular distribution in the brain. Whereas some cell types contain only a few $GABA_A$ receptor subunits, others express most, if not all $GABA_A$ receptor subunits. If all these subunits could randomly coassemble with each other, more than 150.000 $GABA_A$ receptor subtypes with different subunit composition and arrangement could be formed (Burt and Kamatchi, 1991). $GABA_A$ receptors can be, and sometimes are, composed of up to five different subunits. However, due to restrictions imposed during assembly of $GABA_A$ receptors, not all receptors that can be formed theoretically are actually formed in the brain. Nevertheless, from the number of different receptor subtypes so far isolated using subunit-specific antibodies, it was estimated that more than 500 distinct $GABA_A$ receptors probably do exist in the brain (Sieghart and Sperk, 2002). The number of receptors that are relatively abundant, however, is much smaller. Thus, the majority of native receptors are composed of $\alpha$, $\beta$, and $\gamma$ subunits. In minor receptor subtypes, the $\delta$, $\epsilon$, and $\pi$ subunits seem to be able to replace the $\gamma$ subunit in $GABA_A$ receptors, whereas the $\theta$ subunit might be able to replace a $\beta$ subunit. But systematic studies on the composition of $GABA_A$ receptors containing $\epsilon$, $\pi$, or $\theta$ subunits so far are not available (Sieghart and Sperk, 2002).

Evidence is now convincing that receptors composed of $\alpha$, $\beta$, and $\gamma$ subunits contain two $\alpha$, two $\beta$, and one $\gamma$ subunit (Chang *et al.*, 1996; Farrar *et al.*, 1999; Im *et al.*, 1995; Tretter *et al.*, 1997) and that in these receptors a total of four alternating $\alpha$ and $\beta$ subunits are connected by a $\gamma$ subunit (Baumann *et al.*, 2002; Ernst *et al.*, 2003; Tretter *et al.*, 1997). Whether all receptors composed of $\alpha\beta\gamma$ subunits or those composed of $\alpha\beta\delta$, $\alpha\beta\epsilon$, or $\alpha\beta\pi$ subunits exhibit the same subunit stoichiometry and subunit arrangement, presently is not known.

$\rho$ Subunits originally were assumed not to coassemble with other classes of $GABA_A$ receptor subunits (Cutting *et al.*, 1991; Enz and Cutting, 1998). However, it has been demonstrated that these subunits also can assemble with $GABA_A$ $\gamma 2$ or glycine receptor subunits and form functional receptors with properties found in certain cell types of the retina (Pan *et al.*, 2000; Qian and Ripps, 1999), brain stem (Milligan *et al.*, 2004), hippocampus

(Hartmann *et al.*, 2004), or other brain regions (Arakawa and Okada, 1988; Drew *et al.*, 1984; Strata and Cherubini, 1994). In addition, $\rho$ subunits can form homo- as well as hetero-oligomeric channels with other $\rho$ subunits that exhibit properties of the previously characterized $GABA_C$ receptors (Bormann, 2000). Since $\rho$ subunits are structurally part of the family of $GABA_A$ receptor subunits, it was recommended that $\rho$-containing receptors should be classified as a specialized set of the $GABA_A$ receptors (Barnard *et al.*, 1998).

## IV. Pharmacology of $GABA_A$ Receptors

$GABA_A$ receptors not only can be directly activated or inhibited via their GABA binding site but can also be allosterically modulated by benzodiazepines, barbiturates, steroids, anesthetics, convulsants, and many other drugs, the number of which is constantly increasing (Korpi *et al.*, 2002; Sieghart, 1995). Currently, only three distinct binding sites present on $GABA_A$ receptors can be directly investigated by appropriate radioligand binding studies: the GABA/muscimol-, the benzodiazepine-, and the t-butylbicyclophosphorothionate (TBPS)/picrotoxinin-binding site (Sieghart, 1995). Using such studies, compounds competitively interacting with the radioligands and thus, directly binding to the respective sites could be identified. The interaction of all the other drugs with $GABA_A$ receptors can only be investigated by electrophysiology or by studying the allosteric effects of these drugs at the [$^3$H]muscimol-, [$^3$H]benzodiazepine-, or [$^{35}$S]TBPS-binding site. These techniques, however, in most cases do not allow to clarify whether the allosteric effects of different ligands are mediated via the same or distinct binding sites. Therefore, the total number of allosteric binding sites present on $GABA_A$ receptors is not known. Structure–activity studies for most of the allosteric modulators of $GABA_A$ receptors are thus not possible at present, preventing a structurally guided development of novel ligands for the respective binding site.

The aim of this chapter is to provide a short overview on the pharmacology of $GABA_A$ receptors and their subtypes as well as on new developments in this field. A complete coverage of all interactions of drugs with $GABA_A$ receptor is out of the scope of this article. More detailed descriptions on the complex interactions of different drugs with $GABA_A$ receptors have been published previously and are referred to in the text.

### A. GABA Binding Site of $GABA_A$ Receptors

Mutagenesis studies on recombinant $GABA_A$ receptors have identified several amino acid residues on $\alpha$ and $\beta$ subunits that seem to be important for binding of GABA (Fig. 1, compound 1) or muscimol (Fig. 1, compound 2)

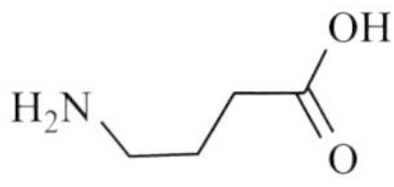

GABA (1) 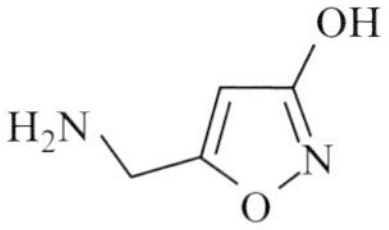 Muscimol (2) 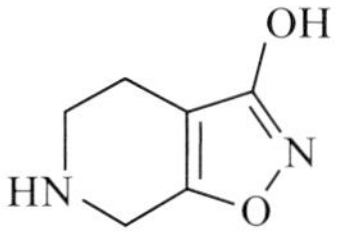 THIP (3) (Gaboxadol)

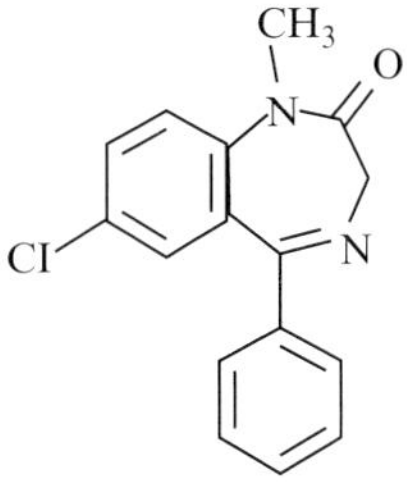

Diazepam (4) 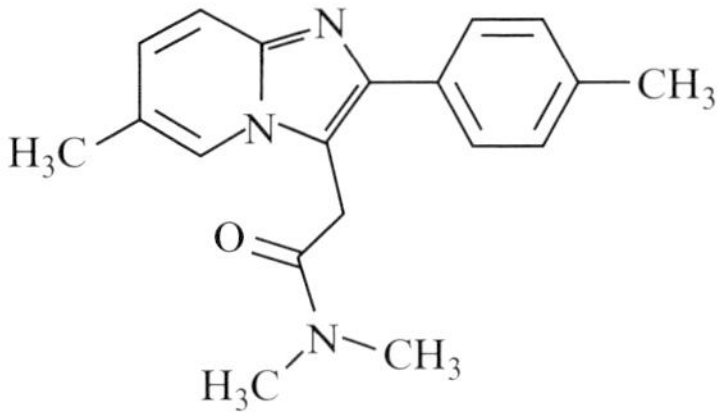 Zolpidem (5) 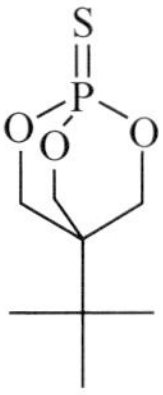 TBPS (6)

**FIGURE 1** GABA$_A$ receptor ligands. Compounds 1–3 are GABA site agonist. Compounds 4 and 5 are benzodiazepine site agonists, and compond 6 is a GABA$_A$ receptor antagonist that inhibits the action of GABA via an allosteric site probably located within the ion channel.

(Smith and Olsen, 1995). It thus was concluded that the GABA binding site of GABA$_A$ receptors is located at the interface of an $\alpha$ and a $\beta$ subunit. Currently, only a few different classes of compounds are known as ligands for the GABA binding site (Frolund *et al.*, 2002). Studies on recombinant GABA$_A$ receptors have indicated that the currently known full agonists (exhibiting an efficacy comparable to GABA) or antagonists at the GABA binding site of these receptors seem not to exhibit a significant receptor subtype selectivity (Adkins *et al.*, 2001; Ebert *et al.*, 1994; Luddens and Korpi, 1995). In addition, the use of these compounds is associated with severe side effects. Full GABA agonists that open all GABA$_A$ receptor associated chloride channels indiscriminately, cause inhibition of most neuronal systems, thus severely interfering with the function of the brain, whereas GABA antagonists precipitate anxiety and convulsions.

However, several partial agonists at the GABA binding site of GABA$_A$ receptors, such as imidazole-4-acetic acid, piperidine-4-sulfonic acid, THIP (4,5,6,7-tetrahydroisoxazolo[5,4-c]pyridin-3-ol), or 4-PIOL (5-(4-piperidyl) isoxazol-3-ol), have been developed that exhibit some receptor subtype-dependent potency and efficacy (Frolund *et al.*, 2002). Thus, THIP (Fig. 1, compound 3) is approximately 10 times more potent at $\alpha4\beta3\delta$ than at $\alpha4\beta3\gamma2S$ receptors. This compound, which is currently developed as Gaboxadol, also seems to exhibit a highly interesting spectrum of *in vivo* actions. For instance, it seems to have potent analgesic effects comparable to that of morphine and seems to improve the quality of sleep (Krogsgaard-Larsen *et al.*, 2004). The full spectrum of pharmacological actions of THIP at different $GABA_A$ receptor subtypes, however, has still not been investigated.

## B. Benzodiazepine Binding Site of $GABA_A$ Receptors

Benzodiazepines, such as diazepam (Fig. 1, compound 4), are the strongest anticonvulsive, muscle relaxant, sedative-hypnotic, and anxiolytic compounds in clinical use (Woods *et al.*, 1992). They enhance the action of GABA on $GABA_A$ receptors by increasing the GABA-induced frequency of opening of the chloride channels (Study and Barker, 1981) and thus, allosterically modulate these receptors. Benzodiazepines and compounds interacting with the benzodiazepine site of $GABA_A$ receptors only can modulate ongoing GABAergic activity. These compounds cannot elicit chloride ion flux in the absence of GABA (Macdonald and Olsen, 1994; Study and Barker, 1981) and thus, exhibit an extremely low degree of toxicity.

Mutagenesis studies have identified several amino acid residues on $\alpha$ and $\gamma 2$ subunits of recombinant $GABA_A$ receptors that seem to be important for binding of benzodiazepines and compounds interacting with the benzodiazepine binding site (Sigel, 2002). It thus was concluded that the benzodiazepine binding site of $GABA_A$ receptors is located at the interface of an $\alpha$ and a $\gamma 2$ subunit.

### *1. Agonists, Antagonists, Inverse Agonists*

Many different classes of compounds interact with the benzodiazepine binding site of $GABA_A$ receptors (Adkins *et al.*, 2001; Atack, 2005; Huang *et al.*, 2000; Korpi *et al.*, 2002; Sieghart, 1995; Teuber *et al.*, 1999). In each of these classes, compounds could be identified that enhanced or reduced the action of GABA on $GABA_A$ receptors. Compounds that enhance the actions of GABA are called allosteric "agonists." These compounds exhibit anxiolytic, anticonvulsant, muscle relaxant, and sedative-hypnotic effects. Compounds that allosterically reduce GABA-induced chloride flux are called "inverse agonists." These compounds have actions opposite to those of "agonists": they are anxiogenic, proconvulsant, enhance vigilance, learning, and memory and are called "inverse agonists." A third class of compounds obviously stabilizes a conformational state that does not directly change GABA-induced chloride flux. These compounds in most cases do not elicit behavioral effects on their own but prevent interaction of "agonists" or "inverse agonists" with these receptors. They are therefore called allosteric "antagonists" (Sieghart, 1995).

The efficacy of compounds for eliciting such effects can be different. Thus, in addition to full agonists or full inverse agonists exhibiting a maximum enhancement or reduction of GABAergic currents, respectively, there are compounds with weaker actions (partial agonists or partial inverse agonists).

The agonist or inverse agonist efficacy of a compound usually is distinct in different receptor subtypes. Thus, a compound can be a "full agonist" at one type of receptor and exhibit different degrees of "partial agonist" activity at other receptor subtypes (Barnard *et al.*, 1998; Hevers and Luddens, 1998; Puia *et al.*, 1991; Wafford *et al.*, 1993). It is even possible that the efficacy of a compound reverses direction at different receptor subtypes: a compound can be a "partial agonist" at one receptor and be an "antagonist" or "partial inverse agonist" at another receptor subtype (Hevers and Luddens, 1998; Puia *et al.*, 1991; Wafford *et al.*, 1993). This explains, for instance, the different spectrum of actions of various clinically used benzodiazepines. Although compounds, such as diazepam, clonazepam, or bromazepam, exhibit a comparable affinity for all $GABA_A$ receptor subtypes composed of $\alpha1\beta\gamma2$, $\alpha2\beta\gamma2$, $\alpha3\beta\gamma2$, or $\alpha5\beta\gamma2$ subunits, their efficacy at individual receptor subtypes is different (Hevers and Luddens, 1998), thus generating their specific anxiolytic, anticonvulsant, muscle relaxant, and sedative-hypnotic activity spectrum (Woods *et al.*, 1992).

### 2. Heterogeneity of the Benzodiazepine Binding Site of $GABA_A$ Receptors

Most of the receptor subtype-selective compounds so far identified interact with the benzodiazepine binding site of $GABA_A$ receptors. Since this site is located at the interface of $\alpha$ and $\gamma$ subunits, its binding properties are influenced by the types of the subunits forming this interface. Since there are 6 different $\alpha$ and 3 different $\gamma$ subunits in the mammalian nervous system, up to 18 different $GABA_A$ receptor-associated benzodiazepine binding sites may exist. Most compounds interacting with the benzodiazepine binding site are inactive or only weakly active at receptors containing $\gamma1$ subunits (Hevers and Luddens, 1998; Puia *et al.*, 1991). Although there seems to be some activity of benzodiazepine ligands at receptors containing $\gamma3$ subunits (Hevers and Luddens, 1998), these receptors exhibit a very low abundance in the brain (Pirker *et al.*, 2000). Thus, the currently prescribed benzodiazepines and most of the structurally unrelated compounds interacting with the benzodiazepine binding site of $GABA_A$ receptors mediate their effects predominantely by interacting with $GABA_A$ receptors composed of $\alpha1\beta\gamma2$, $\alpha2\beta\gamma2$, $\alpha3\beta\gamma2$, or $\alpha5\beta\gamma2$ subunits.

Receptors composed of $\alpha4\beta\gamma2$ or $\alpha6\beta\gamma2$ subunits exhibit a drastically different pharmacology. Most of the classical benzodiazepines, such as diazepam, flunitrazepam, or clonazepam, do not interact with these receptors (Hevers and Luddens, 1998; Sieghart, 1995; Wafford *et al.*, 1996). Imidazobenzodiazepines, such as Ro15–4513 or flumazenil, however, interact with these receptors but also with $\alpha1\beta\gamma2$, $\alpha2\beta\gamma2$, $\alpha3\beta\gamma2$, or $\alpha5\beta\gamma2$ receptors (Huang *et al.*, 2000; Sieghart, 1995; Zhang *et al.*, 1995). Since the selectivity of new compounds aimed to address $\alpha4\beta\gamma2$ or $\alpha6\beta\gamma2$ receptors is only weak (Gu *et al.*, 1993; Huang *et al.*, 2000; Knoflach *et al.*, 1996;

Wong *et al.*, 1993; Zhang *et al.*, 1995), the behavioral effects mediated by these receptors are not known.

### 3. Benzodiazepine Site Ligands with Some $GABA_A$ Receptor Subtype Selectivity

Since most of the benzodiazepine site ligands modulate $\alpha1\beta\gamma2$, $\alpha2\beta\gamma2$, $\alpha3\beta\gamma2$, or $\alpha5\beta\gamma2$ receptors to a more or less similar extent, it is no surprise that the clinical spectrum of action of these compounds is quite similar (Woods *et al.*, 1992). Only some of the drugs in current use, such as the sedative/hypnotic compound zolpidem (Fig. 1, compound 5), exhibit a selectivity for $\alpha1$ subunit containing receptors (Hevers and Luddens, 1998; Sieghart, 1995).

Due to the clinical importance of benzodiazepine-type drugs, a tremendous effort was put into the development of receptor subtype-selective drugs. During the last few years, compounds were developed with a preferential affinity for $\alpha2/\alpha3$, or $\alpha5$ subunit-containing receptors (Huang *et al.*, 1999, 2000; Li *et al.*, 2003; Liu *et al.*, 1996; Quirk *et al.*, 1996; Teuber *et al.*, 1999; Zhang *et al.*, 1995). However, drugs with a selective affinity do not necessarily exhibit a selective efficacy for the respective receptor subtype. Therefore, functional effects of compounds as measured by electrophysiological techniques or fluorescence imaging technologies using voltage sensitive dyes (Adkins *et al.*, 2001; Gonzalez and Tsien, 1997; Gonzalez *et al.*, 1999) in cells expressing recombinant $GABA_A$ receptor subtypes are currently used for developing of compounds with a receptor subtype-selective action.

Such approaches have led to the identification of compounds such as the triazolo[4,3-b]pyridazine L-838,417 (Fig. 2, compound 1), a benzodiazepine site ligand with high affinity to $\alpha1$, $\alpha2$, $\alpha3$, and $\alpha5$ subunit-containing receptors. This compound, however, acts as a partial agonist on $\alpha2$, $\alpha3$, and $\alpha5$-containing receptors and does not enhance the GABA response on $\alpha1$ receptors (McKernan *et al.*, 2000). In animal models, this compound exhibited nonsedating anxiolytic properties, and this also seems to hold true for studies in nonhuman primates (Rowlett *et al.*, 2005).

The compound SL651.498 (Fig. 2, compound 2) exhibits high affinity for receptors containing $\alpha1$ or $\alpha2$ subunits but 10 times lower affinity for receptors containing $\alpha5$ subunits (Griebel *et al.*, 2003). Nevertheless it behaves as a full agonist at recombinant $GABA_A$ receptors containing $\alpha2$ or $\alpha3$ subunits and as a partial agonist at recombinant $GABA_A$ receptors containing $\alpha1$ or $\alpha5$ subunits. SL651.498 produced anxiolytic-like and skeletal muscle relaxant effects similar to those of benzodiazepines but with drastically reduced side effects (Griebel *et al.*, 2003; Licata *et al.*, 2005).

In another attempt, a tricyclic pyridone (Fig. 2, compound 3) with functional selectivity for the $\alpha3$ over the $\alpha1$ containing subtype has been

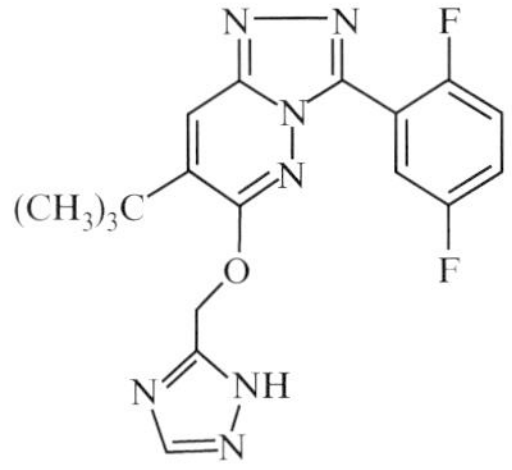

**FIGURE 2** Novel benzodiazepine binding site ligands with selective efficacy for certain $GABA_A$ receptor subtypes.

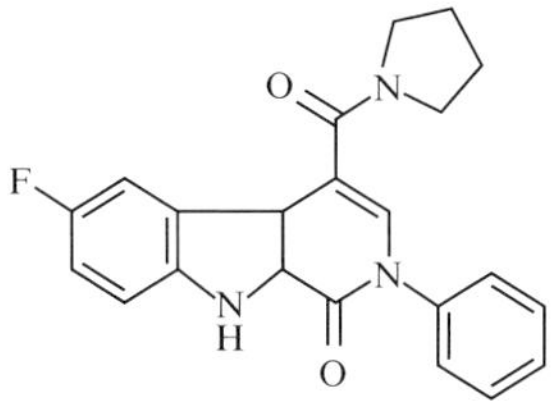

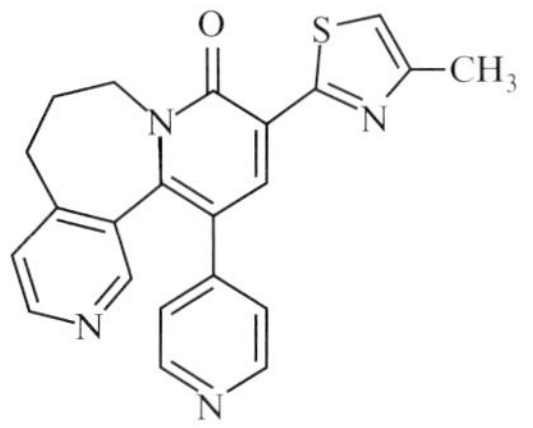

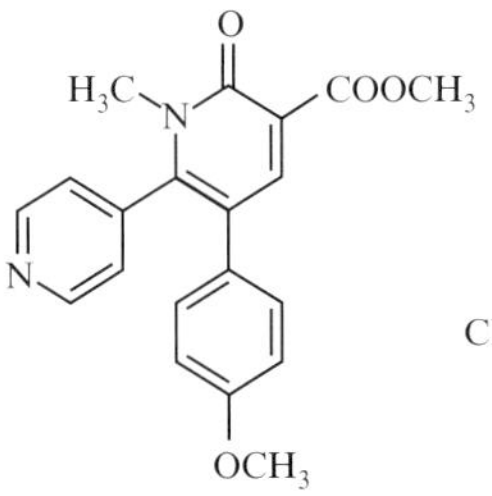

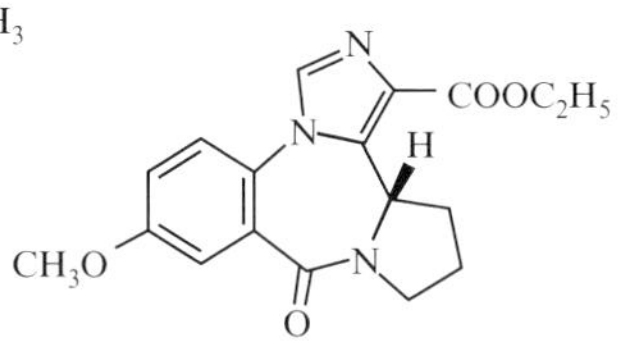

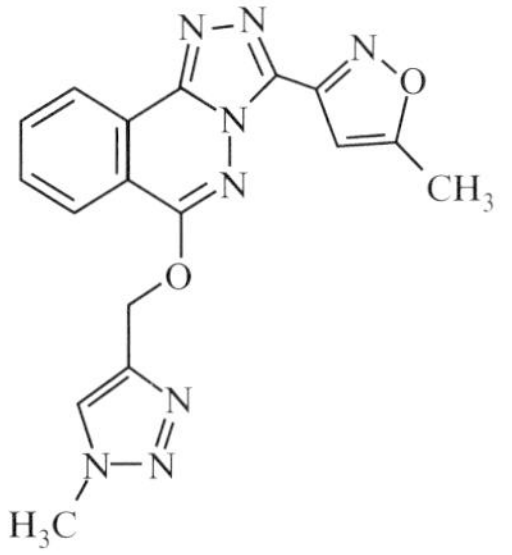

developed that was efficacious in animal models of anxiety and showed no sedation or potentiation of ethanol effects (Crawforth *et al.*, 2004). A compound in the related 3-heteroaryl-2-pyridone class (Fig. 2, compound 4) (Collins *et al.*, 2002) was a selective inverse agonist at α3-containing receptors with minimal efficacy at the α1- and α2-containing receptors. When evaluated in animal models, this compound was found to be anxiogenic, suggesting an important role for α3-containing $GABA_A$ receptors in anxiety (Atack *et al.*, 2005; Whiting, 2003).

Evidence indicated that it is possible to also develop compounds with selective efficacy for α5-containing $GABA_A$ receptors. FG 8094/L-655.708 (Fig. 2, compound 5) was one of the first such compounds developed. It exhibited an affinity for α5 receptors that was 50-fold higher than that to α2 or α3 receptors, 100-fold higher than that to α1, and 200-fold higher than that to α6 receptors (Teuber *et al.*, 1999). This compound acts as a partial inverse agonist on α5-containing receptors (Sternfeld *et al.*, 2004) and its tentative use for cognition enhancement (see later) has been patented. Two other compounds, one of them compound 6 (Fig. 2) (Chambers *et al.*, 2002, 2003; Sternfeld *et al.*, 2004), have been developed with partial inverse agonist properties for α5 receptors but little or no efficacy at other receptor subtypes (Chambers *et al.*, 2002, 2003; Sternfeld *et al.*, 2004). In agreement with the notion that α5-containing receptors might influence learning and memory (see in a later section) these compounds enhance cognition in animals without anxiogenic and convulsive effects (Chambers *et al.*, 2002, 2003; Sternfeld *et al.*, 2004).These data clearly indicate the potential utility of such compounds as cognitive enhancers in disorders such as mild cognitive impairment and Alzheimer's disease.

#### *4. Interaction of Benzodiazepine Site Ligands with Other GABA$_A$ Receptor Binding Sites*

In addition to their interaction with the benzodiazepine binding site located at the α/γ interface of GABA$_A$ receptors, at least some benzodiazepines or benzodiazepine site ligands can also interact with binding sites present on receptors composed of α and β subunits, only (Im *et al.*, 1995, 1998; Khom *et al.*, 2006; Thomet *et al.*, 1999; Walters *et al.*, 2000). Such interactions so far have not been studied extensively and seem to be of low affinity. It can be expected, however, that more thorough investigation of these sites will identify benzodiazepine site ligands with high affinity for these sites and that the properties of the respective binding sites will differ depending on the type of α and β subunits present in the receptors. In addition, receptors composed of αβδ (Hanchar *et al.*, 2005) also seem to be able to bind certain benzodiazepine binding site ligands with high affinity.

## C. TBPS-Binding Site of GABA$_A$ Receptors

TBPS (Fig. 1, compound 6) and picrotoxinin are convulsants that noncompetitively block GABA-gated chloride flux by binding to one or more sites located within or close to the chloride channel (Korpi *et al.*, 2002). The majority of electrophysiological experiments have been performed with picrotoxin, an equimolar mixture of the inactive picrotin and the active compound picrotoxinin, because picrotoxinin exhibits a rapid onset of action (Yoon *et al.*, 1993). TBPS exhibits a slow onset of action in electrophysiological experiments but is much better suited for receptor binding studies, where it exhibits a high affinity for the picrotoxinin binding site (Squires *et al.*, 1983). The fast onset of picrotoxinin inhibition on repetitive GABA application and the slow onset in the absence of GABA suggest that an open channel facilitates the actions of this compound (Inoue and Akaike, 1988). Binding of [$^{35}$S]TBPS can be competitively inhibited by picrotoxinin, pentylenetetrazole, and convulsant barbiturates (Maksay and Simonyi, 1985; Maksay and Ticku, 1985a,b) and presumably also by a variety of insecticides, such as lindane and dieldrin, or by bicyclic cage compounds such as the 4-propyl-4′-ethynylbicycloorthobenzoate EBOB (Korpi *et al.*, 2002).

In addition, binding of [$^{35}$S]TBPS can also be allosterically inhibited by GABA or GABA binding site agonists (Korpi *et al.*, 2002; Sieghart, 1995), in line with the assumption that not only [$^{35}$S]TBPS binding but also its unbinding is facilitated when the channel is open. $GABA_A$ receptor antagonists, such as bicuculline and SR 95531, inhibit these effects of GABA on [$^{35}$S]TBPS binding. Furthermore, compounds that are able to allosterically open the $GABA_A$ receptor associated chloride channel (e.g., barbiturates, etazolate, etomidate, and steroids, see later) are also able to reduce binding of TBPS (Sieghart, 1995). Benzodiazepines inhibited the binding of TBPS only in the presence of micromolar GABA concentrations, in line with the observation that benzodiazepines affect chloride ion conductance only in the presence of GABA. On the other hand, compounds reducing the efficacy of GABA at $GABA_A$ receptors (by reducing the frequency of opening of GABA-induced chloride channels), such as some convulsant $\beta$-carbolines, enhanced TBPS binding (Korpi *et al.*, 2002; Sieghart, 1995). These results are in line with the assumption that the high affinity TBPS binding site might be associated with the "closed" conformation of the chloride channel and might represent TBPS "trapped" in its binding site. In any case, the degree of TBPS binding in the presence of GABA seems to closely reflect the functional state of $GABA_A$ receptors.

## D. Interaction of Barbiturates with $GABA_A$ Receptors

Sedative-hypnotic barbiturates, such as pentobarbital (Fig. 3A, compound 1), phenobarbital, or secobarbital in electrophysiological studies, enhance the actions of GABA by increasing the average channel open duration but have no effect on channel conductance or opening frequency (Study and Barker, 1981). The effects of barbiturates on $GABA_A$ receptors rank in order with their potency as anesthetics (Olsen, 1982) indicating that $GABA_A$ receptors are prime candidates in mediating these effects. At concentrations >50 μM barbiturates are able to directly open $GABA_A$ receptor-associated chloride channels in the absence of GABA (Hevers and Luddens, 1998; Korpi *et al.*, 2002; Sieghart, 1995), and at still higher concentrations they change desensitization of receptors, suggesting the existence of several sites of interaction of barbiturates with $GABA_A$ receptors (Sieghart, 1995). Due to the low affinity of barbiturates, the respective binding sites cannot be investigated directly by receptor binding studies. But sedative-hypnotic barbiturates allosterically enhance [$^3$H]GABA, [$^3$H]muscimol, or [$^3$H]flunitrazepam binding. In contrast to convulsant barbiturates, which allosterically enhance [$^{35}$S]TBPS binding, the sedative-hypnotic barbiturates and some related compounds, such as etomidate (Fig. 3A, compound 2) and etazolate (Fig. 3A, compound 3), seem to allosterically reduce [$^{35}$S]TBPS binding (Sieghart, 1995). These results indicate that the site of action of sedative-hypnotic barbiturates is different from that of GABA, benzodiazepines, or TBPS. Since the modulatory action of pentobarbital can be observed already in homo-oligomeric $GABA_A$ receptors composed of either $\alpha$, $\beta$, $\gamma$, or $\delta$

subunits (Sieghart, 1995), the binding site(s) probably are highly conserved between subunits. Whether etomidate or etazolate exhibit a similar mechanism of action currently is not known.

## E. Interaction of Steroids with GABA$_A$ Receptors

Several steroids, such as the anesthetic alphaxalone (Fig. 3A, compound 4) or the sedative-hypnotic, anxiolytic, and anticonvulsant 3$\alpha$-hydroxylated, 5$\alpha$-, or 5$\beta$-reduced metabolites of progesterone (Fig. 3A, compound 5) and deoxycorticosterone at nM concentrations enhance GABA-stimulated chloride conductance, whereas at >1 μM concentrations these compounds, like barbiturates, produce direct opening of the GABA$_A$

A

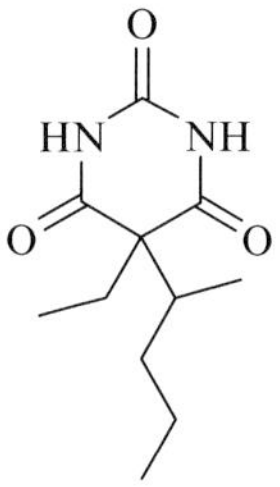

Pentobarbital (1)

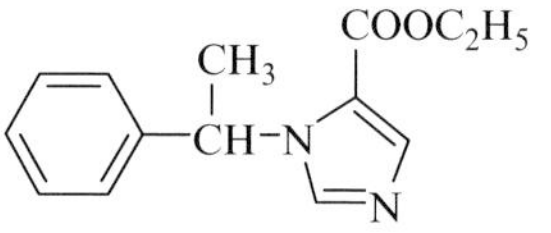

Etomidate (2)

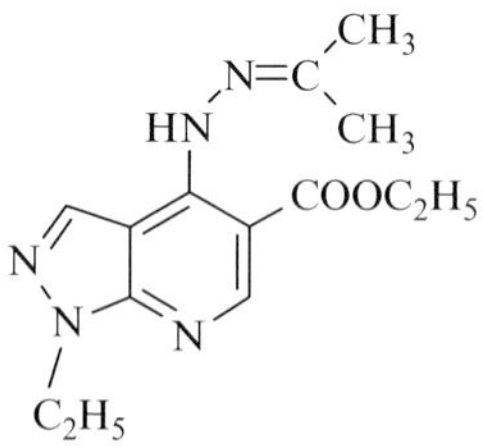

Etazolate (3)

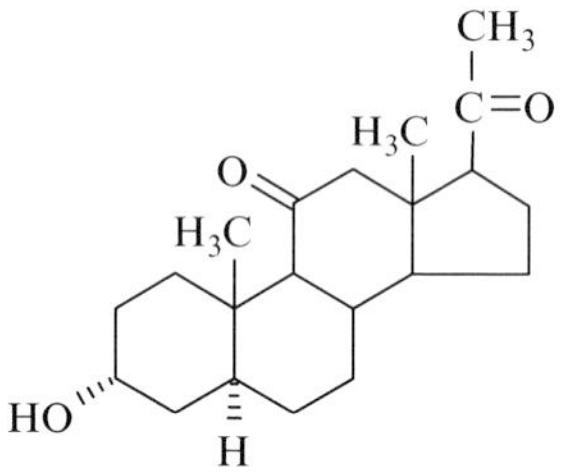

Alphaxalone (4)

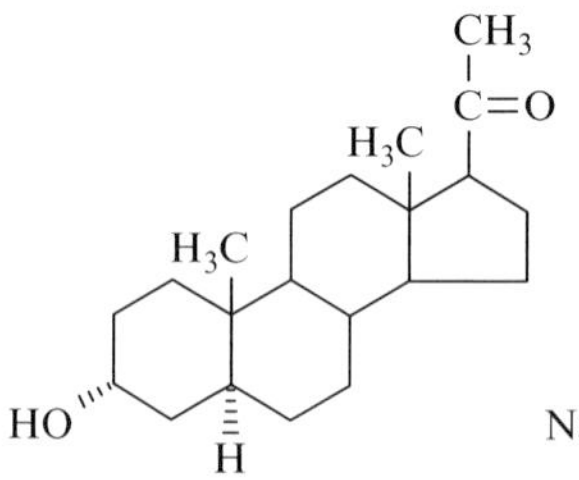

3$\alpha$-OH-5$\alpha$-Pregnane-20-one (5)

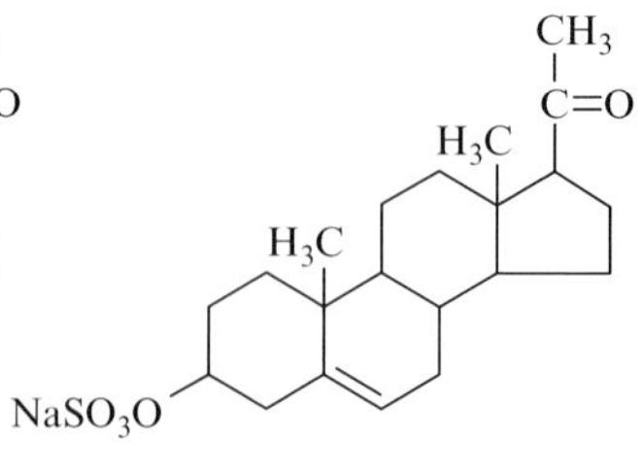

Pregnenolone sulfate (6)

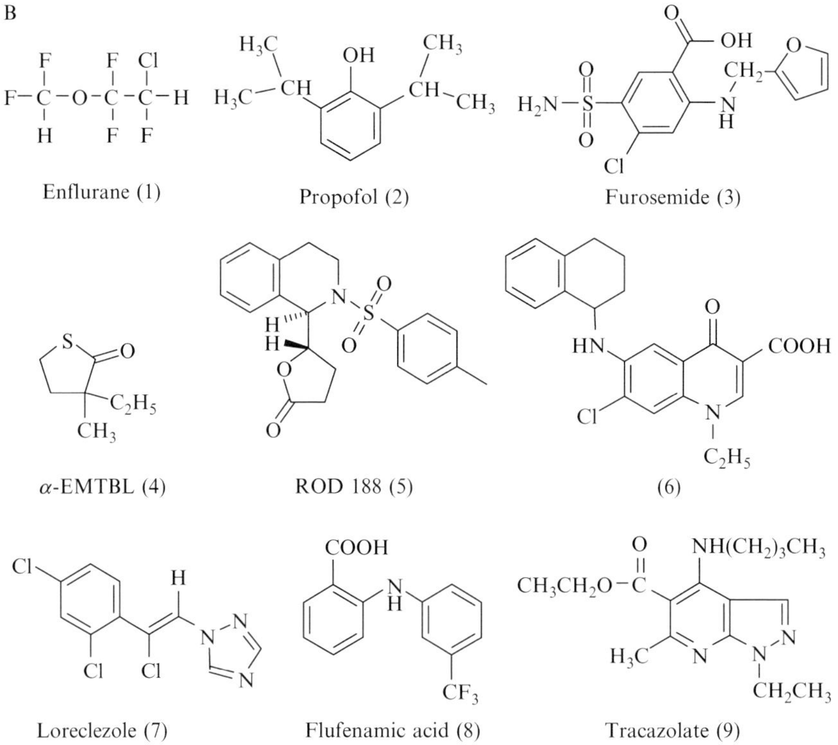

B

Enflurane (1) Propofol (2) Furosemide (3)

α-EMTBL (4) ROD 188 (5) (6)

Loreclezole (7) Flufenamic acid (8) Tracazolate (9)

**FIGURE 3** (A and B) Allosteric modulators of $GABA_A$ receptors acting via allosteric binding sites distinct from the benzodiazepine binding site.

receptor-associated chloride channel (Belelli and Lambert, 2005; Lambert *et al.*, 1995, 2001; Sieghart, 1995). This points to the existence of at least two different steroid binding sites on $GABA_A$ receptors. Steroids active at the $GABA_A$ receptor increase both the frequency and the duration of chloride channel opening (Peters *et al.*, 1988). These steroids enhance [$^3$H]muscimol and [$^3$H]flunitrazepam binding and allosterically reduce [$^{35}$S]TBPS binding. Other experiments indicate that steroids interact with barbiturates in a manner inconsistent with competition with a common binding site (Sieghart, 1995). Together, these experiments provided evidence for a site of action of steroids distinct from the binding sites for GABA, benzodiazepines, barbiturates, and TBPS. The stereoselective action and nM affinity of steroids suggest the existence of a high affinity steroid binding site rather than an unspecific membrane interaction of steroids (Belelli and Lambert, 2005; Lambert *et al.*, 2001; Sieghart, 1995).

The location of the steroid binding sites on $GABA_A$ receptors currently is not known.

In addition to steroids that enhance the actions of GABA on $GABA_A$ receptors, other steroids, such as pregnenolone sulfate (Fig. 3A, compound 6) and dehydroepiandrosterone (DHEAS), act as noncompetitive antagonist at these receptors. These compounds inhibit GABA-induced currents and exhibit excitatory actions on neurons (Lambert *et al.*, 2001; Sieghart, 1995). It is not clear whether the site of action of these two compounds is identical and whether they are interacting with the same binding site(s) as steroids that enhance the action of GABA on $GABA_A$ receptors.

Most studies have indicated that neither potency nor efficacy of neuroactive steroids appear to depend significantly on the subunit composition of receptors (Belelli and Lambert, 2005; Lambert *et al.*, 2001). This conclusion is supported by the finding that neuroactive steroids can modulate homo-oligomeric receptors composed of $\beta$ subunits (Sieghart, 1995) and thus, neither $\alpha$ nor $\gamma$ subunits seem to be necessary for the interaction of steroids with $GABA_A$ receptors. Nevertheless, electrophysiological studies have demonstrated that neurosteroids act differentially at synaptic $GABA_A$ receptors in different brain regions. Whether this heterogeneity is the result of the expression of distinct $GABA_A$ receptor subtypes or is caused by other factors, such as phosphorylation or local steroid metabolism (Belelli and Lambert, 2005; Lambert *et al.*, 2001; Pinna *et al.*, 2000), is not clear.

Evidence, however, seems to indicate that neurosteroids especially stimulate $GABA_A$ receptors such as extrasynaptic $\delta$-containing receptors (Stell *et al.*, 2003). A major role of $\delta$ subunit containing receptors for steroid action is also supported by the observation that the effects of neuroactive steroids are greatly reduced in mice lacking the $\delta$ subunit (Mihalek *et al.*, 1999).

## F. Interaction of Anesthetics with $GABA_A$ Receptors

In addition to the anesthetic steroids, barbiturates, and related compounds, such as etomidate and etazolate mentioned previously, a variety of volatile and other intravenous anesthetics from different chemical classes modulate the $GABA_A$ receptor (Franks and Lieb, 1994; Rudolph and Antkowiak, 2004; Sieghart, 1995). Thus, the volatile anesthetics isoflurane, enflurane (Fig. 3B, compound 1), or halothane at high micromolar or low millimolar concentrations, or the general anesthetics chlormethiazole or propofol (Fig. 3B, compound 2) at low micromolar concentrations enhance GABA-gated chloride currents. At high concentrations these compounds, like barbiturates and steroids, directly open $GABA_A$ receptor associated chloride channels, and these currents can be blocked by picrotoxinin and are sensitive to the competitive GABA antagonist bicuculline (Hevers and

Luddens, 1998; Sieghart, 1995). The anesthetic binding site of GABA$_A$ receptors seems to depend on the type of $\beta$ subunit present in these receptors. Its location, however, has not been unequivocally identified (see in a later section), and it is not clear whether the various anesthetics including barbiturates and steroids mediate their effects via the same or different binding sites. In addition to their interaction with GABA$_A$ receptors, they also affect glutamate and nACh receptors (Franks and Lieb, 1994; Hevers and Luddens, 1998). But GABA$_A$ receptors are the prime candidates for mediating the anesthetic effects of these substances *in vivo*.

## G. Interaction of Other Compounds with GABA$_A$ Receptors

### 1. Interactions Influenced by the Type of $\alpha$ Subunits

*a. Furosemide and Amiloride* Several compounds have been identified that seem to interact with novel, so far unidentified binding sites that are modulated by the type of $\alpha$ subunit present in GABA$_A$ receptors. Thus, for instance, the diuretic furosemide (Fig. 3B, compound 3) exhibits approximately a 100-fold selectivity for $\alpha$6- over $\alpha$1-containing receptors (Korpi *et al.*, 1995). This compound not only blocks $\alpha$6 receptors but also (with less affinity) $\alpha$4 receptors (Knoflach *et al.*, 1996; Korpi and Luddens, 1997). Similarly, the diuretic amiloride (Fisher, 2002) acted as antagonist of GABA$_A$ receptors in an $\alpha$ subunit dependent way by reducing the sensitivity of the receptor to GABA without affecting the maximal current amplitude. In contrast to furosemide, which in addition showed some $\beta$-subunit dependence (see in a later section), amiloride showed no additional dependence on the identity of $\beta$ or $\gamma$ subunits (Fisher, 2002). Its structure could thus be useful for developing drugs targeting this unique modulatory site on GABA$_A$ receptors.

*b. $\gamma$-Butyrolactones* The actions of $\gamma$-butyrolactones, such as $\alpha$-EMTBL (Fig. 3B, compound 4), also seem to be influenced by the $\alpha$ subunit type (El Hadri *et al.*, 2002; Mathews *et al.*, 1994). It was demonstrated that GABA-responses in $\alpha1\beta2\gamma2$-transfected cells or early granule neurons from the cerebellum were potentiated by $\gamma$-butyrolactones whereas those in $\alpha6\beta2\gamma2$ transfected cells or mature granule neurons were not significantly altered (Mathews *et al.*, 1994).

*c. ROD 188* (+)-ROD188 (Fig. 3B, compound 5) shares structural similarity with bicuculline (Razet *et al.*, 2000; Sigel *et al.*, 2001; Thomet *et al.*, 2000) and allosterically stimulated GABA-induced currents in $\alpha1\beta2\gamma2$ and $\alpha1\beta2$ receptors. This indicated that the respective binding site does not require a $\gamma$ subunit. In addition, the effect of this compound was larger in α6 subunit-containing $GABA_A$ receptors (Sigel *et al.*, 2001; Thomet *et al.*, 2000).

*d. Structural Analog of the Fluoroquinolone Antibiotic Norfloxacin* A structural analog of the fluoroquinolone antibiotic norfloxacin was identified (Fig. 3B, compound 6) (Johnstone *et al.*, 2004) that potentiated submaximal GABA currents in HEK-293 cells expressing human α2β2γ2L but not α1β2γ2L $GABA_A$ receptors. This compound seemed to modulate $GABA_A$ receptors via a novel binding site not identical with the sites for TBPS, GABA, benzodiazepines, barbiturates, neuroactive steroids, norfloxacine, or loreclezole and induced anxiolytic effects with a maximum efficacy comparable to the optimal effect of diazepam. Unlike diazepam, however, this compound had no CNS depressant effects in the range of doses tested (Johnstone *et al.*, 2004). Unfortunately, the action of this interesting compound on other receptor subtypes so far has not been investigated.

### 2. Interactions Influenced by the Type of β Subunits

*a. Loreclezole, Etomidate, DMCM, Furosemide* It is widely accepted that the type of the β subunit present in a $GABA_A$ receptor does not significantly influence the GABA, benzodiazepine, barbiturate, propofol, or steroid site pharmacologies of human $GABA_A$ receptor subtypes composed of αβγ subunits (Hadingham *et al.*, 1993; Smith *et al.*, 2004). However, a number of modulators of the $GABA_A$ receptor, for example loreclezole (Fig. 3B, compound 7) (Wafford *et al.*, 1994; Wingrove *et al.*, 1994), etomidate (Belelli *et al.*, 1997), the β-carboline DMCM (Stevenson *et al.*, 1995), or furosemide (Thompson *et al.*, 1999), have been identified that exhibit selectivity for β2/β3 over β1 receptors. In all cases, the potency of the modulator was reduced or abolished when an asparagine at the position 289 in human β2 and 290 in human β3, which is located within the TM2 region of the β subunit, was replaced by serine, (the homologous residue in β1). The replacement of the β1 subunits serine 290 by asparagine produced the converse effect.

*b. Salicylidene Salicylhydrazide* Salicylidene salicylhydrazide was one of the first compounds with a selectivity for receptors containing the β1 subunits (Thompson *et al.*, 2004). This compound partially and selectively inhibited GABA-activated chloride ion channels of β1-containing receptors, and it was demonstrated that mutation of either threonine 255 located within the TM1, or isoleucine 308 located extracellularly just prior to TM3 within the β1 subunit to the β2 counterpart was sufficient to abolish the inhibition (Thompson *et al.*, 2004). However, the converse individual mutations within the β2 subunit did not introduce any inhibition. Thus, different amino acid residues are important for conferring the β2/β3 and β1 selectivity of these compounds. It is not clear whether these residues are located close to the binding sites of these compounds or whether they only are important for transduction of the drug effects.

*c. Nonsteroidal Anti-inflammatory Agents* In a subsequent study, various anti-inflammatory agents including mefenamic acid, flufenamic acid (Fig. 3B, compound 8), meclofenamic acid, tolfenamic acid, niflumic acid, and diflunisal were investigated (Smith *et al.*, 2004). These compounds exhibited varying levels of efficacy and potency at $\beta 2$ or $\beta 3$ subunit-containing receptors, while having antagonist or weak inverse agonist profiles at $\beta 1$-containing receptors. So far, the influence of different $\alpha$ subunits on the effects of these anti-inflammatory agents has not yet been investigated. If such an influence is identified, compounds interacting with the respective binding site might very well be able to address certain $GABA_A$ receptor subtypes and might become lead compounds for the development of more selective compounds with higher affinity and efficacy.

### 3. *Interactions Modulated by Other Subunits*

*a. Tracazolate* The pyrazolopyridine tracazolate (Fig. 3B, compound 9) exhibits anxiolytic and anticonvulsant activity. Compared with the standard benzodiazepine chlordiazepoxide, it was 2 to 20 times less potent as an anxiolytic but interestingly displayed a much larger window of separation between the anxiolytic effect and potential side effects (sedation, motor incoordination, and its interaction with ethanol and barbital) (Patel *et al.*, 1985). It was demonstrated that tracazolate has a unique pharmacological profile on recombinant $GABA_A$ receptors: its potency ($EC_{50}$) is influenced by the nature of the $\beta$ subunit, but more importantly, its intrinsic efficacy, potentiation, or inhibition is determined by the nature of the third subunit ($\gamma$1–3, $\delta$, or $\epsilon$) within the receptor complex (Thompson *et al.*, 2002). The allosteric modulation induced by the binding site mediating the effects of tracazolate seems thus to be especially sensitive to the receptor subunit composition.

*b. Ethanol* Despite the fact that ethanol is the most widely-used psychoactive agent, its actions on brain functions are poorly understood. Several types of receptors and channels have been shown to be functionally altered by ethanol, which include glutamate, serotonin, glycine, and $GABA_A$ receptors and G-protein coupled inwardly rectifying $K^+$ channels (Wallner *et al.*, 2003). Ethanol effects on these targets are seen only at fairly high concentrations (above 60 mM). It was demonstrated that recombinant $\alpha 4\beta 3\delta$ and $\alpha 6\beta 3\delta$ $GABA_A$ receptors are reproducibly enhanced at 3 mM ethanol, a concentration six times lower than the legal blood-alcohol intoxication (driving) limit in most states (0.08% wt/vol or 17.4 mM). In contrast, ethanol required a more than 15-fold higher concentration for activation of $\alpha 4\beta 3\gamma 2$, $\alpha 6\beta 3\gamma 2$, or $\alpha 1\beta 2\gamma 2$ receptors (Wallner *et al.*, 2003). It thus seems unlikely that γ2-containing synaptic receptors are primary ethanol responders, but they might contribute to ethanol toxicity at high concentrations. Surprisingly, ethanol was ten-fold more effective on β3- than on β2-containing α4βδ and α6βδ receptors. Since these receptors presumably are located extrasynaptically, it is possible that ethanol at low concentrations primarily acts via extrasynaptic receptors composed of α4β3δ or α6β3δ (Sundstrom-Poromaa *et al.*, 2002; Wallner *et al.*, 2003 see also Boehm *et al.*, this volume).

*c. Other Compounds* A variety of other compounds, such as avermectin $B_1a$, Ro5-4864, PK8165, PK9084, PK11195, melatonin, polyamines, antidepressants, clozapine, dihydrogenated ergot compounds, carbamazepin, or phenytoin, to name only a few, have been identified that interact with $GABA_A$ receptors and are discussed in previous reviews (Hevers and Luddens, 1998; Korpi *et al.*, 2002; Sieghart, 1995). Similarly, divalent cations, such as $Zn^{2+}$, $Cd^{2+}$, $Ni^{2+}$, $Mn^{2+}$, and $Co^{2+}$, trivalent cations, such as $La^{3+}$ and lanthanides, and chloride ions are able to modulate $GABA_A$ receptors (Korpi *et al.*, 2002; Sieghart, 1995). Several binding sites for the divalent cations were identified on $GABA_A$ receptors (Fisher and Macdonald, 1998; Horenstein and Akabas, 1998; Hosie *et al.*, 2003).

## V. Function of $GABA_A$ Receptor Subtypes in the Brain

The large number of different $GABA_A$ receptor subtypes existing in the brain and the striking segregation of some of these subtypes in functionally different neuronal populations raise the possibility that a selective modulation of certain receptor subtypes will precipitate quite specific pharmacological effects and will make it possible to study the function of the respective receptors in the brain. So far, however, no pharmacological tools are available that can address a certain receptor subtype with a sufficiently high selectivity.

Attempts to investigate the function of $GABA_A$ receptor subtypes by generating mouse lines in which the genes for certain receptor subunits were inactivated did not yield clear-cut results due to adaptive changes in development and function of the brain caused by the lacking receptors (Rudolph and Mohler, 2004; Sieghart and Ernst, 2005). A combined molecular genetic and pharmacological approach (Rudolph *et al.*, 1999), however, for the first time provided information on the function of some major $GABA_A$ receptor subtypes. This approach was based on the introduction of a point mutation into specific α subunit-types of $GABA_A$ receptors that rendered the respective receptors insensitive to allosteric modulation by diazepam without significantly changing the function and distribution of these receptors. In these animals, therefore, those effects of diazepam normally mediated by the respective receptors are lost and can be identified by comparing diazepam effects in wild-type and mutated animals. Using this approach, it was demonstrated that $GABA_A$ receptors containing $\alpha 1$ subunits mediate the sedative, anterograde amnesic, and partly the anticonvulsant actions of diazepam (Crestani *et al.*, 2000; McKernan *et al.*, 2000; Rudolph *et al.*, 1999). These data are in line with the predominantly sedative effects of $\alpha 1$-selective compounds such as zolpidem (Crestani *et al.*, 2000).

Using a similar approach, it was demonstrated that receptors containing $\alpha 2$ subunits seem to mediate the anxiolytic, muscle relaxant, and hypnotic effects of diazepam, whereas $\alpha 3$-containing receptors seem to have a weak function in muscle relaxation (Rudolph and Mohler, 2004; Sieghart and Ernst, 2005). However, the observation that an inverse agonist selective for $\alpha 3$-containing receptors precipitates anxiety (Atack *et al.*, 2005) and that an agonist possibly selective for $\alpha 3$-containing receptors (Langen *et al.*, 2005) exhibits anxiolytic effects, strongly argues for an involvement of these receptors in anxiety (Wafford *et al.*, 2004; Whiting, 2003). Further experiments will have to clarify this discrepancy.

A point mutation that eliminates the interaction of diazepam with receptors containing $\alpha 5$ subunits seems to eliminate the memory impairing effects of diazepam (Crestani *et al.*, 2002; Yee *et al.*, 2004). Similarly, it was demonstrated that $\alpha 5$ subunit-deficient mice exhibit increased abilities in learning and memory tasks (Collinson *et al.*, 2002). This is in line with the observation that a selective partial inverse agonists of $GABA_A$ receptors containing $\alpha 5$ subunits exhibited cognition enhancing properties without exhibiting convulsant, proconvulsant, or anxiogenic activity (Chambers *et al.*, 2004).

An approach similar to that used for unraveling the function of $GABA_A$ receptors containing different $\alpha$ subunits was also used for studying the function of receptors containing different $\beta$ subunits. Thus, the point mutation $\beta 2$(Asn265Ser) that renders $\beta 2$ subunit-containing $GABA_A$ receptors less selective to the intravenous anesthetic etomidate (Belelli *et al.*, 1997; Hill-Venning *et al.*, 1997) was introduced into the $\beta 2$ subunit gene of a mouse (Reynolds *et al.*, 2003). As with the histidine mutations in the $\alpha$ subunits, this single amino acid switch is also effectively silent with regards to normal GABAergic function, but receptors containing this mutation no longer were sensitive to the sedative, ataxic, and hypothermic effects of etomidate. This indicates that these effects are mediated by receptors containing the $\beta 2$ subunit. This point mutation, however, did not impair the anesthetic effects of etomidate indicating that these effects are mediated via receptors containing other $\beta$ subunits.

The equivalent mutation $\beta 3$(Asn265Met) in the $\beta 3$ subunit of mice has also been generated, and experiments indicated that the righting reflex after etomidate is profoundly affected in this mouse. In addition, the anesthetic effect of etomidate was abolished by this point mutation (Jurd *et al.*, 2003). These results indicate that the $\beta 3$-containing receptors are the primary mediators of the anesthetic effects of etomidate.

## VI. GABA$_A$ Receptor Structure

The GABA$_A$ receptor is a member of the superfamily of pentameric ligand-gated ion channels that also includes the nACh receptor, the 5-hydroxytryptamine type 3 receptor, and the glycine receptor. So far, no receptor belonging to this superfamily has been characterized structurally by X-ray crystallography. In 2001, however, the X-ray crystallographic structure of a soluble remote homolog of the N-terminal domain of nACh receptor subunits, the acetylcholine binding protein (AChBP), has been published (Brejc *et al.*, 2001). This protein forms homopentamers that resemble the nACh receptor extracellular domain. Its crystal structure, featuring a novel fold of modified immunoglobuline-like topology, was then used to construct comparative models of the extracellular domain of other superfamily members including the GABA$_A$ receptor (Ernst *et al.*, 2003). Modeling a pentameric receptor extracellular domain consisting of two $\alpha$, two $\beta$, and one $\gamma$ subunit results in a single (absolute) subunit arrangement (Fig. 4) in which amino acid residues known to contribute to ligand bindig sites and interfaces are correctly positioned in the respective subunits (Ernst *et al.*, 2003).

As has been established previously, there are two binding pockets for GABA in GABA$_A$ receptors, formed at the extracellular interface between adjacent $\alpha$ and $\beta$ subunits. The pockets are formed by six so-called "loops," termed loop A, B, and C of the $\beta$ subunit at the plus (principle) side and D, E,

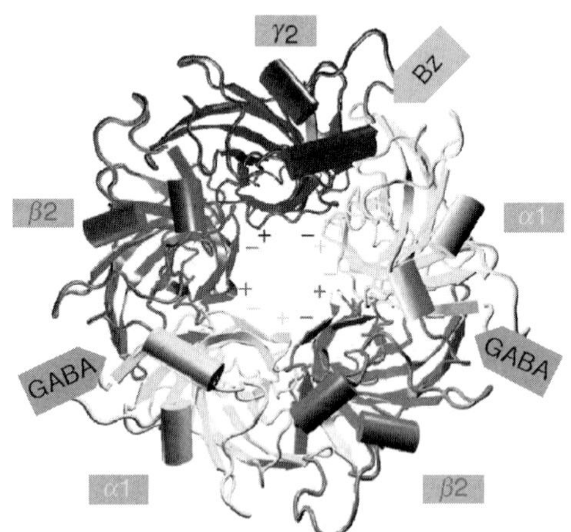


**FIGURE 4** Model structure of GABA$_A$ receptor extracellular domains. The absolute arrangement for $\alpha 1$, $\beta 2$, and $\gamma 2$-containing GABA$_A$ receptors is shown, view from the extracellular site. The + and − sides of the subunits are identified on the inner circumference of the channel. Labels indicate the interfaces at which the benzodiazepine binding site or the two GABA binding sites are located. Taken from Ernst *et al.* (2003), with permission. (See Color Insert.)

and F of the $\alpha$ subunit at the minus (complementary) side (Ernst *et al.*, 2003). It should be noted that this terminology has been established for the ligand-binding segments of pentameric ligand-gated ion channel prior to the publication of the AChBP crystal structure, and not all of them are loops in the structural sense.

The same picture of a pocket framed by the "loops" also emerged for the binding site of benzodiazepine ligands, which is localized in the extracellular domain at the $\alpha$–$\gamma$ interface, and thus consists of loops A, B, and C of the $\alpha$ subunit and loops D and E of the $\gamma$ subunit (Ernst *et al.*, 2003). These three-dimensional (3D) models of the binding sites have nicely confirmed what has been suspected on the basis of mutagenesis experiments and have been used to some degree to attempt docking studies of selected ligands (Kucken *et al.*, 2003). The homology between $GABA_A$ receptors and AChBP is too low, however, to expect that subtype differences in the binding sites will be modeled properly, but the models can be used as good guides for the overall architecture of the binding sites. For instance, the 3D arrangement of the "loops" narrows down on choices for possible subsites of agonistic and antagonistic substances (Ernst *et al.*, 2003).

Following the release of the AChBP structure, cryo-EM images of the electric fish organ nACh receptor in the open and closed state (Unwin, 1995) have been analyzed by fitting the core of the AChBP X-ray structure into the two sets of EM-density maps (Unwin *et al.*, 2002). The ACh-bound state turned out to be pseudosymmetrical, with all subunits in the conformation that corresponds with the HEPES bound conformation of AChBP subunits. The ACh-free (resting) state, on the other hand, was found to be conformationally asymmetrical. The extracellular domain of the two $\alpha$ subunits, which form the plus sides of the ACh pockets is in a conformation distinct from the $\beta$, $\gamma$, and $\delta$ subunits extracellular domain (Unwin *et al.*, 2002).

The cryo-EM atomic structure of the transmembrane domain of the nACh receptor in the resting state was published in 2003 (Miyazawa *et al.*, 2003) consisting of five bundles of four $\alpha$-helices. Shortly thereafter, a first model combining the extracellular and transmembrane domains of the nACh receptor has been discussed (Unwin, 2003), which later was published in a refined version and released with the protein data bank identifier 2BG9 (Unwin, 2005). Thus, the structure of the combined extracellular and transmembrane domains of the nACh receptors can now also be used as a template to model the corresponding structures of the $GABA_A$ receptor.

Such studies have been performed (Ernst *et al.*, 2005), providing important information on the overall organization of the extracellular and transmembrane domain of $GABA_A$ receptors. The structure (1OED; PDB, http://www.rcsb.org/pdb/) of the nAChR transmembrane fragments in the resting state, and thus, also that of the $GABA_A$ receptor and of other members of the superfamily, is loosely packed suggesting that the interface between subunits of this receptor family contains additional "cavities" beyond the ones found extracellularly (Ernst *et al.*, 2005; Sieghart and Ernst, 2005). These are located at the junction between the extracellular and "transmembrane" domain (the latter is not entirely inserted in the membrane) and extend into the subunit junction inside the lipid bilayer (Fig. 5). In some models, these cavities of the helical domain appear to communicate with their extracellular counterparts (Ernst *et al.*, 2005). Thus, it might be that the interface between subunits contains a continuous groove that might allow conformational mobility of the receptor but could also provide multiple independent binding sites.

Another type of cavity is found to be contained inside each of the subunits (Fig. 5), surrounded by the four helices that make up the transmembrane domain (Ernst *et al.*, 2005; Sieghart and Ernst, 2005). These latter

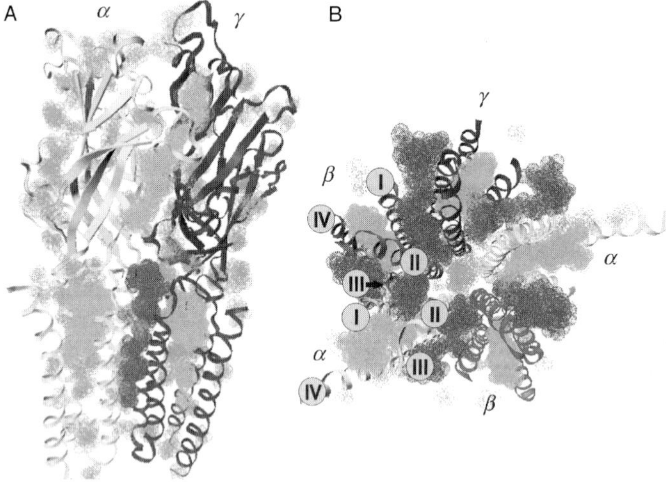


**FIGURE 5** Solvent-accessible space contained in $GABA_A$ receptor models. Two views of a $GABA_A$ receptor model are shown to illustrate the pockets found by pocket-finding algorithms. The left view shows a dimer from the outside of the pore, the right view is from extracellular, with the $\beta$-folded domain invisible. The protein is shown in ribbon representation, the putative pockets identified with PASS are shown in dotted space filling representation. Clusters of connected solvent accessible volumes that may correspond to drug binding pockets are highlighted by colors: pink for the space associated with the subunit-interface of the $\beta$-folded domain, purple for the large cavity present at the subunit interface at the junction between the $\beta$-folded and the helical domain that extends into the interface of the helical domains, and green for the cavity that is present inside each of the four-helix bundles that form the helical domain of each subunit. Additional smaller clusters are shown in pale gray. It should be noted that because of the high uncertainty in side-chain positions, the total volume, shape, and electrostatic properties of the pockets varies considerably among models; in some models some of the pockets may even be missing. Within the uncertainty of the method, it is also possible that there is significant communication between "pink" and "purple" as well as between "green" and "purple pockets." For this illustration, a representative model was used whose properties correspond to what the majority of models display. Figure was taken from Ernst *et al.* (2005), *Mol. Pharmacol.* 68, 1291–1300, with permission. (See Color Insert.)

cavities are also found in models based on unrelated proteins (Bertaccini and Trudell, 2001), and those formed by the $\alpha$ subunits are thought to correspond to the long-proposed "anesthetic pockets" for the volatile anesthetics that are defined by a serine residue in the TM2 of the $\alpha$ subunit (Nishikawa *et al.*, 2002).

Altogether, the qualitative features of this structure go well with what is known about the structure of this domain in various receptors. Due to alignment ambiguities in two of the helical segments, however, certain specific interpretations of homology models based on the nAChR structure are still subject to debate (Lobo *et al.*, 2004). Using multiple alignments and proper interpretation of chemical restraints, such as hydrophobic packing, however, a favored alignment could be selected that agrees with a number of additional experimental observations (Ernst *et al.*, 2005). The loose packing of the four-helix bundle seen in structures of the transmembrane domain of the nACh receptor (Unwin, 2005) also explains the high accessibility of individual amino acid residues in the putative transmembrane helices (Akabas, 2004; Williams and Akabas, 2002) that was observed in studies using the substituted cysteine accessibility method (SCAM) and was originally interpreted as evidence against a helical transmembrane motif (Cascio, 2004). In addition, the observed conformational flexibility (Akabas, 2004) in this domain also is very consistent with a loosely packed highly mobile structure.

The occurrence of multiple pockets at subunit interfaces as well as "inside" of the four-helix bundle of individual subunits explains the large number of proposed "separate" allosterically interacting modulatory sites discussed previously. Depending on the functional state of the receptors, drugs might be able to bind into one or several of these pockets and by that stabilize or induce distinct conformations of the receptor that finally cause a change in chloride flux. Mutagenesis studies have already identified several segments that are essential for the action of certain modulatory drugs and that can now be examined in the light of 3D models. For instance, the TM2 segment of the $\beta$ subunit, that is homologous to that of the $\alpha$ subunit, which contributes a serine residue to the putative volatile anesthetics pocket in $GABA_A$ receptors, is known to be responsible for the $\beta$-subtype selectivity of loreclezole, etomidate, and $\beta$-carboline action (see in an earlier section).

Loss or change of a drug effect on mutation in a segment that mediates subtype specific drug action could be due to drug binding or due to the segment being crucial for the transduction of the drug effect. This question can, at least in principle, be addressed by a combined approach of identifying pocket forming segments in structural models and subsequent mutagenesis and SCAM studies. For instance, $\beta$2Met286C has been shown to be protected by propofol from covalent modification by cystein reagents in a concentration-dependent manner, a strong hint toward a binding site near this residue (Bali and Akabas, 2004). In homology models of $GABA_A$ receptors, this residue indeed is part of a putative pocket (Ernst *et al.*, 2005).

The models of the $GABA_A$ receptor, thus, are not only consistent with most experimental data but could also explain experimental observations and propose the location of putative drug binding sites. These models can now be used to design new experiments for clarification of pharmacological and structural questions as well as for shedding light on conformational changes during binding of agonists, gating and allosteric modulation of these receptors. Overall, these experiments will lead to an improvement in the accuracy of the models and finally pave the way for a structure-based drug design.

## Acknowledgments

Work in the author's laboratory was supported by the Austrian Science Fund.

## References

Adkins, C. E., Pillai, G. V., Kerby, J., Bonnert, T. P., Haldon, C., McKernan, R. M., Gonzalez, J. E., Oades, K., Whiting, P. J., and Simpson, P. B. (2001). alpha4beta3delta $GABA_A$ receptors characterized by fluorescence resonance energy transfer-derived measurements of membrane potential. *J. Biol. Chem.* **276**, 38934–38939.

Akabas, M. H. (2004). $GABA_A$ receptor structure-function studies: A reexamination in light of new acetylcholine receptor structures. *Int. Rev. Neurobiol.* **62**, 1–43.

Arakawa, T., and Okada, Y. (1988). Excitatory and inhibitory action of GABA on synaptic transmission in slices of guinea pig superior colliculus. *Eur. J. Pharmacol.* **158**, 217–224.

Atack, J. R. (2005). The benzodiazepine binding site of $GABA_A$ receptors as a target for the development of novel anxiolytics. *Expert Opin. Investig. Drugs* **14**, 601–618.

Atack, J. R., Hutson, P. H., Collinson, N., Marshall, G., Bentley, G., Moyes, C., Cook, S. M., Collins, I., Wafford, K., McKernan, R. M., and Dawson, G. R. (2005). Anxiogenic properties of an inverse agonist selective for alpha3 subunit-containing $GABA_A$ receptors. *Br. J. Pharmacol.* **144**, 357–366.

Bali, M., and Akabas, M. H. (2004). Defining the propofol binding site location on the $GABA_A$ receptor. *Mol. Pharmacol.* **65**, 68–76.

Barnard, E. A., Skolnick, P., Olsen, R. W., Mohler, H., Sieghart, W., Biggio, G., Braestrup, C., Bateson, A. N., and Langer, S. Z. (1998). International Union of Pharmacology. XV. Subtypes of $\gamma$-aminobutyric $acid_A$ receptors: Classification on the basis of subunit structure and receptor function. *Pharmacol. Rev.* **50**, 291–313.

Baumann, S. W., Baur, R., and Sigel, E. (2002). Forced subunit assembly in alpha1beta2-gamma2 $GABA_A$ receptors: Insight into the absolute arrangement. *J. Biol. Chem.* **277**, 46020–46025.

Belelli, D., and Lambert, J. J. (2005). Neurosteroids: Endogenous regulators of the $GABA_A$ receptor. *Nat. Rev. Neurosci.* **6**, 565–575.

Belelli, D., Lambert, J. J., Peters, J. A., Wafford, K., and Whiting, P. J. (1997). The interaction of the general anesthetic etomidate with the gamma-aminobutyric acid type A receptor is influenced by a single amino acid. *Proc. Natl. Acad. Sci. USA* **94**, 11031–11036.

Berridge, K. C., and Pecina, S. (1995). Benzodiazepines, appetite, and taste palatability. *Neurosci. Biobehav. Rev.* **19**, 121–131.

Bertaccini, E., and Trudell, J. R. (2001). Molecular modeling of ligand-gated ion channels: Progress and challenges. *Int. Rev. Neurobiol.* **48**, 141–166.

Bormann, J. (2000). The 'ABC' of GABA receptors. *Trends Pharmacol. Sci.* **21**, 16–19.

Brejc, K., van Dijk, W. J., Klaassen, R. V., Schuurmans, M., van der Oost, J., Smit, A. B., and Sixma, T. K. (2001). Crystal structure of an ACh-binding protein reveals the ligand-binding domain of nicotinic receptors. *Nature* **411**, 269–276.

Burt, D. R., and Kamatchi, G. L. (1991). $GABA_A$ receptor subtypes: From pharmacology to molecular biology. *FASEB J.* **5**, 2916–2923.

Cascio, M. (2004). Structure and function of the glycine receptor and related nicotinicoid receptors. *J. Biol. Chem.* **279**, 19383–19386.

Chambers, M. S., Atack, J. R., Bromidge, F. A., Broughton, H. B., Cook, S., Dawson, G. R., Hobbs, S. C., Maubach, K. A., Reeve, A. J., Seabrook, G. R., Wafford, K., and MacLeod, A. M. (2002). 6,7-Dihydro-2-benzothiophen-4(5H)-ones: A novel class of $GABA_A$ alpha5 receptor inverse agonists. *J. Med. Chem.* **45**, 1176–1179.

Chambers, M. S., Atack, J. R., Broughton, H. B., Collinson, N., Cook, S., Dawson, G. R., Hobbs, S. C., Marshall, G., Maubach, K. A., Pillai, G. V., Reeve, A. J., and MacLeod, A. M. (2003). Identification of a novel, selective $GABA_A$ alpha5 receptor inverse agonist which enhances cognition. *J. Med. Chem.* **46**, 2227–2240.

Chambers, M. S., Atack, J. R., Carling, R. W., Collinson, N., Cook, S. M., Dawson, G. R., Ferris, P., Hobbs, S. C., O'Connor, D., Marshall, G., Rycroft, W., and Macleod, A. M. (2004). An orally bioavailable, functionally selective inverse agonist at the benzodiazepine site of $GABA_A$ alpha5 receptors with cognition enhancing properties. *J. Med. Chem.* **47**, 5829–5832.

Chang, Y., Wang, R., Barot, S., and Weiss, D. S. (1996). Stoichiometry of a recombinant $GABA_A$ receptor. *J. Neurosci.* **16**, 5415–5424.

Collins, I., Moyes, C., Davey, W. B., Rowley, M., Bromidge, F. A., Quirk, K., Atack, J. R., McKernan, R. M., Thompson, S. A., Wafford, K., Dawson, G. R., Pike, A., *et al.* (2002). 3-Heteroaryl-2-pyridones: Benzodiazepine site ligands with functional selectivity for alpha 2/alpha 3-subtypes of human $GABA_A$ receptor-ion channels. *J. Med. Chem.* **45**, 1887–1900.

Collinson, N., Kuenzi, F. M., Jarolimek, W., Maubach, K. A., Cothliff, R., Sur, C., Smith, A., Otu, F. M., Howell, O., Atack, J. R., McKernan, R. M., Seabrook, G. R., *et al.* (2002). Enhanced learning and memory and altered GABAergic synaptic transmission in mice lacking the alpha 5 subunit of the $GABA_A$ receptor. *J. Neurosci.* **22**, 5572–5580.

Cooper, S. J. (1989). Benzodiazepines and appetite: Recent pre-clinical advances and their clinical implications. *Human Psychopharmacol.* **4**, 81–89.

Crawforth, J., Atack, J. R., Cook, S. M., Gibson, K. R., Nadin, A., Owens, A. P., Pike, A., Rowley, M., Smith, A. J., Sohal, B., Sternfeld, F., Wafford, K., *et al.* (2004). Tricyclic pyridones as functionally selective human $GABA_A$ alpha 2/3 receptor-ion channel ligands. *Bioorg. Med. Chem. Lett.* **14**, 1679–1682.

Crestani, F., Martin, J. R., Mohler, H., and Rudolph, U. (2000). Mechanism of action of the hypnotic zolpidem *in vivo*. *Br. J. Pharmacol.* **131**, 1251–1254.

Crestani, F., Keist, R., Fritschy, J.-M., Benke, D., Vogt, K., Prut, L., Bluthmann, H., Mohler, H., and Rudolph, U. (2002). Trace fear conditioning involves hippocampal alpha5 $GABA_A$ receptors. *Proc. Natl. Acad. Sci. USA* **99**, 8980–8985.

Cutting, G. R., Lu, L., O'Hara, B. F., Kasch, L. M., Montrose-Rafizadeh, C., Donovan, D. M., Shimada, S., Antonarakis, S. E., Guggino, W. B., Uhl, G. R., and Kazazian, H. H., Jr. (1991). Cloning of the gamma-aminobutyric acid (GABA) rho 1 cDNA: A GABA receptor subunit highly expressed in the retina. *Proc. Natl. Acad. Sci. USA* **88**, 2673–2677.

Drew, C. A., Johnston, G. A., and Weatherby, R. P. (1984). Bicuculline-insensitive GABA receptors: Studies on the binding of (−)-baclofen to rat cerebellar membranes. *Neurosci. Lett.* **52**, 317–321.

Ebert, B., Wafford, K. A., Whiting, P. J., Krogsgaard-Larsen, P., and Kemp, J. A. (1994). Molecular pharmacology of gamma-aminobutyric acid type A receptor agonists and partial agonists in oocytes injected with different alpha, beta, and gamma receptor subunit combinations. *Mol. Pharmacol.* **46**, 957–963.

El Hadri, A., Abouabdellah, A., Thomet, U., Baur, R., Furtmuller, R., Sigel, E., Sieghart, W., and Dodd, R. H. (2002). N-Substituted 4-amino-3,3-dipropyl-2(3H)-furanones: New positive allosteric modulators of the $GABA_A$ receptor sharing electrophysiological properties with the anticonvulsant loreclezole. *J. Med. Chem.* **45**, 2824–2831.

Enz, R., and Cutting, G. R. (1998). Molecular composition of $GABA_C$ receptors. *Vision Res.* **38**, 1431–1441.

Ernst, M., Brauchart, D., Boresch, S., and Sieghart, W. (2003). Comparative modeling of $GABA_A$ receptors: Limits, insights, future developments. *Neuroscience* **119**, 933–943.

Ernst, M., Bruckner, S., Boresch, S., and Sieghart, W. (2005). Comparative models of $GABA_A$ receptor extracellular and transmembrane domains: Important insights in pharmacology and function. *Mol. Pharmacol.* **68**, 1291–1300.

Farrar, S. J., Whiting, P. J., Bonnert, T. P., and McKernan, R. M. (1999). Stoichiometry of a ligand-gated ion channel determined by fluorescence energy transfer. *J. Biol. Chem.* **274**, 10100–10104.

Fisher, J. L. (2002). Amiloride inhibition of gamma-aminobutyric acid(A) receptors depends upon the alpha subunit subtype. *Mol. Pharmacol.* **61**, 1322–1328.

Fisher, J. L., and Macdonald, R. L. (1998). The role of an alpha subtype M2-M3 His in regulating inhibition of $GABA_A$ receptor current by zinc and other divalent cations. *J. Neurosci.* **18**, 2944–2953.

Franks, N. P., and Lieb, W. R. (1994). Molecular and cellular mechanisms of general anaesthesia. *Nature* **367**, 607–614.

Fritschy, J. M., Benke, D., Mertens, S., Oertel, W. H., Bachi, T., and Mohler, H. (1992). Five subtypes of type A gamma-aminobutyric acid receptors identified in neurons by double and triple immunofluorescence staining with subunit-specific antibodies. *Proc. Natl. Acad. Sci. USA* **89**, 6726–6730.

Fritschy, J. M., Kiener, T., Bouilleret, V., and Loup, F. (1999). GABAergic neurons and $GABA_A$-receptors in temporal lobe epilepsy. *Neurochem. Int.* **34**, 435–445.

Frolund, B., Ebert, B., Kristiansen, U., Liljefors, T., and Krogsgaard-Larsen, P. (2002). $GABA_A$ receptor ligands and their therapeutic potentials. *Curr. Top. Med. Chem.* **2**, 817–832.

Gonzalez, J. E., and Tsien, R. Y. (1997). Improved indicators of cell membrane potential that use fluorescence resonance energy transfer. *Chem. Biol.* **4**, 269–277.

Gonzalez, J. E., Oades, K., Leychkis, Y., Harootunian, A., and Negulescu, P. A. (1999). Cell-based assays and instrumentation for screening ion-channel targets. *Drug. Discov. Today* **4**, 431–439.

Griebel, G., Perrault, G., Simiand, J., Cohen, C., Granger, P., Depoortere, H., Francon, D., Avenet, P., Schoemaker, H., Evanno, Y., Sevrin, M., George, P., *et al.* (2003). SL651498, a $GABA_A$ receptor agonist with subtype-selective efficacy, as a potential treatment for generalized anxiety disorder and muscle spasms. *CNS Drug Rev.* **9**, 3–20.

Gu, Z. Q., Wong, G., Dominguez, C., de Costa, B. R., Rice, K. C., and Skolnick, P. (1993). Synthesis and evaluation of imidazo[1,5-a][1,4]benzodiazepine esters with high affinities and selectivities at "diazepam-insensitive" benzodiazepine receptors. *J. Med. Chem.* **36**, 1001–1006.

Hadingham, K. L., Wingrove, P. B., Wafford, K. A., Bain, C., Kemp, J. A., Palmer, K. J., Wilson, A. W., Wilcox, A. S., Sikela, J. M., Ragan, C. I., and Whiting, P. J. (1993). Role of the beta subunit in determining the pharmacology of human gamma-aminobutyric acid type A receptors. *Mol. Pharmacol.* **44**, 1211–1218.

Hanchar, H. J., Chutsrinopkun, P., Meera, P., Supavilai, P., Sieghart, W., Wallner, M., and Olsen, R. W. (2006). Ethanol potently and competitively inhibits binding of the alcohol antagonist Ro 15–4513 to $\alpha_4/\alpha_6\beta_3\delta$ $GABA_A$ receptors. *Proc. Natl. Acad. Sci. USA* (in press).

Hartmann, K., Stief, F., Draguhn, A., and Frahm, C. (2004). Ionotropic GABA receptors with mixed pharmacological properties of $GABA_A$ and $GABA_C$ receptors. *Eur. J. Pharmacol.* **497**, 139–146.

Hevers, W., and Luddens, H. (1998). The diversity of $GABA_A$ receptors: Pharmacological and electrophysiological properties of $GABA_A$ channel subtypes. *Mol. Neurobiol.* **18**, 35–86.

Hill-Venning, C., Belelli, D., Peters, J. A., and Lambert, J. J. (1997). Subunit-dependent interaction of the general anaesthetic etomidate with the gamma-aminobutyric acid type A receptor. *Br. J. Pharmacol.* **120**, 749–756.

Horenstein, J., and Akabas, M. H. (1998). Location of a high affinity $Zn^{2+}$ binding site in the channel of alpha1beta1 gamma-aminobutyric acidA receptors. *Mol. Pharmacol.* **53**, 870–877.

Hosie, A. M., Aronstein, K., Sattelle, D. B., and ffrench-Constant, R. H. (1997). Molecular biology of insect neuronal GABA receptors. *Trends Neurosci.* **20**, 578–583.

Hosie, A. M., Dunne, E. L., Harvey, R. J., and Smart, T. G. (2003). Zinc-mediated inhibition of $GABA_A$ receptors: Discrete binding sites underlie subtype specificity. *Nat. Neurosci.* **6**, 362–399.

Huang, Q., Cox, E. D., Gan, T., Ma, C., Bennett, D. W., McKernan, R. M., and Cook, J. M. (1999). Studies of molecular pharmacophore/receptor models for $GABA_A$/benzodiazepine receptor subtypes: Binding affinities of substituted beta-carbolines at recombinant alpha x beta 3 gamma 2 subtypes and quantitative structure-activity relationship studies via a comparative molecular field analysis. *Drug Des. Discov.* **16**, 55–76.

Huang, Q., He, X., Ma, C., Liu, R., Yu, S., Dayer, C. A., Wenger, G. R., McKernan, R., and Cook, J. M. (2000). Pharmacophore/receptor models for $GABA_A$/BzR subtypes (alpha1beta3gamma2, alpha5beta3gamma2, and alpha6beta3gamma2) via a comprehensive ligand-mapping approach. *J. Med. Chem.* **43**, 71–95.

Im, H. K., Im, W. B., Carter, D. B., and McKinley, D. D. (1995). Interaction of beta-carboline inverse agonists for the benzodiazepine site with another site on $GABA_A$ receptors. *Br. J. Pharmacol.* **114**, 1040–1044.

Im, H. K., Im, W. B., Pregenzer, J. F., Stratman, N. C., VonVoigtlander, P. F., and Jacobsen, E. J. (1998). Two imidazoquinoxaline ligands for the benzodiazepine site sharing a second low affinity site on rat $GABA_A$ receptors but with the opposite functionality. *Br. J. Pharmacol.* **123**, 1490–1494.

Im, W. B., Pregenzer, J. F., Binder, J. A., Dillon, G. H., and Alberts, G. L. (1995). Chloride channel expression with the tandem construct of alpha 6-beta 2 $GABA_A$ receptor subunit requires a monomeric subunit of alpha 6 or gamma 2. *J. Biol. Chem.* **270**, 26063–26066.

Inoue, M., and Akaike, N. (1988). Blockade of gamma-aminobutyric acid-gated chloride current in frog sensory neurons by picrotoxin. *Neurosci. Res.* **5**, 380–394.

Izquierdo, I., and Medina, J. H. (1991). $GABA_A$ receptor modulation of memory: The role of endogenous benzodiazepines. *Trends Pharmacol. Sci.* **12**, 260–265.

Johnstone, T. B., Hogenkamp, D. J., Coyne, L., Su, J., Halliwell, R. F., Tran, M. B., Yoshimura, R. F., Li, W. Y., Wang, J., and Gee, K. W. (2004). Modifying quinolone antibiotics yields new anxiolytics. *Nat. Med.* **10**, 31–32.

Jurd, R., Arras, M., Lambert, S., Drexler, B., Siegwart, R., Crestani, F., Zaugg, M., Vogt, K. E., Ledermann, B., Antkowiak, B., and Rudolph, U. (2003). General anesthetic actions *in vivo* strongly attenuated by a point mutation in the $GABA_A$ receptor beta3 subunit. *FASEB J.* **17**, 250–252.

Khom, S., Baburin, I., Timin, E. N., Hohaus, A., Sieghart, W., and Hering, S. (2006). Pharmacological properties of $GABA_A$ receptors containing gamma1 subunits. *Mol. Pharmacol.* **69**, 640–649.

Knoflach, F., Benke, D., Wang, Y., Scheurer, L., Luddens, H., Hamilton, B. J., Carter, D. B., Mohler, H., and Benson, J. A. (1996). Pharmacological modulation of the diazepam-insensitive recombinant gamma-aminobutyric acidA receptors alpha 4 beta 2 gamma 2 and alpha 6 beta 2 gamma 2. *Mol. Pharmacol.* **50**, 1253–1261.

Korpi, E. R., and Luddens, H. (1997). Furosemide interactions with brain $GABA_A$ receptors. *Br. J. Pharmacol.* **120**, 741–748.

Korpi, E. R., Kuner, T., Seeburg, P. H., and Luddens, H. (1995). Selective antagonist for the cerebellar granule cell-specific gamma-aminobutyric acid type A receptor. *Mol. Pharmacol.* **47**, 283–289.

Korpi, E. R., Grunder, G., and Luddens, H. (2002). Drug interactions at $GABA_A$ receptors. *Prog. Neurobiol.* **67**, 113–159.

Krogsgaard-Larsen, P., Frolund, B., Liljefors, T., and Ebert, B. (2004). $GABA_A$ agonists and partial agonists: THIP (Gaboxadol) as a non-opioid analgesic and a novel type of hypnotic. *Biochem. Pharmacol.* **68**, 1573–1580.

Kucken, A. M., Teissere, J. A., Seffinga-Clark, J., Wagner, D. A., and Czajkowski, C. (2003). Structural requirements for imidazobenzodiazepine binding to $GABA_A$ receptors. *Mol. Pharmacol.* **63**, 289–296.

Lambert, J. J., Belelli, D., Hill-Venning, C., and Peters, J. A. (1995). Neurosteroids and $GABA_A$ receptor function. *Trends Pharmacol. Sci.* **16**, 295–303.

Lambert, J. J., Harney, S. C., Belelli, D., and Peters, J. A. (2001). Neurosteroid modulation of recombinant and synaptic $GABA_A$ receptors. *Int. Rev. Neurobiol.* **46**, 177–205.

Langen, B., Egerland, U., Bernoster, K., Dost, R., Unverferth, K., and Rundfeldt, C. (2005). Characterization in rats of the anxiolytic potential of ELB139 [1-(4-chlorophenyl)-4-piperidin-1-yl-1,5-dihydro-imidazol-2-on], a new agonist at the benzodiazepine binding site of the $GABA_A$ receptor. *J. Pharmacol. Exp. Ther.* **314**, 717–724.

Laurie, D. J., Seeburg, P. H., and Wisden, W. (1992). The distribution of 13 $GABA_A$ receptor subunit mRNAs in the rat brain. II. Olfactory bulb and cerebellum. *J. Neurosci.* **12**, 1063–1076.

Li, X., Cao, H., Zhang, C., Furtmueller, R., Fuchs, K., Huck, S., Sieghart, W., Deschamps, J., and Cook, J. M. (2003). Synthesis, *in vitro* affinity, and efficacy of a bis 8-ethynyl-4H-imidazo[1,5a]-[1,4]benzodiazepine analogue, the first bivalent alpha5 subtype selective BzR/$GABA_A$ antagonist. *J. Med. Chem.* **46**, 5567–5570.

Licata, S. C., Platt, D. M., Cook, J. M., Sarma, P. V., Griebel, G., and Rowlett, J. K. (2005). Contribution of $GABA_A$ receptor subtypes to the anxiolytic-like, motor, and discriminative stimulus effects of benzodiazepines: Studies with the functionally-selective ligand SL651498. *J. Pharmacol. Exp. Ther.* **313**, 1118–1125.

Liu, R., Hu, R. J., Zhang, P., Skolnick, P., and Cook, J. M. (1996). Synthesis and pharmacological properties of novel 8-substituted imidazobenzodiazepines: High-affinity, selective probes for alpha 5-containing $GABA_A$ receptors. *J. Med. Chem.* **39**, 1928–1934.

Lobo, I. A., Mascia, M. P., Trudell, J. R., and Harris, R. A. (2004). Channel gating of the glycine receptor changes accessibility to residues implicated in receptor potentiation by alcohols and anesthetics. *J. Biol. Chem.* **279**, 33919–33927.

Luddens, H., and Korpi, E. R. (1995). GABA antagonists differentiate between recombinant $GABA_A$/benzodiazepine receptor subtypes. *J. Neurosci.* **15**, 6957–6962.

Macdonald, R. L., and Olsen, R. W. (1994). $GABA_A$ receptor channels. *Annu. Rev. Neurosci.* **17**, 569–602.

Maksay, G., and Simonyi, M. (1985). Benzodiazepine anticonvulsants accelerate and beta-carboline convulsants decelerate the kinetics of [$^{35}$S]TBPS binding at the chloride ionophore. *Eur. J. Pharmacol.* **117**, 275–278.

Maksay, G., and Ticku, M. K. (1985a). GABA, depressants and chloride ions affect the rate of dissociation of $^{35}$S-t-butylbicyclophosphorothionate binding. *Life Sci.* **37**, 2173–2180.

Maksay, G., and Ticku, M. K. (1985b). Dissociation of [$^{35}$S]t-butylbicyclophosphorothionate binding differentiates convulsant and depressant drugs that modulate GABAergic transmission. *J. Neurochem.* **44**, 480–486.

Mathews, G. C., Bolos-Sy, A. M., Holland, K. D., Isenberg, K. E., Covey, D. F., Ferrendelli, J. A., and Rothman, S. M. (1994). Developmental alteration in $GABA_A$ receptor structure and physiological properties in cultured cerebellar granule neurons. *Neuron* **13**, 149–158.

McKernan, R. M., Rosahl, T. W., Reynolds, D. S., Sur, C., Wafford, K. A., Atack, J. R., Farrar, S., Myers, J., Cook, G., Ferris, P., Garrett, L., Bristow, L., *et al.* (2000). Sedative but not anxiolytic properties of benzodiazepines are mediated by the $GABA_A$ receptor alpha1 subtype. *Nat. Neurosci.* **3**, 587–592.

Mihalek, R. M., Banerjee, P. K., Korpi, E. R., Quinlan, J. J., Firestone, L. L., Mi, Z. P., Lagenaur, C., Tretter, V., Sieghart, W., Anagnostaras, S. G., Sage, J. R., Fanselow, M. S., *et al.* (1999). Attenuated sensitivity to neuroactive steroids in gamma-aminobutyrate type A receptor delta subunit knockout mice. *Proc. Natl. Acad. Sci. USA* **96**, 12905–12910.

Milligan, C. J., Buckley, N. J., Garret, M., Deuchars, J., and Deuchars, S. A. (2004). Evidence for inhibition mediated by coassembly of $GABA_A$ and $GABA_C$ receptor subunits in native central neurons. *J. Neurosci.* **24**, 7241–7250.

Miyazawa, A., Fujiyoshi, Y., and Unwin, N. (2003). Structure and gating mechanism of the acetylcholine receptor pore. *Nature* **423**, 949–955.

Nayeem, N., Green, T. P., Martin, I. L., and Barnard, E. A. (1994). Quaternary structure of the native $GABA_A$ receptor determined by electron microscopic image analysis. *J. Neurochem.* **62**, 815–818.

Nishikawa, K., Jenkins, A., Paraskevakis, I., and Harrison, N. L. (2002). Volatile anesthetic actions on the $GABA_A$ receptors: Contrasting effects of alpha 1(S270) and beta 2(N265) point mutations. *Neuropharmacology* **42**, 337–345.

Nutt, D. J., Glue, P., and Lawson, C. (1990). The neurochemistry of anxiety: An update. *Prog. Neuropsychopharmacol. Biol. Psychiatry* **14**, 737–752.

Olsen, R. W. (1982). Drug interactions at the GABA receptor-ionophore complex. *Annu. Rev. Pharmacol. Toxicol.* **22**, 245–277.

Olsen, R. W., and Avoli, M. (1997). GABA and epileptogenesis. *Epilepsia* **38**, 399–407.

Pan, Z. H., Zhang, D., Zhang, X., and Lipton, S. A. (2000). Evidence for coassembly of mutant $GABA_C$ rho1 with $GABA_A$ gamma2S, glycine alpha1 and glycine alpha2 receptor subunits *in vitro*. *Eur. J. Neurosci.* **12**, 3137–3145.

Patel, J. B., Malick, J. B., Salama, A. I., and Goldberg, M. E. (1985). Pharmacology of pyrazolopyridines. *Pharmacol. Biochem. Behav.* **23**, 675–680.

Paulsen, O., and Moser, E. I. (1998). A model of hippocampal memory encoding and retrieval: GABAergic control of synaptic plasticity. *Trends Neurosci.* **21**, 273–278.

Persohn, E., Malherbe, P., and Richards, J. G. (1992). Comparative molecular neuroanatomy of cloned $GABA_A$ receptor subunits in the rat CNS. *J. Comp. Neurol.* **326**, 193–216.

Peters, J. A., Kirkness, E. F., Callachan, H., Lambert, J. J., and Turner, A. J. (1988). Modulation of the $GABA_A$ receptor by depressant barbiturates and pregnane steroids. *Br. J. Pharmacol.* **94**, 1257–1269.

Pinna, G., Uzunova, V., Matsumoto, K., Puia, G., Mienville, J. M., Costa, E., and Guidotti, A. (2000). Brain allopregnanolone regulates the potency of the $GABA_A$ receptor agonist muscimol. *Neuropharmacology* **39**, 440–448.

Pirker, S., Schwarzer, C., Wieselthaler, A., Sieghart, W., and Sperk, G. (2000). $GABA_A$ receptors: Immunocytochemical distribution of 13 subunits in the adult rat brain. *Neuroscience* **101**, 815–850.

Pratt, J. A. (1992). The neuroanatomical basis of anxiety. *Pharmacol. Ther.* **55**, 149–181.

Puia, G., Vicini, S., Seeburg, P. H., and Costa, E. (1991). Influence of recombinant gamma-aminobutyric acid-A receptor subunit composition on the action of allosteric modulators of gamma-aminobutyric acid-gated Cl- currents. *Mol. Pharmacol.* **39**, 691–696.

Qian, H., and Ripps, H. (1999). Response kinetics and pharmacological properties of heteromeric receptors formed by coassembly of GABA rho- and gamma 2-subunits. *Proc. R. Soc. Lond. B. Biol. Sci.* **266**, 2419–2425.

Quirk, K., Blurton, P., Fletcher, S., Leeson, P., Tang, F., Mellilo, D., Ragan, C. I., and McKernan, R. M. (1996). [$^3$H]L-655,708, a novel ligand selective for the benzodiazepine site of $GABA_A$ receptors which contain the $\alpha5$ subunit. *Neuropharmacology* **35**, 1331–1335.

Razet, R., Thomet, U., Furtmuller, R., Chiaroni, A., Sigel, E., Sieghart, W., and Dodd, R. H. (2000). 5-[1′-(2′-N-Arylsulfonyl-1′,2′,3′,4′-tetrahydroisoquinolyl)]-4, 5-dihydro-2(3H)-furanones: Positive allosteric modulators of the $GABA_A$ receptor with a new mode of action. *J. Med. Chem.* **43**, 4363–4366.

Reynolds, D. S., Rosahl, T. W., Cirone, J., O'Meara, G. F., Haythornthwaite, A., Newman, R. J., Myers, J., Sur, C., Howell, O., Rutter, A. R., Atack, J., Macaulay, A. J., *et al.* (2003). Sedation and anesthesia mediated by distinct $GABA_A$ receptor isoforms. *J. Neurosci.* **23**, 8608–8617.

Rowlett, J. K., Platt, D. M., Lelas, S., Atack, J. R., and Dawson, G. R. (2005). Different $GABA_A$ receptor subtypes mediate the anxiolytic, abuse-related, and motor effects of benzodiazepine-like drugs in primates. *Proc. Natl. Acad. Sci. USA* **102**, 915–920.

Rudolph, U., and Antkowiak, B. (2004). Molecular and neuronal substrates for general anaesthetics. *Nat. Rev. Neurosci.* **5**, 709–720.

Rudolph, U., and Mohler, H. (2004). Analysis of $GABA_A$ receptor function and dissection of the pharmacology of benzodiazepines and general anesthetics through mouse genetics. *Annu. Rev. Pharmacol. Toxicol.* **44**, 475–498.

Rudolph, U., Crestani, F., Benke, D., Brunig, I., Benson, J. A., Fritschy, J. M., Martin, J. R., Bluethmann, H., and Mohler, H. (1999). Benzodiazepine actions mediated by specific gamma-aminobutyric acid(A) receptor subtypes. *Nature* **401**, 796–800.

Sarter, M., Schneider, H. H., and Stephens, D. N. (1988). Treatment strategies for senile dementia: Antagonist beta-carbolines. *Trends Neurosci.* **11**, 13–17.

Schofield, P. R., Darlison, M. G., Fujita, N., Burt, D. R., Stephenson, F. A., Rodriguez, H., Rhee, L. M., Ramachandran, J., Reale, V., Glencorse, T. A., Seeburg, P. H., and Barnard, E. A. (1987). Sequence and functional expression of the $GABA_A$ receptor shows a ligand-gated receptor super-family. *Nature* **328**, 221–227.

Schuske, K., Beg, A. A., and Jorgensen, E. M. (2004). The GABA nervous system in *C. elegans*. *Trends Neurosci.* **27**, 407–414.

Sieghart, W. (1995). Structure and pharmacology of $\gamma$-aminobutyric $acid_A$ receptor subtypes. *Pharmacol. Rev.* **47**, 181–234.

Sieghart, W., and Ernst, M. (2005). Heterogeneity of $GABA_A$ receptors: Revived interest in the development of subtype-selective drugs. *Curr. Med. Chem. Cent. Nerv. Syst. Agents* **5**, 217–242.

Sieghart, W., and Sperk, G. (2002). Subunit composition, distribution and function of $GABA_A$ receptor subtypes. *Curr. Top. Med. Chem.* **2**, 795–816.

Sigel, E. (2002). Mapping of the benzodiazepine recognition site on $GABA_A$ receptors. *Curr. Top. Med. Chem.* **2**, 833–839.

Sigel, E., and Buhr, A. (1997). The benzodiazepine binding site of $GABA_A$ receptors. *Trends Pharmacol. Sci.* **18**, 425–429.

Sigel, E., Baur, R., Furtmueller, R., Razet, R., Dodd, R. H., and Sieghart, W. (2001). Differential cross talk of ROD compounds with the benzodiazepine binding site. *Mol. Pharmacol.* **59**, 1470–1477.

Simon, J., Wakimoto, H., Fujita, N., Lalande, M., and Barnard, E. A. (2004). Analysis of the set of $GABA_A$ receptor genes in the human genome. *J. Biol. Chem.* **279**, 41422–41435.

Smith, A. J., Oxley, B., Malpas, S., Pillai, G. V., and Simpson, P. B. (2004). Compounds exhibiting selective efficacy for different beta subunits of human recombinant gamma-aminobutyric acid A receptors. *J. Pharmacol. Exp. Ther.* **311**, 601–609.

Smith, G. B., and Olsen, R. W. (1995). Functional domains of $GABA_A$ receptors. *Trends Pharmacol. Sci.* **16**, 162–168.

Somogyi, P., Tamas, G., Lujan, R., and Buhl, E. H. (1998). Salient features of synaptic organisation in the cerebral cortex. *Brain Res. Brain Res. Rev.* **26**, 113–135.

Sperk, G., Schwarzer, C., Tsunashima, K., Fuchs, K., and Sieghart, W. (1997). $GABA_A$ receptor subunits in the rat hippocampus I: Immunocytochemical distribution of 13 subunits. *Neuroscience* **80**, 987–1000.

Squires, R. F., Casida, J. E., Richardson, M., and Saederup, E. (1983). [35S]t-butylbicyclophosphorothionate binds with high affinity to brain-specific sites coupled to gamma-aminobutyric acid-A and ion recognition sites. *Mol. Pharmacol.* **23**, 326–336.

Stell, B. M., Brickley, S. G., Tang, C. Y., Farrant, M., and Mody, I. (2003). Neuroactive steroids reduce neuronal excitability by selectively enhancing tonic inhibition mediated by delta subunit-containing $GABA_A$ receptors. *Proc. Natl. Acad. Sci. USA* **100**, 14439–14444.

Sternfeld, F., Carling, R. W., Jelley, R. A., Ladduwahetty, T., Merchant, K. J., Moore, K. W., Reeve, A. J., Street, L. J., O'Connor, D., Sohal, B., Atack, J. R., Cook, S., *et al.* (2004). Selective, orally active gamma-aminobutyric acidA alpha5 receptor inverse agonists as cognition enhancers. *J. Med. Chem.* **47**, 2176–2179.

Stevenson, A., Wingrove, P. B., Whiting, P. J., and Wafford, K. A. (1995). beta-Carboline gamma-aminobutyric acidA receptor inverse agonists modulate gamma-aminobutyric acid via the loreclezole binding site as well as the benzodiazepine site. *Mol. Pharmacol.* **48**, 965–969.

Strata, F., and Cherubini, E. (1994). Transient expression of a novel type of GABA response in rat CA3 hippocampal neurones during development. *J. Physiol.* **480**(Pt 3), 493–503.

Study, R. E., and Barker, J. L. (1981). Diazepam and (–)-pentobarbital: Fluctuation analysis reveals different mechanisms for potentiation of gamma-aminobutyric acid responses in cultured central neurons. *Proc. Natl. Acad. Sci. USA* **78**, 7180–7184.

Sundstrom-Poromaa, I., Smith, D. H., Gong, Q. H., Sabado, T. N., Li, X., Light, A., Wiedmann, M., Williams, K., and Smith, S. S. (2002). Hormonally regulated alpha(4)beta (2)delta $GABA_A$ receptors are a target for alcohol. *Nat. Neurosci.* **5**, 721–722.

Teuber, L., Watjens, F., and Jensen, L. H. (1999). Ligands for the benzodiazepine binding site: A survey. *Curr. Pharm. Des.* **5**, 317–343.

Thomet, U., Baur, R., Scholze, P., Sieghart, W., and Sigel, E. (1999). Dual mode of stimulation by the beta-carboline ZK 91085 of recombinant $GABA_A$ receptor currents: Molecular determinants affecting its action. *Br. J. Pharmacol.* **127**, 1231–1239.

Thomet, U., Baur, R., Razet, R., Dodd, R. H., Furtmuller, R., Sieghart, W., and Sigel, E. (2000). A novel positive allosteric modulator of the $GABA_A$ receptor: The action of (+)-ROD188. *Br. J. Pharmacol.* **131**, 843–850.

Thompson, S. A., Arden, S. A., Marshall, G., Wingrove, P. B., Whiting, P. J., and Wafford, K. A. (1999). Residues in transmembrane domains I and II determine gamma-aminobutyric acid type A receptor subtype-selective antagonism by furosemide. *Mol. Pharmacol.* **55**, 993–999.

Thompson, S.-A., Wingrove, P. B., Connelly, L., Whiting, P. J., and Wafford, K. A. (2002). Tracazolate reveals a novel type of allosteric interaction with recombinant gamma-aminobutyric acid(A) receptors. *Mol. Pharmacol.* **61**, 861–869.

Thompson, S. A., Wheat, L., Brown, N. A., Wingrove, P. B., Pillai, G. V., Whiting, P. J., Adkins, C., Woodward, C. H., Smith, A. J., Simpson, P. B., Collins, I., and Wafford, K. A. (2004). Salicylidene salicylhydrazide, a selective inhibitor of beta 1-containing $GABA_A$ receptors. *Br. J. Pharmacol.* **142**, 97–106.

Tretter, V., Ehya, N., Fuchs, K., and Sieghart, W. (1997). Stoichiometry and assembly of a recombinant $GABA_A$ receptor subtype. *J. Neurosci.* **17**, 2728–2737.

Turek, F. W., and Van Reeth, O. (1988). Altering the mammalian circadian clock with the short-acting benzodiazepine, triazolam. *Trends Neurosci.* **11**, 535–541.

Unwin, N. (1995). Acetylcholine receptor channel imaged in the open state. *Nature* **373**, 37–43.

Unwin, N. (2003). Structure and action of the nicotinic acetylcholine receptor explored by electron microscopy. *FEBS Lett* **555**, 91–95.

Unwin, N. (2005). Refined structure of the nicotinic acetylcholine receptor at 4A resolution. *J. Mol. Biol.* **346**, 967–989.

Unwin, N., Miyazawa, A., Li, J., and Fujiyoshi, Y. (2002). Activation of the nicotinic acetylcholine receptor involves a switch in conformation of the [alpha] subunits. *J. Mol. Biol.* **319**, 1165–1176.

Wafford, K. A., Bain, C. J., Whiting, P. J., and Kemp, J. A. (1993). Functional comparison of the role of gamma subunits in recombinant human gamma-aminobutyric acidA/ benzodiazepine receptors. *Mol. Pharmacol.* **44**, 437–442.

Wafford, K. A., Bain, C. J., Quirk, K., McKernan, R. M., Wingrove, P. B., Whiting, P. J., and Kemp, J. A. (1994). A novel allosteric modulatory site on the $GABA_A$ receptor beta subunit. *Neuron* **12**, 775–782.

Wafford, K. A., Thompson, S. A., Thomas, D., Sikela, J., Wilcox, A. S., and Whiting, P. J. (1996). Functional characterization of human gamma-aminobutyric acidA receptors containing the alpha 4 subunit. *Mol. Pharmacol.* **50**, 670–678.

Wafford, K. A., Macaulay, A. J., Fradley, R., O'Meara, G. F., Reynolds, D. S., and Rosahl, T. W. (2004). Differentiating the role of gamma-aminobutyric acid type A ($GABA_A$) receptor subtypes. *Biochem. Soc. Trans.* **32**, 553–556.

Wagner, S., Castel, M., Gainer, H., and Yarom, Y. (1997). GABA in the mammalian suprachiasmatic nucleus and its role in diurnal rhythmicity. *Nature* **387**, 598–603.

Wallner, M., Hanchar, H. J., and Olsen, R. W. (2003). Ethanol enhances alpha 4 beta 3 delta and alpha 6 beta 3 delta gamma-aminobutyric acid type A receptors at low concentrations known to affect humans. *Proc. Natl. Acad. Sci. USA* **100**, 15218–15223.

Walters, R. J., Hadley, S. H., Morris, K. D., and Amin, J. (2000). Benzodiazepines act on $GABA_A$ receptors via two distinct and separable mechanisms. *Nat. Neurosci.* **3**, 1274–1281.

Whiting, P. J. (2003). The $GABA_A$ receptor gene family: New opportunities for drug development. *Curr. Opin. Drug. Discov. Devel.* **6**, 648–657.

Williams, D. B., and Akabas, M. H. (2002). Structural evidence that propofol stabilizes different $GABA_A$ receptor states at potentiating and activating concentrations. *J. Neurosci.* **22**, 7417–7424.

Wingrove, P. B., Wafford, K. A., Bain, C., and Whiting, P. J. (1994). The modulatory action of loreclezole at the gamma-aminobutyric acid type A receptor is determined by a single amino acid in the beta 2 and beta 3 subunit. *Proc. Natl. Acad. Sci. USA* **91**, 4569–4573.

Wisden, W., Laurie, D. J., Monyer, H., and Seeburg, P. H. (1992). The distribution of 13 $GABA_A$ receptor subunit mRNAs in the rat brain. I. Telencephalon, diencephalon, mesencephalon. *J. Neurosci.* **12**, 1040–1062.

Wong, G., Koehler, K. F., Skolnick, P., Gu, Z. Q., Ananthan, S., Schonholzer, P., Hunkeler, W., Zhang, W., and Cook, J. M. (1993). Synthetic and computer-assisted analysis of the structural requirements for selective, high-affinity ligand binding to diazepam-insensitive benzodiazepine receptors. *J. Med. Chem.* **36**, 1820–1830.

Woods, J. H., Katz, J. L., and Winger, G. (1992). Benzodiazepines: Use, abuse, and consequences. *Pharmacol. Rev.* **44**, 151–347.

Yee, B. K., Hauser, J., Dolgov, V. V., Keist, R., Mohler, H., Rudolph, U., and Feldon, J. (2004). GABA receptors containing the alpha5 subunit mediate the trace effect in aversive and appetitive conditioning and extinction of conditioned fear. *Eur. J. Neurosci.* 20, 1928–1936.

Yoon, K. W., Covey, D. F., and Rothman, S. M. (1993). Multiple mechanisms of picrotoxin block of GABA-induced currents in rat hippocampal neurons. *J. Physiol.* **464**, 423–439.

Zhang, W., Koehler, K. F., Zhang, P., and Cook, J. (1995). Development of a comprehensive pharmacophore model for the benzodiazepine receptor. Harwood Academic Publishers GmbH.

**Rasmus Prætorius Clausen*, Karsten Madsen†, Orla Miller Larsson†, Bente Frølund*, Povl Krogsgaard-Larsen*, and Arne Schousboe†**

*Department of Medicinal Chemistry
The Danish University of Pharmaceutical Sciences
2 Universitetsparken
DK-2100 Copenhagen, Denmark

†Department of Pharmacology and Pharmacotherapy
The Danish University of Pharmaceutical Sciences
DK-2100 Copenhagen, Denmark

# Structure–Activity Relationship and Pharmacology of $\gamma$-Aminobutyric Acid (GABA) Transport Inhibitors

## I. Chapter Overview

Intervention in transport of $\gamma$-aminobutyric acid (GABA) has for more than 3 decades been the aim of extensive research, and a very large number of transport inhibitors have been characterized. The group of GABA uptake inhibitors includes competitive substrate-related GABA analogs of low-molecular weight displaying great variance in pharmacological profile as well as inhibitors based on these substrate-related inhibitors but modified with lipophilic aromatic side chains. The latter display both competitive, mixed type and noncompetitive inhibition kinetics and are often highly GAT1 selective. While much is known about inhibition of the cloned GABA transporter GAT1 due to the existence of selective, potent, and blood–brain barrier penetrating GAT1 inhibitors, little is known about the role and therapeutic potential of the other transporter subtypes. Despite extensive variation in the lipophilic aromatic part of these inhibitors there

*Advances in Pharmacology, Volume 54* 1054-3589/06 $35.00

DOI: 10.1016/S1054-3589(06)54011-6

continues to be a need for potent and selective inhibitors of other transporter subtypes. However, compounds targeting GAT2/BGT-1 have recently appeared and *in vivo* administration of such compounds has pointed to an important role of this transporter subtype in seizure control. The inhibition kinetics of GABA uptake inhibitors has not been reported very thoroughly and is difficult to predict. Since the inhibition kinetics could affect the nature of GABA uptake intervention, such information will be of considerable interest.

## II. The GABAergic Synapses

GABAergic neurotransmission is the most abundant part of inhibitory neurotransmission in the central nervous system (CNS) and abnormalities in the GABAergic system have been linked to a number of CNS disorders, such as epilepsy, anxiety, sleep disorders, and pain (Lloyd and Morselli, 1987). Therefore, many of the key proteins involved in GABA neurotransmission have been the aim of extensive research with the ultimate purpose of finding new therapeutic possibilities. These key proteins include the GABA receptors, metabolic enzymes and transporters, and within all three protein classes the efforts continue to provide clinically relevant compounds.

The GABA neurotransmission event is terminated following vesicular release of GABA into the synapse and subsequent binding to receptors by uptake of GABA into the presynaptic nerve ending or surrounding astrocytes via high-affinity GABA transporters. Uptake into the GABAergic neuron allows reuse of GABA by vesicular uptake from the cytosol of the neuron. When transported into surrounding glia cells, GABA is metabolized via GABA-transaminase and subsequent oxidation to succinate, and it may be either fully oxidized or converted to glutamine which can reenter the neuron and ultimately regenerate GABA (Waagepetersen *et al.*, 2003). However, it is believed that the major fraction of the glial pathway leads to degradation of GABA instead of reuse (Schousboe *et al.*, 2004). The GABA transporters have been recognized as therapeutic targets since uptake inhibitors would slow down termination of neurotransmission thereby compensating for GABA hypoactivity (Schousboe *et al.*, 1983). This is believed to be the mechanism underlying the therapeutic beneficial effects in epileptic disorders of (*R*)-*N*-[4,4-bis(3-methyl-2-thienyl)but-3-en-1-yl]nipecotic acid (Tiagabine), the only GABA transport inhibitor that has been approved as a drug (Braestrup *et al.*, 1990). It has long been speculated that highly glia-selective compounds would present a therapeutic advantage (Schousboe *et al.*, 1983), given the degradative GABA pathway in glial cells, and this has been supported by the notion that inhibitors with higher potency at glial uptake are anticonvulsive while some selective neuronal inhibitors are proconvulsive (White *et al.*, 2002).

Although GABA uptake inhibitors have been primarily developed against epileptic disorders, there is increasing evidence that GABA transport inhibitors could be applied in other disorders. Thus, several studies indicate that GABA uptake inhibitors could be applied in the treatment of anxiety, abuse, and sleep disorders, and clinical trials probing the application of Tiagabine in these disorders are ongoing (Todorov *et al.*, 2005; Zwanzger and Rupprecht, 2005).

## III. Transporter Heterogeneity, Nomenclature, and Function

So far, five different GABA transporter subtypes with high affinity for GABA have been cloned. Apart from the vesicular GABA transporter the nomenclature of the remaining four transporters has been quite confusing (Table I). GAT1 is the same transporter in human, rat, and mouse, but the mouse GAT2 corresponds to the betaine/GABA transporter (BGT-1) in human and rat. Furthermore, mouse GAT3 and GAT4 are homologous to GAT2 and GAT3 in human and rat, respectively.

Although the nomenclature of man and rat seems more descriptive and straightforward, the mouse nomenclature will be used since much of the pharmacology described here has been characterized using cells expressing the mouse transporters.

The $K_M$ of GABA is approximately the same at GAT1, GAT3, and GAT4, whereas the $K_M$ at GAT2 is at least threefold higher (Bolvig *et al.*, 1999).

When the GAT1 transporter was cloned it was originally believed to be the neuronal transporter (Guastella *et al.*, 1990), whereas GAT3 and GAT4 were expected to account for glial transport (Borden *et al.*, 1992).

GAT1 is predominately expressed in presynaptic axons and to a lesser extent in distal astrocytic processes. GAT2 is located primarily in dendrites in extrasynaptic regions near glutamatergic neurons and also in the soma. GAT3 is expressed in the leptomeninges and distal astrocytic processes and the axons and dendrites of neurons primarily in extra-synaptic regions.

**TABLE I** Summary of Cloned GAT Subtypes from Different Species and Their Inter-species Homologs (Schousboe and Kanner, 2002)

| *Species* | *Nomenclature* | | | |
|---|---|---|---|---|
| Mouse | GAT1 | GAT2 | GAT3 | GAT4 |
| Human | GAT1 | BGT-1 | NC | GAT3 |
| Rat | GAT1 | BGT-1 | GAT2 | GAT3 |

NC, not cloned.

GAT4 is exclusively located to distal astrocytic processes within the synapses (Borden, 1996; Conti *et al.*, 1998, 1999, 2004; Durkin *et al.*, 1995; Minelli *et al.*, 1996; Pietrini *et al.*, 1994; Radian *et al.*, 1990; Zhu and Ong, 2004).

The mRNAs for GAT1 and GAT4 are, in general, differentially distributed within the brain between neurons and astrocytes. Based on results from Northern blot studies, GAT1 appears to be more abundant than GAT4 in the CNS (Durkin *et al.*, 1995). Although GAT3 is present in the cerebral cortex, GAT1 and GAT4 mediate the largest uptake of GABA (Conti *et al.*, 1998). The large and subtle differences in pharmacological, physiological, or subcellular localization that exist between the GABA transporter subtypes can have a profound effect on the fine tuning of extracellular GABA levels. These differences complicate the search for glia-selective compounds, and explain why this endeavor has not been very successful.

## IV. Structure–Activity Relationship of GABA Uptake Inhibitors

The GABA uptake inhibitors can be divided into two groups: (1) small substrate-related analogs of GABA and $\beta$-alanine (Fig. 1) and (2) GABA and $\beta$-alanine analogs containing aromatic lipophilic side chains (Fig. 2). This division based on the chemical structure reflects some important pharmacological differences.

### A. Substrate-Related Inhibitors

In general, the small-sized GABA analogs, such as nipecotic acid, (1*S*,3*R*)-3-aminocyclohexanecarboxylic acid (ACHC), and (*S*)-2,4-diaminobutyric acid (DABA), are competitive inhibitors that are often substrates (Schousboe *et al.*, 1983). They have been important pharmacological tools rather than therapeutic candidates since they are substrates and because they do not readily penetrate the blood–brain barrier (BBB) by passive diffusion owing to the high polarity at physiological pH. In a few cases, BBB penetration has been observed when there is a small ratio between the ionized (zwitterionic) and the unionized state of the compounds (I/U ratio) determined by the $pK_a$ difference between the basic amino and the acidic group (Krogsgaard-Larsen *et al.*, 1983, 2000).

The small-sized inhibitors have been a fruitful source for selective uptake inhibitors without receptor activity and inhibitors displaying variance in subtype and cellular pharmacological profiles (Table II). Following the initial discovery of a GABA transport system (Iversen and Neal, 1968), muscimol was recognized as an unselective naturally occurring GABA analog interacting with both GABA receptors and transporters but not metabolic enzymes. These interactions were separated by modifying the chemical

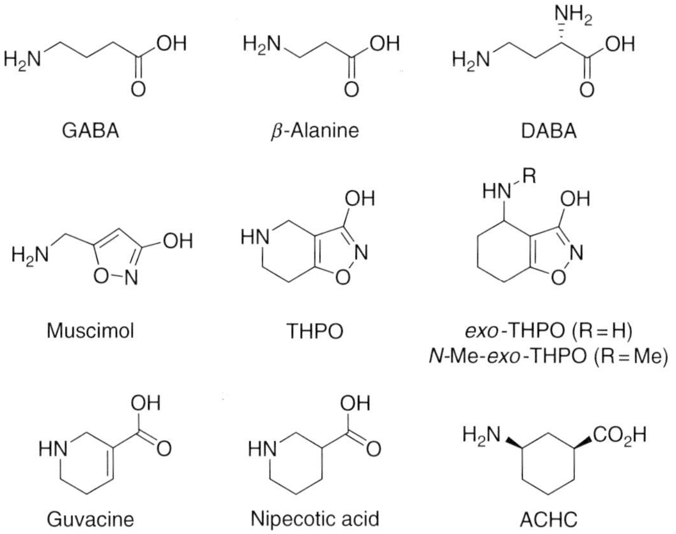

GABA $\beta$-Alanine DABA

Muscimol THPO *exo*-THPO (R = H) *N*-Me-*exo*-THPO (R = Me)

Guvacine Nipecotic acid ACHC

**FIGURE 1** Substrate-related GABA uptake inhibitors.

structure of muscimol into the rigid GABA analog 4,5,6,7-tetrahydroisothiazolo[5,4-*c*]pyridin-3-ol (THIP) and the equally rigid $\beta$-alanine analog 4,5,6,7-tetrahydroisoxazolo[4,5-*c*]pyridin-3-ol (THPO) (Krogsgaard-Larsen and Johnston, 1975; Krogsgaard-Larsen *et al.*, 2000). THIP, which is today known to be a super-agonist at $\delta$-subunit–containing $GABA_A$ receptors (Adkins *et al.*, 2001), was characterized as a specific receptor agonist with no measurable uptake inhibition (Krogsgaard-Larsen *et al.*, 1983), whereas THPO had essentially lost its affinity to the receptor binding site and displayed increased uptake inhibitory properties (Krogsgaard-Larsen *et al.*, 1975). The retro-bioisosteric conversion of the isoxazolol group into a carboxyl group enabled the discovery of two very potent substrate inhibitors of GABA uptake, namely nipecotic acid and guvacine (Krogsgaard-Larsen *et al.*, 1975) with no detectable GABA receptor affinity. Like muscimol, these two compounds are naturally occurring and have proven to be lead structures in the development of highly potent GABA uptake inhibitors.

The existence of at least two different transport systems was evidenced very early by the complementary substrate inhibitory effects of DABA/ACHC and $\beta$-alanine, reflecting the neuronal and glial transport systems, respectively (Iversen and Kelly, 1975; Neal and Bowery, 1977). A highly glia-selective compound was discovered by further modification of THPO. Moving the amino group of THPO to an *exo*-cyclic position gives 3-hydroxy-4-amino-4,5,6,7-tetrahydro-1,2-benzisoxazole (*exo*-THPO), and within a small series of *N*-alkylated *exo*-THPO derivatives, the mono-methylated

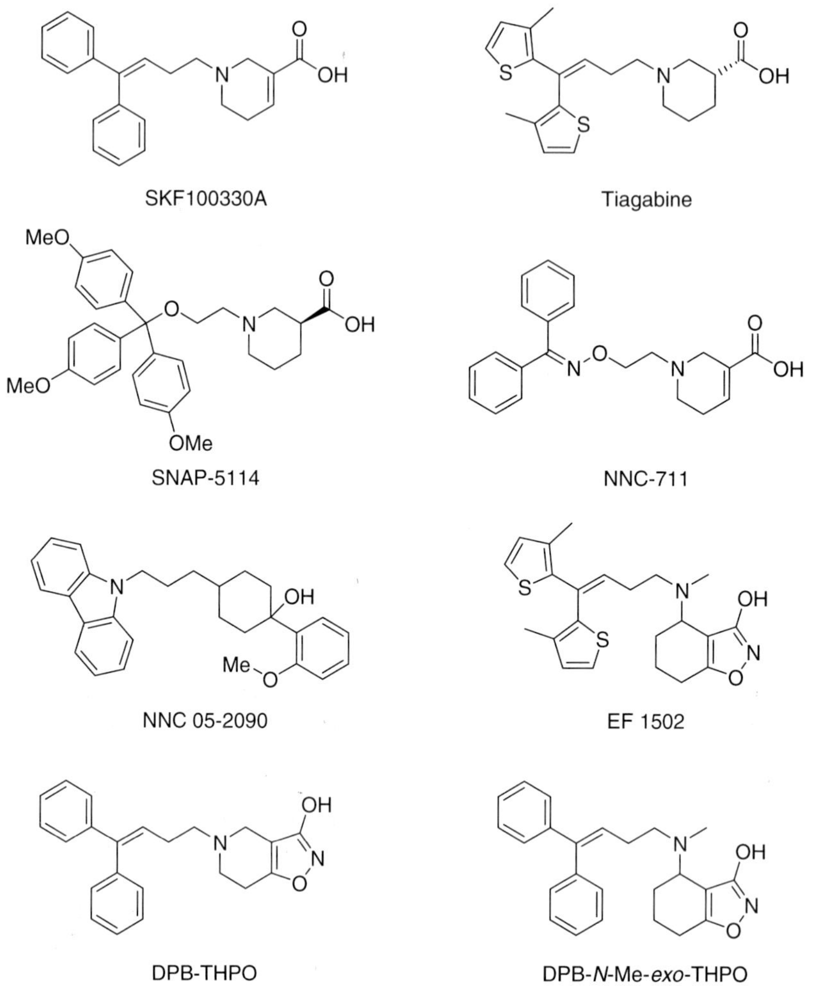

SKF100330A

Tiagabine

SNAP-5114

NNC-711

NNC 05-2090

EF 1502

DPB-THPO

DPB-*N*-Me-*exo*-THPO

**FIGURE 2** Lipophilic aromatic GABA uptake inhibitors.

compound *N*-methyl-*exo*-THPO proved to be the most selective inhibitor for glial vs neuronal GABA uptake reported yet (Falch *et al.*, 1999).

Many of the small-sized inhibitors have turned out to display a varying profile at the four GABA transporter subtypes cloned (Table II). Although GABA is recognized by all subtypes, it has itself a reduced potency at GAT2 (BGT-1) compared to the other transporters. Nipecotic acid and guvacine interact well with all subtypes except GAT2 (BGT-1), while their flexible parental structure $\beta$-alanine is GAT3/GAT4 selective. It has been difficult to use the subtype pharmacological profiles to explain the neuronal vs glial specificity of the compounds. Thus, other transport systems may exist,

**TABLE II** [$^3$H]GABA Uptake Inhibition ($IC_{50}$, μM) into Synaptosomes, Cultured Cortex Astrocytes and Neurons, and Cells Transfected with Cloned GABA Transporters (GAT1–4)

| | *Synaptosomes* | *Neurons* | *Astrocytes* | *GAT1* | *GAT2* | *GAT3* | *GAT4* |
|---|---|---|---|---|---|---|---|
| GABA | 10 | 23[a] | 46[a] | 17[a] | 51[a] | 15[a] | 17[a] |
| Nipecotic acid | 5 | 16 | 12 | 24 | 2350 | 113 | 159 |
| Guvacine | 12 | 29 | 32 | 39 | 1420 | 228 | 378 |
| DABA | 27 | 1000 | >5000 | 128 | 528 | 300 | 710 |
| ACHC | 8 | 200 | 700 | 132 | 1070 | >1000 | >10,000 |
| *β*-Alanine | >10,000 | 1666 | 843 | 2920 | 1100 | 66 | 110 |
| *N*-Me-*exo*-THPO | 63 | 423 | 28 | 450 | >3000 | >3000 | >3000 |
| *exo*-THPO | 181 | 883 | 208 | 1000 | 3000 | >3000 | >3000 |
| Tiagabine | 0.067 | 0.36 | 0.18 | 0.8 | 300 | >300 | 800 |
| SNAP-5114 | ND | ND | ND | >30 | 22 | 20 | 6.6 |
| NNC-05 2090 | ND | ND | ND | 19 | 1.4 | 41 | 15 |
| EF1502 | 0.87 | 2 | 2 | 7 | 26 | >300 | >300 |
| (*R*)-EF1502 | 0.48 | 0.65 | 1.5 | 4 | 22 | >150 | >150 |
| (*S*)-EF1502 | >100 | >100 | >100 | 120 | 34 | >150 | >150 |

[a]$K_M$ value.

Sources: Data from Borden *et al.* (1995), Schousboe *et al.* (1979), and White *et al.* (2002). Reprinted with permission from Elsevier Bolvig *et al.* (1999), Borden (1996), Clausen *et al.* (2005), Larsson *et al.* (1983), and Schousboe *et al.* (1978). Reprinted with permission from Ali *et al.* (1985) and Falch *et al.* (1999). Copyright (1985, 1999) American Chemical Society. Reprinted with permission from Macmillan Publishers Ltd. Nature, Thomsen *et al.* (1997), copyright (1997).

ND, not determined.

differences could exist in transporter environments in different cell types, or it could be a consequence of an altered pharmacology in transporter heteromeric assemblies. However, these issues have not been addressed.

## B. Lipophilic Aromatic Inhibitors

Nipecotic acid and guvacine have been important lead structures for the development of a large number of GABA uptake inhibitors. The development was initiated by the discovery that introduction of the lipophilic diaromatic side chain 4,4-diphenylbut-3-en-1-yl (DPB) at these compounds gave very potent GABA uptake inhibitors, such as *N*-4,4-diphenylbut-3-en-1-yl-nipecotic acid (SKF89976A) and *N*-4,4-diphenylbut-3-en-1-yl-guvacine (SKF 100330A), that are orally active (Ali *et al.*, 1985; Yunger *et al.*, 1984). The introduction of the smaller methyl and ethyl N-substituents led to decreased potency. This transformation had some important consequences for the properties of the compounds. In contrast to the small inhibitors, the lipophilic aromatic analogs were able to penetrate the BBB as viewed by their anticonvulsive properties when given orally or intraperitoneally (Ali *et al.*, 1985). Obviously, this observation greatly expanded the possibility of therapeutic application of GABA uptake inhibition. Furthermore, these compounds are no longer substrates (Larsson *et al.*, 1988) and their inhibition kinetics is often observed to be other than competitive.

Following this discovery, a very large number of analogs based on nipecotic acid and guvacine containing aromatic side chains have been synthesized and characterized (Andersen *et al.*, 1993, 1994, 1999, 2001a,b; Dhar *et al.*, 1994; Knutsen *et al.*, 1999; Pavia *et al.*, 1992).

In general, the aromatic lipophilic analogs of guvacine often display a pronounced GAT1 preference (Borden *et al.*, 1994). As mentioned previously, this may be due to the high level of GAT1 expression in the assays employed in the development of these compounds, and potentially some of the less active compounds in these assays could have significant activity at other subtypes than GAT1.

The remaining aromatic compounds are rather unselective, and extensive variation in the lipophilic aromatic part has only led to modestly selective compounds (Borden, 1996). Thus, compounds like Tiagabine and 1-(2-(((diphenylmethylene)amino)oxy)ethyl)-1,2,5,6-tetrahydro-3-pyridinecarboxylic (NNC-711) are highly GAT1 selective compounds, while (*S*)-1-[2-[tris(4-methoxyphenyl)methoxy]ethyl]-3-piperidinecarboxylic acid (SNAP-5114) is a GAT4 preferring compound with significant activity at GAT2 and GAT3 (Dhar *et al.*, 1994). When considering the diminished potency of GABA at GAT2, SNAP-5114 might actually inhibit GAT2–4 equally well, thereby limiting the application as a GAT4 specific pharmacological tool. A GAT2 selective compound was reported (Thomsen *et al.*, 1997). This compound, 1-(3-(9*H*-carbazol-9-yl)-1-propyl)-4-(2-methoxyphenyl)-4-piperidinol (NNC 05-2090), however, still has activity at the other transporter subtypes. Since most of the aromatic lipophilic inhibitors are based on nipecotic acid or guvacine, it is interesting that NNC 05-2090, which is devoid of an acidic moiety, is not based on a structural GABA analog. However, this also raises the question whether this compound could affect other neurotransmitter systems not related to GABA.

We reported the development of (*RS*)-4-[*N*-[1,1-bis(3-methyl-2-thienyl) but-1-en-4-yl]-*N*-methylamino]-4,5,6,7-tetrahydrobenzo[*d*]isoxazol-3-ol (EF1502; Clausen *et al.*, 2005), a novel lipophilic diaromatic GABA uptake inhibitor based on *N*-Me-*exo*-THPO substituted with the side chain from Tiagabine, which surprisingly turned out to be equally effective at inhibiting GAT1 and GAT2. Resolution of the enantiomers revealed that while GAT1 activity was dependent on the stereochemistry of the GABA-resembling moiety, whereas the enantiomers were equally potent at GAT2-mediated uptake. This renders (*S*)-EF1502 a GAT2 selective compound with no measurable activity at GAT3 and GAT4. *In vivo* pharmacological characterization disclosed that EF1502 not only was a potent anticonvulsant but also potentiated the anticonvulsive effect of Tiagabine in a synergistic manner. For the first time an important functional role of GAT2/BGT-1 in the CNS (White *et al.*, 2005) was evidenced since selective GAT1 inhibitors only displayed an additive effect. The synergistic effect was absent in the rotarod model, and it therefore seems likely that EF1502 could improve the therapeutic application of Tiagabine by enhancing anticonvulsive properties but not adverse effects. These results underline the need for highly selective inhibitors for other subtypes than GAT1 to establish the functional roles at the different subtypes in the CNS, and to obtain novel clinical candidates in the treatment of disorders where GABA is believed to play an important role.

EF1502 was part of larger series of lipophilic aromatic analogs of *exo*-THPO. Most of these compounds were not very glia selective, the highest selectivity being tenfold. However, they were all very potent in the synaptosome GABA transport assay (Table III), which is notable given the low activity of the parent *exo*-THPO. It is interesting that side chains, such as 4,4-diphenylbut-1-yl that reduces the activity of nipecotic acid, could potentiate *exo*-THPO dramatically giving inhibitors much more potent than nipecotic acid.

## V. Kinetics of GABA Uptake Inhibitors

While the inhibitory effect of small GABA analogs has proven largely competitive so far, it is less evident which type of inhibition the lipophilic derivatives display. Furthermore, very few of the lipophilic aromatic inhibitors have been characterized with respect to their kinetic behavior as transport inhibitors. This is surprising since the kinetics could affect the nature of termination of neurotransmission. A competitive inhibitor will inhibit transport at low-GABA concentrations, which could increase GABA-mediated tonic inhibition, but since vesicular release of GABA leads to high local concentrations of GABA, the inhibitor could be rendered ineffective until the GABA concentration had decreased to a certain level where the inhibitor again would exert its function. A strictly noncompetitive inhibitor would block GABA transport regardless of the GABA concentration. It is difficult to predict the kinetics of the lipophilic uptake inhibitors since they have structural amino acid elements that can overlap with GABA and lipophilic elements, which do not overlap with GABA.

Tiagabine behaves both as a competitive and a mixed-type inhibitor on synaptosomal uptake depending on whether the preparation is preincubated with the inhibitor (Braestrup *et al.*, 1990). The DPB substituted THPO and *N*-Me-*exo*-THPO compounds were competitive and noncompetitive inhibitors, respectively at GAT1 (Sarup *et al.*, 2003), although sharing very similar

**TABLE III** [$^{3}$H]GABA Uptake Inhibition ($IC_{50}$, μM) into Rat Synaptosomes, Cultured Rat Cortex Astrocytes and Neurons, and Cells Transfected with Cloned Mouse GABA Transporters (GAT1–4)

*Exo*-THPO = 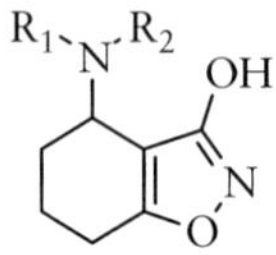 Nip =

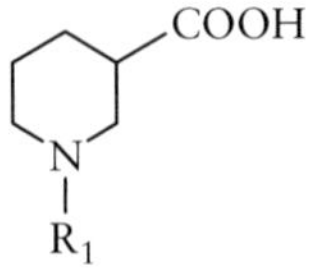

| *Compound* | | *Exo-THPO* | | | *Nip*[a] |
|---|---|---|---|---|---|
| $R_1$ | $R_2$ | *Synaptosomes* | *Astrocytes* | *Neurons* | *Synaptosomes* |
| 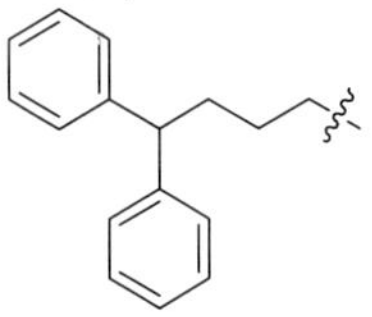 | H | 0.22 | 0.5 | 3 | 27%[b] |
| | Me | 0.41 | 1.7 | 17 | 27%[b] |
| 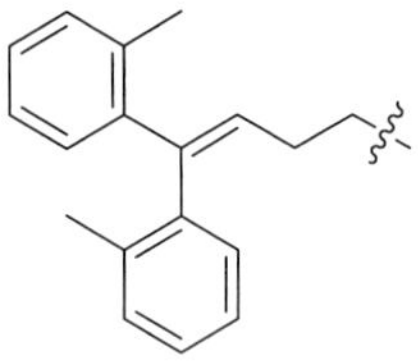 | H | 0.3 | 2 | 12 | 0.08 |
| | Me | 0.7 | 8 | 5 | 0.08 |
| 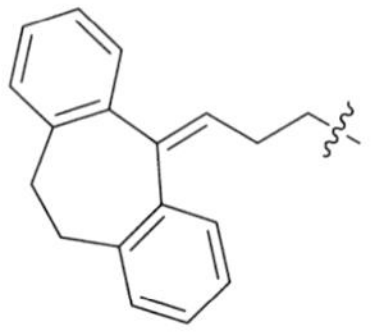 | H | 0.76 | 7 | 80 | 13.6 |
| | Me | 1.1 | 3 | 7.5 | 13.6 |
| 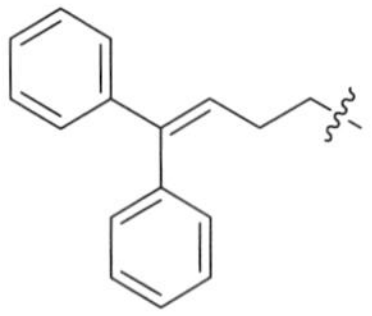 | H | 0.14 | 0.6 | 1.4 | 0.33 |
| | Me | 0.37 | 2 | 5 | 0.33 |

(continues)

**TABLE III** (*continued*)

| *Compound* | | *Exo-THPO* | | | *Nip*[a] |
|---|---|---|---|---|---|
| *R*$_1$ | *R*$_2$ | *Synaptosomes* | *Astrocytes* | *Neurons* | *Synaptosomes* |
| [structure] | H | 0.17 | 2 | 4 | 0.09 |
| | Me | 0.87 | 2 | 2 | 0.09 |

[a]Inhibition of GABA uptake into synaptosomes by nipecotic acid derivatives.
[b]Inhibition at 10 μM.
Comparison of lipophilic aromatic GABA uptake inhibitors based on *exo*-THPO and nipecotic acid.
Sources: Data reprinted with permission from Ali *et al.* (1985) and Andersen *et al.* (1993, 2001a). Copyright (1985, 1993, 2001) American Chemical Society. Reprinted with permission from Elsevier Clausen *et al.* (2005).

recognition elements. Also EF1502 was a noncompetitive inhibitor of both GAT1 and GAT2 mediated transport (White *et al.*, 2005). It was observed in one study that mutation of tyrosine140 in GAT1 to phenylalanine or tryptophan abolished the affinity of GABA, however, the lipophilic inhibitor SKF100330A still had some affinity on the Y140F mutant determined by the ability to inhibit sodium-dependent charge movements induced by voltage jumps in patch-clamp experiments, albeit at higher concentrations (Bismuth *et al.*, 1997). It therefore seems that the type of inhibition can depend on the extent to which the GABA recognition site contributes to the binding of the inhibitor. The picture can be further complicated if the inhibitor has varying affinities to different states in the transport cycle.

## VI. Reevaluation of Lipophilic Aromatic GABA Uptake Inhibitors

We have now reevaluated some lipophilic GABA uptake inhibitors (Fig. 3) previously reported (Andersen *et al.*, 1993, 1999, 2001a) with respect to inhibitory effects on GABA uptake in cultured astrocytic and neuronal cell cultures from cortex as well as cells expressing the cloned GABA transporters from mouse GAT1–4. The results will be discussed in the following.

### A. Methods

#### *1. Materials*

Newborn mice and 15-day-old mouse embryos were obtained from Taconic Europe (Ry, Denmark). Plastic tissue culture dishes were purchased from NUNC A/S (Roskilde, Denmark) and fetal calf serum (FCS) and

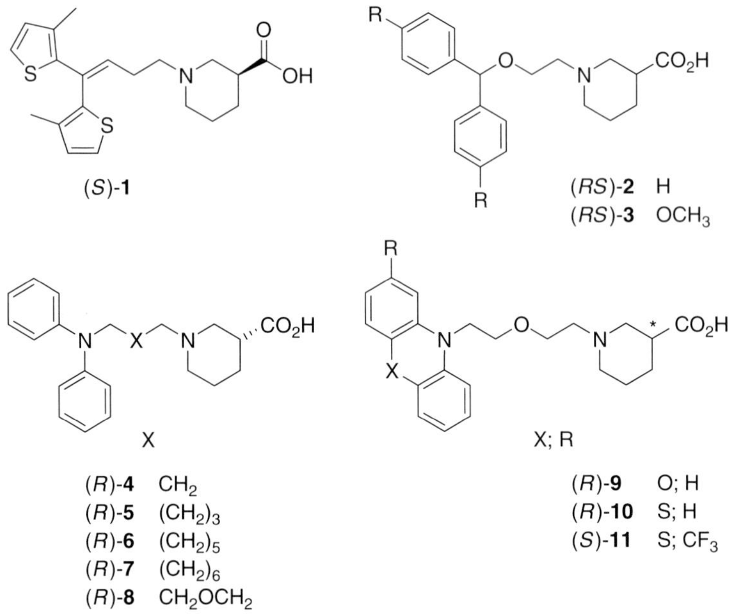

(*S*)-**1**

| | R |
|---|---|
| (*RS*)-**2** | H |
| (*RS*)-**3** | $OCH_3$ |

| | X |
|---|---|
| (*R*)-**4** | $CH_2$ |
| (*R*)-**5** | $(CH_2)_3$ |
| (*R*)-**6** | $(CH_2)_5$ |
| (*R*)-**7** | $(CH_2)_6$ |
| (*R*)-**8** | $CH_2OCH_2$ |

| | X; R |
|---|---|
| (*R*)-**9** | O; H |
| (*R*)-**10** | S; H |
| (*S*)-**11** | S; $CF_3$ |

**FIGURE 3** Series of lipophilic aromatic GABA uptake inhibitors.

Blasticidin-S from Invitrogen (Carlsbad, USA). Poly-D-lysine (molecular weight 300,000), trypsin, soybean trypsin inhibitor, dibutyryl cyclic AMP (dBcAMP), DNase, cytosine arabinoside, penicillin/streptomycin, and amino acids were obtained from Sigma-Aldrich (St. Louis, USA). [$^3$H]GABA (3.5 TBq/mmol) was from PerkinElmer (MA, USA). Several GABA uptake inhibitors were generously provided by Novo Nordisk A/S. All other chemicals were of the purest grade available from regular commercial sources.

### 2. *Primary Cell Cultures*

Primary cell cultures of astrocytes were prepared from the neopallium from newborn mice essentially as described earlier (Hertz *et al.*, 1989b). Dissociated tissue was cultured in a slightly modified Dulbeccos minimum essential medium (DMEM) supplemented with 20% (v/v) FCS as defined previously (Hertz *et al.*, 1982) and plated onto 96-well multidishes. During the course of the 3 weeks the serum concentration was weekly lowered to 15% and finally 10%. During the last week the cell culture medium was supplemented with 0.25 mM dbcAMP in order to obtain a well-differentiated stellate phenotype of the astrocytes (Hertz *et al.*, 1982).

Cerebral cortical neurons were obtained from 15-day-old mouse embryos and were prepared as described previously (Hertz *et al.*, 1989a). After dissociation of the tissue by a mild trypsinization and trituration in a DNase solution containing soybean trypsin inhibitor, cells were plated onto poly-D-lysine-coated 96-well multidishes. Cells were cultured in DMEM supplemented with 10% FBS. To prevent astroglial profilation cytosine arabinoside were added to a final concentration of 20 μM, 48 h after preparation (Hertz *et al.*, 1989a).

### 3. Stable Cell Lines

The four cell lines of stably transfected HEK-293 cells expressing mGAT1–4 were prepared using an expression vector pIRES (CLONETECH, Palo Alto, CA). The expression vectors were modified to contain the enzyme Blasticidin-S deaminase, a set of primers and the cDNA of GAT1–4, for further detail see White *et al.* (2002). The cell lines were cultured in modified Dulbecco's medium supplemented with 5 μg/ml Blasticidin-S, penicillin/streptomycin, and 10% calf serum and plated onto 96-well multidishes.

### 4. [$^3$H]GABA Uptake

The uptake of [$^3$H]GABA in cultured astrocytes, neurons, and recombinant cell systems was investigated essentially as described previously (Larsson *et al.*, 1981). The incubations were carried out at 37 °C in phosphate buffered saline containing [$^3$H]GABA (1 μCi/ml) and 1 μM GABA and increasing concentrations of inhibitor. The incubations were terminated after 3 min using an Elx50 automated strip washer (BioTek, Vermont, USA).

The cells were solubilized directly in Microscint-20$^{TM}$. Radioactivity was counted in a TopCount microplate scintillation counter from Packard (Boston, MA, USA). $IC_{50}$ values were determined by nonlinear regression analysis using Prism 3.0 (GraphPad software, CA, USA).

### 5. Kinetic Analysis

The kinetic analysis was performed roughly as [$^3$H]GABA uptake except the [$^3$H]GABA was 2 μCi/ml. The inhibitor was tested at four different concentrations, and the concentration of GABA at each inhibitor concentration was varied over the range 0–800 μM. The nonspecific binding was measured to every concentration of GABA. The protein content was determined as an average of eight wells and measured using PIERCE micro BSA assay. The kinetic parameters were calculated by fitting the uptake velocities and applied substrate concentrations to the following equation: $[(V_{max} \cdot S)/(K_m + S)] + k \cdot S$ using a nonlinear regression analysis employing SigmaPlot 2002 (Chicago, IL, USA).

## B. Results and Discussions

In general, it was observed that the activity of the compounds mainly resided on GAT1 as previously observed for several of the potent inhibitors of synaptosomal uptake (Table IV). However, compounds like 3 and 7 with

**TABLE IV** [$^3$H]GABA Uptake Inhibition ($IC_{50}$, μM) into Synaptosomes, Cultured Cortex Astrocytes and Neurons, and Cells Transfected with Cloned Mouse or Rat GABA Transporter Subtypes (Mouse Nomenclature GAT1–4)

| | *GABA uptake inhibition* | | | | | | |
|---|---|---|---|---|---|---|---|
| | *Synaptosomes* | *Neurons* | *Astrocytes* | *GAT1* | *GAT2* | *GAT3* | *GAT4* |
| GABA | ND | 23 | 46 | 17 | 51 | 15 | 17 |
| Tiagabine | 0.067 | 0.36 | 0.18 | 0.8 | 300 | >300 | 800 |
| (*S*)-**1** | 0.21 | 5.4 | 3.8 | 3.0 | 355 | >1000 | >1000 |
| (*RS*)-**2** | 1.37 | 6.9 | 5.2 | 10 | 856 | >1000 | >1000 |
| (*RS*)-**3** | >3 | 18 | 11 | 35 | 359 | 218 | 175 |
| (*R*)-**4** | >9 | 79 | 99 | 235 | 722 | >1000 | >1000 |
| (*R*)-**5** | 1.38 | 0.67 | 12 | 4.9 | 286 | 578 | 476 |
| (*R*)-**6** | 0.23 | 1.8 | 12 | 4.2 | 117 | 213 | 202 |
| (*R*)-**7** | 1.29 | 13 | 11 | 12 | 77 | 168 | 104 |
| (*R*)-**8** | 0.09 | 0.19 | 17 | 1.3 | 622 | 591 | >1000 |
| (*R*)-**9** | 14.6 | 384 | 595 | 741 | 543 | >1000 | 901 |
| (*R*)-**10** | 0.31 | 0.37 | 5.0 | 1.9 | 126 | 124 | >1000 |
| (*S*)-**11** | 0.10 | 0.66 | 3.5 | 1.9 | 98 | 33 | 95 |

Sources: Data from present study reprinted with permission from Andersen *et al.* (1993, 1999, 2001a). Copyright (1993, 1999, 2001) American Chemical Society.

relatively low activity were less selective. Compound **9** turned out to be vaguely GAT2-preferring, although this compound displays very low activity. When comparing the activity of compounds **4–7**, it is interesting to observe how the increasing chain length between the amino group and the diaromatic moiety affects the pharmacological profile. Thus, **4** is relatively inactive on all subtypes, while compound **5** containing two carbons more in the chain seems to have reached an optimal length for GAT1 activity. By increasing the chain length further, the inhibitory effects at the other subtypes also increases, thereby diminishing the GAT1-preference. The transporters therefore appear to share pharmacophore elements that can be reached by increasing the chain length pointing to the possibility of finding inhibitors with preference for other than GAT1 in some of the previous described series of GABA uptake inhibitors that has not been characterized on the cloned transporter subtypes.

The Michaelis–Menten kinetics of three compounds (**3**, **7**, and **11**) having pronounced activity on several subtypes were evaluated (Tables V and VI). Thus, the kinetics of GAT1 and GAT4 activity of compound **3** were investigated and while GAT1 activity proved to be competitive, the GAT4 activity was uncompetitive. Due to the significant activity on all subtypes, the kinetics of compound **7** was investigated on GAT1–4 and proved to be a noncompetitive inhibitor at GAT1–3, but uncompetitive at GAT4. Compound **11** was characterized on GAT1, GAT3, and GAT4 and was a

**TABLE V** Kinetic Data on the Inhibition of [$^3$H]GABA Uptake into Cells Transfected with Cloned Mouse GABA Transporters (GAT1–4) by Compounds 3, 7, and 11

| *Compound* | | *Concentration/(μM)* | $V_{max}$ ± *SEM* | $K_m$ ± *SEM* | $r^2$ |
|---|---|---|---|---|---|
| (*RS*)-3 | GAT1 | 0 | 5.26 ± 0.24 | 23.76 ± 4.54 | 0.99 |
| | | 20 | 5.06 ± 0.08 | 50.6 ± 3.0 | 0.99 |
| | | 40 | 6.19 ± 0.29 | 57.5 ± 8.6 | 0.99 |
| | | 72 | 5.05 ± 0.15 | 72.1 ± 7.4 | 0.99 |
| (*RS*)-3 | GAT4 | 0 | 5.47 ± 0.14 | 16.67 ± 1.98 | 0.99 |
| | | 50 | 0.71 ± 0.06 | 4.40 ± 1.87 | 0.98 |
| | | 100 | 0.35 ± 0.02 | 3.61 ± 1.27 | 0.99 |
| | | 200 | 0.158 ± 0.006 | 1.48 ± 0.37 | 0.99 |
| (*R*)-7 | GAT1 | 0 | 8.41 ± 0.31 | 34.0 ± 5.1 | 0.99 |
| | | 6 | 6.63 ± 0.10 | 36.2 ± 2.2 | 0.99 |
| | | 12 | 3.94 ± 0.22 | 28.1 ± 6.4 | 0.99 |
| | | 24 | 2.86 ± 0.06 | 39.9 ± 3.3 | 0.99 |
| (*R*)-7 | GAT2 | 0 | 16.39 ± 0.14 | 185.4 ± 4.4 | 0.99 |
| | | 50 | 13.73 ± 0.12 | 173.4 ± 4.3 | 0.99 |
| | | 90 | 8.31 ± 0.10 | 168.4 ± 5.7 | 0.99 |
| | | 180 | 5.94 ± 0.14 | 200.8 ± 12.2 | 0.99 |
| (*R*)-7 | GAT3 | 0 | 3.12 ± 0.17 | 14.87 ± 3.64 | 0.99 |
| | | 90 | 1.21 ± 0.02 | 10.53 ± 0.81 | 0.99 |
| | | 170 | 1.38 ± 0.04 | 9.94 ± 1.29 | 0.99 |
| | | 340 | 0.38 ± 0.05 | 7.01 ± 4.42 | 0.96 |
| (*R*)-7 | GAT4 | 0 | 4.19 ± 0.10 | 13.59 ± 1.43 | 0.99 |
| | | 50 | 2.78 ± 0.06 | 11.5 ± 1.8 | 0.99 |
| | | 90 | 0.94 ± 0.04 | 6.66 ± 1.42 | 0.99 |
| | | 180 | 0.26 ± 0.03 | 2.37 ± 1.77 | 0.96 |
| (*S*)-**11** | GAT1 | 0 | 7.52 ± 0.27 | 24.7 ± 3.8 | 0.99 |
| | | 1 | 8.05 ± 0.25 | 58.5 ± 6.6 | 0.99 |
| | | 2 | 7.90 ± 0.13 | 82.5 ± 4.43 | 0.99 |
| | | 4 | 8.89 ± 0.30 | 201.1 ± 18.1 | 0.99 |
| (*S*)-**11** | GAT3 | 0 | 5.04 ± 0.45 | 11.7 ± 5.0 | 0.98 |
| | | 20 | 5.14 ± 0.14 | 30.5 ± 3.3 | 0.99 |
| | | 40 | 3.52 ± 0.09 | 40.8 ± 3.9 | 0.99 |
| | | 64 | 3.75 ± 0.19 | 71.0 ± 12.7 | 0.99 |
| (*S*)-**11** | GAT4 | 0 | 10.05 ± 0.31 | 18.6 ± 2.5 | 0.99 |
| | | 50 | 6.56 ± 0.48 | 17.7 ± 5.8 | 0.98 |
| | | 100 | 4.42 ± 0.38 | 20.5 ± 7.6 | 0.98 |
| | | 200 | 2.57 ± 0.38 | 13.3 ± 9.2 | 0.96 |

competitive inhibitor at GAT1, mixed-type at GAT3, and noncompetitive at GAT4. The results emphasize how the lipophilic diaromatic inhibitors display very varying inhibition kinetics with no obvious correlation to individual subtypes or chemical structures. The differences in kinetics may ultimately lead to variance in the nature of GABA uptake inhibition.

**TABLE VI** Inhibition Kinetics of Compounds 3, 7, and 11 on Mouse GABA Transporter Subtypes GAT1–4

| | *GAT1* | *GAT2* | *GAT3* | *GAT4* |
|---|---|---|---|---|
| 3 | Competitive | ND | ND | Uncompetitive |
| 7 | Noncompetitive | Noncompetitive | Noncompetitive | Uncompetitive |
| 11 | Competitive | ND | Mixed type | Noncompetitive |

ND, not determined.

## VII. Conclusions

Termination of GABAergic neurotransmission is mediated by transporters in both neuronal and glial cells, and the development of transporter inhibitors has been the aim of extensive research for more than 3 decades. Application of the transport inhibitor, Tiagabine, in the treatment of epilepsy has been approved, but it is likely that applications in other disorders can be demonstrated.

A very large number of derivatives of nipecotic acid and guvacine containing lipophilic aromatic side chains have been synthesized with the aim of finding suitable anticonvulsive compounds. These have typically been characterized pharmacologically in a neuronal-type synaptosome assay, which seems to probe the GAT1 activity of the compounds. Consequently, many of these compounds are very potent and selective GAT1 inhibitors such as Tiagabine. Compounds with a comparable potency and selectivity at other subtypes have not been developed despite extensive variation in the aromatic side chain. Thus, there continues to be a need for potent and selective inhibitors in order to establish the role of the other transporter subtypes and therapeutic potential of such inhibitors. The kinetic characteristics of GABA uptake inhibitors are not well described and for most of the uptake inhibitors the kinetic characteristics are unknown. Since the kinetics of the inhibitor could be important for mechanism underlying the termination of neurotransmission this is an issue that should be addressed in the future.

## Acknowledgments

Novo Nordisk A/S is gratefully acknowledged for supplying a series of GABA uptake inhibitors. The work was supported by the Lundbeck Foundation and the Danish Medical Research Council (22-04-0723 & 22-03-0250).

## References


Adkins, C. E., Pillai, G. V., Kerby, J., Bonnert, T. P., Haldon, C., McKernan, R. M., Gonzalez, J. E., Oades, K., Whiting, P. J., and Simpson, P. B. (2001). $\alpha4\beta3\delta$ $GABA_A$ receptors characterized by fluorescence resonance energy transfer-derived measurements of membrane potential. *J. Biol. Chem.* **276**(42), 38934–38939.

Ali, F. E., Bondinell, W. E., Dandridge, P. A., Frazee, J. S., Garvey, E., Girard, G. R., Kaiser, C., Ku, T. W., Lafferty, J. J., and Moonsammy, G. I. (1985). Orally active and potent inhibitors of gamma-aminobutyric acid uptake. *J. Med. Chem.* **28**(5), 653–660.

Andersen, K. E., Braestrup, C., Gronwald, F. C., Jørgensen, A. S., Nielsen, E. B., Sonnewald, U., Sørensen, P. O., Suzdak, P. D., and Knutsen, L. J. (1993). The synthesis of novel GABA uptake inhibitors. 1. Elucidation of the structure-activity studies leading to the choice of (*R*)-1-[4,4-bis(3-methyl-2-thienyl)-3-butenyl]-3-piperidinecarboxylic acid (tiagabine) as an anticonvulsant drug candidate. *J. Med. Chem.* **36**(12), 1716–1725.

Andersen, K. E., Begtrup, M., Chorghade, M. S., Lee, E. C., Lau, J., Lundt, B. F., Petersen, H., Sørensen, P. O., and Thøgersen, H. (1994). The synthesis of novel GABA uptake inhibitors. 2. Synthesis of 5-hydroxytiagabine, a human metabolite of the GABA reuptake inhibitor Tiagabine. *Tetrahedron* **50**(29), 8699–8710.

Andersen, K. E., Sørensen, J. L., Huusfeldt, P. O., Knutsen, L. J., Lau, J., Lundt, B. F., Petersen, H., Suzdak, P. D., and Swedberg, M. D. (1999). Synthesis of novel GABA uptake inhibitors. 4. Bioisosteric transformation and successive optimization of known GABA uptake inhibitors leading to a series of potent anticonvulsant drug candidates. *J. Med. Chem.* **42**(21), 4281–4291.

Andersen, K. E., Sørensen, J. L., Lau, J., Lundt, B. F., Petersen, H., Huusfeldt, P. O., Suzdak, P. D., and Swedberg, M. D. (2001a). Synthesis of novel $\gamma$-aminobutyric acid (GABA) uptake inhibitors. 5. Preparation and structure-activity studies of tricyclic analogues of known GABA uptake inhibitors. *J. Med. Chem.* **44**(13), 2152–2163.

Andersen, K. E., Lau, J., Lundt, B. F., Petersen, H., Huusfeldt, P. O., Suzdak, P. D., and Swedberg, M. D. B. (2001b). Synthesis of novel GABA uptake inhibitors. Part 6: Preparation and evaluation of *N*-O asymmetrically substituted nipecotic acid derivatives. *Bioorg. Med. Chem.* **9**(11), 2773–2785.

Bismuth, Y., Kavanaugh, M. P., and Kanner, B. I. (1997). Tyrosine 140 of the $\gamma$-aminobutyric acid transporter GAT-1 plays a critical role in neurotransmitter recognition. *J. Biol. Chem.* **272**(26), 16096–16102.

Bolvig, T., Larsson, O. M., Pickering, D. S., Nelson, N., Falch, E., Krogsgaard-Larsen, P., and Schousboe, A. (1999). Action of bicyclic isoxazole GABA analogues on GABA transporters and its relation to anticonvulsant activity. *Eur. J. Pharmacol.* **375**, 367–374.

Borden, L. A. (1996). GABA transporter heterogeneity: Pharmacology and cellular localization. *Neurochem. Int.* **29**(4), 335–356.

Borden, L. A., Smith, K. E., Hartig, P. R., Branchek, T. A., and Weinshank, R. L. (1992). Molecular heterogeneity of the $\gamma$-aminobutyric acid (GABA) transport system. Cloning of two novel high affinity GABA transporters from rat brain. *J. Biol. Chem.* **267**(29), 21098–21104.

Borden, L. A., Murali Dhar, T. G., Smith, K. E., Weinshank, R. L., Branchek, T. A., and Gluchowski, C. (1994). Tiagabine, SK&F 89976-A, CI-966, and NNC-711 are selective for the cloned GABA transporter GAT-1. *Eur. J. Pharmacol.* **269**(2), 219–224.

Borden, L. A., Smith, K. E., Vaysse, P. J., Gustafson, E. L., Weinshank, R. L., and Branchek, T. A. (1995). Re-evaluation of GABA transport in neuronal and glial cell cultures: Correlation of pharmacology and mRNA localization. *Receptors Channels* **3**, 129–146.

Braestrup, C., Nielsen, E. B., Sonnewald, U., Knutsen, L. J. S., Andersen, K. E., Jansen, J. A., Frederiksen, K., Andersen, P. H., Mortensen, A., and Suzdak, P. D. (1990). (*R*)-*N*-[4,4-Bis

(3-methyl-2-thienyl)but-3-en-1-yl]nipecotic acid binds with high-affinity to the brain γ-aminobutyric acid uptake carrier. *J. Neurochem.* **54**(2), 639–647.

Clausen, R. P., Moltzen, E. K., Perregaard, J., Lenz, S. M., Sanchez, C., Falch, E., Frolund, B., Bolvig, T., Sarup, A., and Larsson, O. M. (2005). Selective inhibitors of GABA uptake: Synthesis and molecular pharmacology of 4-*N*-methylamino-4,5,6,7-tetrahydrobenzo[*d*] isoxazol-3-ol analogues. *Bioorg. Med. Chem.* **13**(3), 895–908.

Conti, F., Melone, M., De Biasi, S., Minelli, A., Brecha, N. C., and Ducati, A. (1998). Neuronal and glial localization of GAT-1, a high-affinity γ-aminobutyric acid plasma membrane transporter, in human cerebral cortex: With a note on its distribution in monkey cortex. *J. Comp. Neurol.* **396**(1), 51–63.

Conti, F., Zuccarello, L. V., Barbaresi, P., Minelli, A., Brecha, N. C., and Melone, M. (1999). Neuronal, glial, and epithelial localization of γ-aminobutyric acid transporter 2, a high-affinity gamma-aminobutyric acid plasma membrane transporter, in the cerebral cortex and neighboring structures. *J. Comp. Neurol.* **409**(3), 482–494.

Conti, F., Minelli, A., and Melone, M. (2004). GABA transporters in the mammalian cerebral cortex: Localization, development and pathological implications. *Brain Res. Brain Res. Rev.* **45**(3), 196–212.

Dhar, T. G., Borden, L. A., Tyagarajan, S., Smith, K. E., Branchek, T. A., Weinshank, R. L., and Gluchowski, C. (1994). Design, synthesis and evaluation of substituted triarylnipecotic acid derivatives as GABA uptake inhibitors: Identification of a ligand with moderate affinity and selectivity for the cloned human GABA transporter GAT-3. *J. Med. Chem.* **37**(15), 2334–2342.

Durkin, M. M., Smith, K. E., Borden, L. A., Weinshank, R. L., Branchek, T. A., and Gustafson, E. L. (1995). Localization of messenger RNAs encoding three GABA transporters in rat brain: An *in situ* hybridization study. *Brain Res. Mol. Brain Res.* **33**(1), 7–21.

Falch, E., Perregaard, J., Frølund, B., Søkilde, B., Buur, A., Hansen, L. M., Frydenvang, K., Brehm, L., Bolvig, T., Larsson, O. M., Sanchez, C., White, H. S., *et al.* (1999). Selective inhibitors of glial GABA uptake: Synthesis, absolute stereochemistry, and pharmacology of the enantiomers of 3-hydroxy-4-amino-4,5,6,7-tetrahydro-1,2-benzisoxazole (*exo*-THPO) and analogues. *J. Med. Chem.* **42**(26), 5402–5414.

Guastella, J., Nelson, N., Nelson, H., Czyzyk, L., Keynan, S., Miedel, M. C., Davidson, N., Lester, H. A., and Kanner, B. I. (1990). Cloning and expression of a rat brain GABA transporter. *Science* **249**, 1303–1306.

Hertz, E., Yu, A. C. H., Hertz, L., Juurlink, B. H. J., and Schousboe, A. (1989a). Preparation of primary cultures of mouse cortical neurons. *In* "A Dissection and Tissue Culture Manual of the Nervous System" (A. Shahar, J. de Vellis, A. Vernadakis, and B. Haber, Eds.), pp. 183–186. Alan R. Liss, Inc., New York.

Hertz, L., Juurlink, B. H. J., Fosmark, H., and Schousboe, A. (1982). Astrocytes in primary cultures. *In* "Neuroscience Approached Through Cell Culture" (S. E. Pfeiffer, Ed.), pp. 175–186. CRC Press, Boca Raton, Florida.

Hertz, L., Juurlink, B. H. J., Hertz, E., Fosmark, H., and Schousboe, A. (1989b). Preparation of primary cultures of mouse (rat) astrocytes. *In* "A Dissection and Tissue Culture Manual of the Nervous System" (A. Shahar, J. de Vellis, A. Vernadakis, and B. Haber, Eds.), pp. 105–108. Alan R. Liss, Inc., New York.

Iversen, L. L., and Kelly, J. S. (1975). Uptake and metabolism of γ-aminobutyric acid by neurons and glial cells. *Biochem. Pharmacol.* **24**(9), 933–938.

Iversen, L. L., and Neal, M. J. (1968). Uptake of [$^3$H]GABA by slices of rat cerebral cortex. *J. Neurochem.* **15**(10), 1141–1149.

Knutsen, L. J., Andersen, K. E., Lau, J., Lundt, B. F., Henry, R. F., Morton, H. E., Naerum, L., Petersen, H., Stephensen, H., Suzdak, P. D., Swedberg, M. D., Thomsen, C., and Sørensen, P. O. (1999). Synthesis of novel GABA uptake inhibitors. 3. Diaryloxime and diarylvinyl ether derivatives of nipecotic acid and guvacine as anticonvulsant agents. *J. Med. Chem.* **42**(18), 3447–3462.

Krogsgaard-Larsen, P., and Johnston, G. A. R. (1975). Inhibition of GABA uptake in rat brain slices by nipecotic acid, various isoxazoles and related compounds. *J. Neurochem.* **25**(6), 797–802.

Krogsgaard-Larsen, P., Johnston, G. A. R., Curtis, D. R., Game, C. J., and McCulloch, R. M. (1975). Structure and biological activity of a series of conformationally restricted analogues of GABA. *J. Neurochem.* **25**(6), 803–809.

Krogsgaard-Larsen, P., Mikkelsen, H., Jacobsen, P., Falch, E., Curtis, D. R., Peet, M. J., and Leah, J. D. (1983). 4,5,6,7-Tetrahydroisothiazolo[5,4-*c*]pyridin-3-ol and related analogues of THIP. Synthesis and biological activity. *J. Med. Chem.* **26**(6), 895–900.

Krogsgaard-Larsen, P., Frølund, B., and Frydenvang, K. (2000). GABA uptake inhibitors. Design, molecular pharmacology and therapeutic aspects. *Curr. Pharm. Des.* **6**(12), 1193–1209.

Larsson, O. M., Thorbek, P., Krogsgaard-Larsen, P., and Schousboe, A. (1981). Effect of homo-beta-proline and other heterocyclic GABA analogues on GABA uptake in neurons and astroglial cells and on GABA receptor binding. *J. Neurochem.* **37**, 1509–1516.

Larsson, O. M., Johnston, G. A., and Schousboe, A. (1983). Differences in uptake kinetics of cis-3-aminocyclohexane carboxylic acid into neurons and astrocytes in primary cultures. *Brain Res.* **260**, 279–285.

Larsson, O. M., Falch, E., Krogsgaard-Larsen, P., and Schousboe, A. (1988). Kinetic characterization of inhibition of $\gamma$-aminobutyric acid uptake into cultured neurons and astrocytes by 4,4-diphenyl-3-butenyl derivatives of nipecotic acid and guvacine. *J. Neurochem.* **50**(3), 818–823.

Lloyd, K. G., and Morselli, P. L. (1987). Psychopharmacology of GABAergic drugs. *In* "Psychopharmacology: The Third Generation of Progress" (H. Y. Meltzer, Ed.), pp. 183–195. Raven Press, New York.

Minelli, A., DeBiasi, S., Brecha, N. C., Zuccarello, L. V., and Conti, F. (1996). GAT-3, a high-affinity GABA plasma membrane transporter, is localized to astrocytic processes, and it is not confined to the vicinity of GABAergic synapses in the cerebral cortex. *J. Neurosci.* **16**(19), 6255–6264.

Neal, M. J., and Bowery, N. G. (1977). Cis-3-aminocyclohexanecarboxylic acid: A substrate for the neuronal GABA transport system. *Brain Res.* **138**(1), 169–174.

Pavia, M. R., Lobbestael, S. J., Nugiel, D., Mayhugh, D. R., Gregor, V. E., Taylor, C. P., Schwarz, R. D., Brahce, L., and Vartanian, M. G. (1992). Structure-activity studies on benzhydrol-containing nipecotic acid and guvacine derivatives as potent, orally-active inhibitors of GABA uptake. *J. Med. Chem.* **35**(22), 4238–4248.

Pietrini, G., Suh, Y. J., Edelmann, L., Rudnick, G., and Caplan, M. J. (1994). The axonal gamma-aminobutyric acid transporter GAT-1 is sorted to the apical membranes of polarized epithelial cells. *J. Biol. Chem.* **269**(6), 4668–4674.

Radian, R., Ottersen, O. P., Storm-Mathisen, J., Castel, M., and Kanner, B. I. (1990). Immunocytochemical localization of the GABA transporter in rat brain. *J. Neurosci.* **10**(4), 1319–1330.

Sarup, A., Larsson, O. M., Bolvig, T., Frølund, B., Krogsgaard-Larsen, P., and Schousboe, A. (2003). Effects of 3-hydroxy-4-amino-4,5,6,7-tetrahydro-1,2-benzisoxazol (*exo*-THPO) and its *N*-substituted analogs on GABA transport in cultured neurons and astrocytes and by the four cloned mouse GABA transporters. *Neurochem. Int.* **43**(4–5), 445–451.

Schousboe, A., and Kanner, B. I. (2002). GABA transporters: Functional and pharmacological properties. *In* "Glutamate and GABA Receptors and Transporters: Structure, Function and Pharmacology" (J. Egebjerg, A. Schousboe, and P. Krogsgaard-Larsen, Eds.), pp. 337–349. Taylor and Francis, London.

Schousboe, A., Krogsgaard-Larsen, P., Svenneby, G., and Hertz, L. (1978). Inhibition of the high-affinity, net uptake of GABA into cultured astrocytes by beta-proline, nipecotic acid and other compounds. *Brain Res.* **153**, 623–626.

Schousboe, A., Thorbek, P., Hertz, L., and Krogsgaard-Larsen, P. (1979). Effects of GABA analogues of restricted conformation on GABA transport in astrocytes and brain cortex slices and on GABA receptor binding. *J. Neurochem.* **33**, 181–189.

Schousboe, A., Larsson, O. M., Wood, J. D., and Krogsgaard-Larsen, P. (1983). Transport and metabolism of $\gamma$-aminobutyric acid in neurons and glia: Implications for epilepsy. *Epilepsia* **24**(5), 531–538.

Schousboe, A., Sarup, A., Bak, L. K., Waagepetersen, H. S., and Larsson, O. M. (2004). Role of astrocytic transport processes in glutamatergic and GABAergic neurotransmission. *Neurochem. Int.* **45**(4), 521–527.

Thomsen, C., Sørensen, P. O., and Egebjerg, J. (1997). 1-(3-(9*H*-carbazol-9-yl)-1-propyl)-4-(2-methoxyphenyl)-4-piperidinol, a novel subtype selective inhibitor of the mouse type II GABA-transporter. *Br. J. Pharmacol.* **120**(6), 983–985.

Todorov, A. A., Kolchev, C. B., and Todorov, A. B. (2005). Tiagabine and gabapentin for the management of chronic pain. *Clin. J. Pain* **21**(4), 358–361.

Waagepetersen, H. S., Sonnewald, U., and Schousboe, A. (2003). Compartmentation of glutamine, glutamate, and GABA metabolism in neurons and astrocytes: Functional implications. *Neuroscientist* **9**(5), 398–403.

White, H. S., Sarup, A., Bolvig, T., Kristensen, A. S., Petersen, G., Nelson, N., Pickering, D. S., Larsson, O. M., Frølund, B., Krogsgaard-Larsen, P., and Schousboe, A. (2002). Correlation between anticonvulsant activity and inhibitory action on glial $\gamma$-aminobutyric acid uptake of the highly selective mouse $\gamma$-aminobutyric acid transporter 1 inhibitor 3-hydroxy-4-amino-4,5,6,7-tetrahydro-1,2-benzisoxazole and its *N*-alkylated analogs. *J. Pharmacol. Exp. Ther.* **302**(2), 636–644.

White, H. S., Watson, W. P., Hansen, S. L., Slough, S., Perregaard, J., Sarup, A., Bolvig, T., Petersen, G., Larsson, O. M., Clausen, R. P., Frølund, B., Falch, E., *et al.* (2005). First demonstration of a functional role for central nervous system betaine/$\gamma$-aminobutyric acid transporter (mGAT2) based on synergistic anticonvulsant action among inhibitors of mGAT1 and mGAT2. *J. Pharmacol. Exp. Ther.* **312**(2), 866–874.

Yunger, L. M., Fowler, P. J., Zarevics, P., and Setler, P. E. (1984). Novel inhibitors of $\gamma$-aminobutyric acid (GABA) uptake: Anticonvulsant actions in rats and mice. *J. Pharmacol. Exp. Ther.* **228**(1), 109–115.

Zhu, X. M., and Ong, W. Y. (2004). A light and electron microscopic study of betaine/GABA transporter distribution in the monkey cerebral neocortex and hippocampus. *J. Neurocytol.* **33**(2), 233–240.

Zwanzger, P., and Rupprecht, R. (2005). Selective GABAergic treatment for panic? Investigations in experimental panic induction and panic disorder. *J. Psychiatry Neurosci.* **30**(3), 167–175.

**Graham A. R. Johnston*, Jane R. Hanrahan[†], Mary Chebib[†], Rujee K. Duke*, and Kenneth N. Mewett***

*Department of Pharmacology, The University of Sydney
NSW, 2006, Australia

[†]Faculty of Pharmacy, The University of Sydney
NSW, 2006, Australia

# Modulation of Ionotropic GABA Receptors by Natural Products of Plant Origin

## I. Chapter Overview

There is now an impressive array of natural products of plant origin that are known to influence the function of ionotropic receptors for GABA. The major chemical classes of such natural products are flavonoids, terpenoids, phenols, and polyacetylenic alcohols. While it was the interaction of flavonoids with benzodiazepine modulatory sites on $GABA_A$ receptors that led to the great interest in flavonoids as positive modulators of such receptors, many of the interactions between flavonoids and $GABA_A$ receptors do not involve classical flumazenil-sensitive benzodiazepine sites. There are significant synergistic interactions between some of these positive modulators, for example, between substances isolated from *Valeriana officinalis*. Thus, the sleep inducing effects of hesperidin are potentiated by 6-methylapigenin, while the sedating and sleep inducing effects of valerenic acid are dramatically potentiated when co-administered with the flavonoid glycoside linarin.

*Advances in Pharmacology, Volume 54*

1054-3589/06 $35.00
DOI: 10.1016/S1054-3589(06)54012-8

The discovery of second order positive modulators adds an exciting new dimension to the concept of allosteric modulation of $GABA_A$ receptors. Second order positive modulators act only in conjunction with a specific first order positive modulator. The dietary flavonoids apigenin and (−)-epigallocatechin gallate, under conditions in which they have no direct action on the activation of $GABA_A$ receptors by GABA, have been shown to enhance the first order positive modulatory action of diazepam. The complexity of the interactions between active constituents of herbal preparations indicates that functional assays are vital for the quality control of such preparations. Understanding such complexity is likely to provide greater insight into the mechanisms underlying the allosteric modulation of ionotropic GABA receptors.

## II. Introduction

Natural products of plant origin represent a rich diversity in chemical structures that has led to the discovery of important therapeutic agents. There is now an impressive array of natural products that are known to influence the function of ionotropic receptors for GABA, the major inhibitory neurotransmitter in the brain. Many of the chemicals first used to study ionotropic GABA receptors are of plant origin including the antagonists bicuculline (from *Dicentra cucullaria*) (Curtis *et al.*, 1970) and picrotoxin (from *Anamirta cocculus*) (Jarboe *et al.*, 1968) and the agonist muscimol (from *Amanita muscaria*) (Johnston *et al.*, 1968). We now know that a wide range of plant-derived flavonoids, terpenes, and related substances modulate the function of ionotropic GABA receptors. Such GABA modulators have been found in fruit (e.g., grapefruit), vegetables (e.g., onions), various beverages (including tea, red wine, and whiskey), and in herbal preparations (such as *Ginkgo biloba* and *Ginseng*). These substances are known to cross the blood–brain barrier and are thus able to influence brain function.

There is increasing community acceptance of herbal medicines and functional foods. The occurrence of substances that could modulate GABA receptor function in such preparations may underlie some of the actions that herbal medicines and functional foods may have on brain function. There is a widely held view that "natural substances" are inherently safer than "unnatural substances," that is, synthetic chemicals. In fact, many of the most toxic chemicals are natural products and the majority of therapeutic agents are synthetic. It is the molecular structure and dose that determine the effects of substances on human health, not whether they are of natural or synthetic origin (Topliss *et al.*, 2002). In the present context, it is the chemical diversity of natural substances and their effects on brain function that are important both to provide a rational basis for the understanding of the effects of dietary chemicals and herbal products and to lead to the development of new therapeutic agents and strategies.

This review is directed toward the effects of some natural products of plant origin on the function of ionotropic GABA receptors. GABA itself is an important plant constituent, widely studied as a metabolite involved in responses to stress (Bouche and Fromm, 2004), but it may also have a role as a signaling molecule (Bouche *et al.*, 2003) and in regulating pollen tube growth and guidance (Yang, 2003). The presence of GABA can be a confounding factor in the bioactivity-guided fractionation of extracts of traditional medicinal plants using GABA/benzodiazepine binding assays (Misra, 1998). Furthermore, the use of benzodiazepine binding assays appears unwise in view of the discovery of an increasing number of agents that modulate ionotropic GABA receptors independently of classical flumazenil-sensitive benzodiazepine sites (Johnston, 2005).

## III. Ionotropic GABA Receptors

Ionotropic receptors for the inhibitory neurotransmitter GABA are found on most, if not all, neurons in the central nervous system (CNS) (Chebib and Johnston, 2000). They are ligand-gated ion channels that mediate fast neurotransmission via a central pore constituted by five surrounding protein subunits that on activation by GABA is permeant to chloride ions. They belong to the nicotinicoid superfamily of ligand-gated ion channels (Le Novere and Changeux, 2001) that includes nicotinic acetylcholine, strychnine-sensitive glycine, and $5HT_3$ receptors. The family of ionotropic GABA receptors is divided into two subfamilies, $GABA_A$ and $GABA_C$ receptors on the basis of their ability to form endogenous functional heteromeric and homomeric receptors, respectively, and differences in their physiological and pharmacological properties (Chebib and Johnston, 2000).

The heteromeric $GABA_A$ receptors are made up of different protein subunits (e.g., a common makeup involves two $\alpha1$, two $\beta2$, and one $\gamma2$ subunits). There are 16 different subunits comprising the $GABA_A$ receptor family: $\alpha1-6$, $\beta1-3$, $\gamma1-3$, $\delta$, $\epsilon$, $\pi$, and $\theta$ (Whiting, 2003). In addition, there are splice variants of many of these subunits. While the potential structural diversity of $GABA_A$ receptors is huge, studies of native $GABA_A$ receptors suggest that there may be fewer than 20 widely occurring $GABA_A$ receptor subtype combinations (McKernan and Whiting, 1996; Whiting, 2003). There is less diversity in the homomeric $GABA_C$ receptors in that they are made up exclusively of either $\rho1$, $\rho2$, or $\rho3$ subunits, although "pseudoheteromeric" $GABA_C$ receptors have been described (Johnston *et al.*, 2003).

## A. $GABA_A$ Receptors as Therapeutic Targets

Enhancing the action of GABA on $GABA_A$ receptors is a key property of several classes of important therapeutic agents including the benzodiazepines, barbiturates, and many general anesthetics. With advances in our understanding of the molecular diversity of $GABA_A$ receptors, there is an urgent need for the development of agents acting on subtypes of these receptors. The potential therapeutic market for subtype selective modulators of $GABA_A$ receptors is huge with particular emphasis on the treatment of anxiety, cognitive disorders, epilepsy, insomnia, and schizophrenia.

Heritable mutations are known to occur across the nicotinicoid superfamily of ligand-gated ion channels including $GABA_A$ receptors (Vafa and Schofield, 1998). For example, Angelman syndrome, a neurodevelopmental disorder characterized by severe mental retardation, epilepsy, and delayed motor development, has been associated with deletions of $GABA_A$ receptor $\beta3$ subunits (Holopainen *et al.*, 2001). Heritable mutations in $GABA_A$ receptor subunits are strongly implicated in idiopathic generalized epilepsies (Jones-Davis and Macdonald, 2003). GABA systems are known to play an important role in sleep, and modulators of $GABA_A$ receptors are widely used to promote restful sleep (Gottesmann, 2002).

The subunit composition of $GABA_A$ receptors influences the effects of modulators. The therapeutically useful properties of benzodiazepines (anxiolytic, anticonvulsant, sedative, and muscle-relaxant effects) may result from actions on different $GABA_A$ receptor subtypes. Studies of mice deficient in particular $\alpha$ subunits suggest that the $\alpha1$-$GABA_A$ subunit is responsible for the sedative properties of benzodiazepines, while the $\alpha2$-$GABA_A$ subunit is responsible for the anxiolytic properties (McKernan *et al.*, 2000). The $\delta$ subunit has been shown to confer significantly increased sensitivity to ethanol at $GABA_A$ receptors (Wallner *et al.*, 2003).

Agents that enhance the action of GABA on $GABA_A$ receptors are known as positive modulators (Johnston, 1996) and are generally considered to involve action at allosteric sites on $GABA_A$ receptors remote from the GABA recognition sites (orthosteric sites). Such allosteric sites are highly valued as targets for the development of subtype specific drugs, since there is generally greater diversity between receptor subtypes in amino acid sequence at allosteric sites than at orthosteric sites (Christopoulos, 2002). Agents that reduce the action of GABA on $GABA_A$ receptors are known as negative allosteric modulators (once known as "inverse agonists," since they have the opposite actions to those of the classical benzodiazepines). Agents that block the actions of both positive and negative allosteric modulators are known as neutralizing allosteric modulators, for example, the classical benzodiazepine "antagonist" flumazenil (Johnston, 1996).

The discovery of second order positive modulators adds an exciting new dimension to the concept of allosteric modulation of $GABA_A$ receptors

(Campbell *et al.*, 2004). While it is known that some first order positive modulators interact positively with each other, for example, ethanol and neurosteroids (Akk and Steinbach, 2003), second order positive modulators act only in conjunction with a specific first order positive modulator. The dietary flavonoids apigenin and (−)-epigallocatechin gallate, under conditions in which they have no direct effect on the activation of $GABA_A$ receptors by GABA, have been shown to enhance the first order positive modulatory action of diazepam. The second order modulatory action of these flavonoids appears to be specific for first order benzodiazepine modulators as it is not observed with first order modulators such as allopregnanolone or pentobarbitone. Such second order modulation may result from alteration in the coupling of benzodiazepine allosteric sites with the orthosteric GABA sites on $GABA_A$ receptors. The second order modulation of a primary modulator may represent a novel form of drug action that is unlikely to be restricted to the modulation of $GABA_A$ receptors (Campbell *et al.*, 2004). In addition to offering increased chemical diversity of agents acting on $GABA_A$ receptors, second order allosteric modulators offer further possibilities in that they could influence the action of endogenous first order modulators and also offer the opportunity of reducing the dose needed of a drug acting as a first order modulator such as a benzodiazepine.

### B. $GABA_C$ Receptors as Therapeutic Targets

There is evidence for functional $GABA_C$ receptors in the retina, spinal cord, superior colliculus, pituitary, and gastrointestinal tract. Given the lower abundance and less widespread distribution of $GABA_C$ receptors in the CNS compared to $GABA_A$ receptors, $GABA_C$ receptors may be a more selective drug target than $GABA_A$ receptors (Johnston *et al.*, 2003). The major indications for drugs acting on $GABA_C$ receptors are in the treatment of visual, sleep, and cognitive disorders. Agents acting on $GABA_C$ receptors may be useful for the treatment of myopia (Froestl *et al.*, 2004). A study has linked $GABA_C$ receptors to Alzheimer's disease by providing evidence that the stimulation of $GABA_C$ receptors has a neuroprotective action against amyloid $\beta$ protein (Liu *et al.*, 2005).

## IV. Flavonoids

Flavonoids are responsible for many of the brilliant colors of fruits and vegetables and are important constituents of red wine, green tea, and many herbal preparations. Fruits, vegetables, and beverages, such as tea and red wine, are major sources of flavonoids in our diet (Aherne and O'Brien, 2002). It has been estimated that the average daily intake of flavonoids is 1–2 g (Havsteen, 2002). Many flavonoids are polyphenolic and are thus strongly antioxidant (Heim *et al.*, 2002). They have a wide variety of biological activities and are being studied intensively as anticancer agents (Le Marchand, 2002) and for their effects on the vascular system (Woodman and Chan, 2004). More than 5000 different flavonoids have been described.

Flavonoids have a range of activities on $GABA_A$ receptors (Marder and Paladini, 2002) and have been described as a "new family of benzodiazepine receptor ligands" (Medina *et al.*, 1997). They were first linked to $GABA_A$ receptors when three isoflavans isolated from bovine urine were shown to inhibit diazepam binding to brain membranes (Luk *et al.*, 1983). The most potent compound was 3′,7-dihydroxyisoflavan (Fig. 1) with an $IC_{50}$ of 45 μM. These isoflavans were most probably derived from plant sources in the bovine diet. Subsequently many flavonoids directly isolated from plants were shown to influence benzodiazepine binding (Marder and Paladini, 2002).

A low-affinity benzodiazepine site is emerging as a possible target for the modulatory action of some flavonoids. This site is insensitive to flumazenil and has been described on a wide range of $GABA_A$ receptors including those made up of only $\alpha1\beta2$ subunits (Walters *et al.*, 2000).

## A. Amentoflavone

The biflavonoid amentoflavone (Fig. 1) has one of the most potent actions of any plant-derived flavonoid in displacing benzodiazepine binding to rat brain membranes with a nM affinity comparable to that of diazepam (Nielsen *et al.*, 1988). Further studies on amentoflavone, however, illustrate the difficulties in investigating flavonoid actions—the variety of effects, the lack of selectivity, the need for functional assays, and the mismatch between *in vitro* and *in vivo* findings.

Amentoflavone was isolated from Karmelitter Geist®, an alcoholic tincture of various plants used to treat anxiety and epilepsy. However, it was concluded that amentoflavone could not be responsible for any pharmacological effects of the plant extract as amentoflavone did not influence flunitrazepam binding in the brain *in vivo* following i.v. administration to mice (Nielsen *et al.*, 1988). It was suggested that amentoflavone was either rapidly metabolized or did not cross the blood–brain barrier, but a study does indicate that amentoflavone does cross the blood–brain barrier (Gutmann *et al.*, 2002).

Amentoflavone occurs in a variety of herbal preparations including St John's wort (Baureithel *et al.*, 1997). It can be extracted from *Ginkgo biloba* but is removed from herbal preparations of *Ginkgo* such as EGb 761 (Hanrahan *et al.*, 2003). A comprehensive battery of *in vitro* binding assays has shown that amentoflavone influences a variety of G-protein–coupled receptors for serotonin, dopamine, and opioids at nM concentrations while

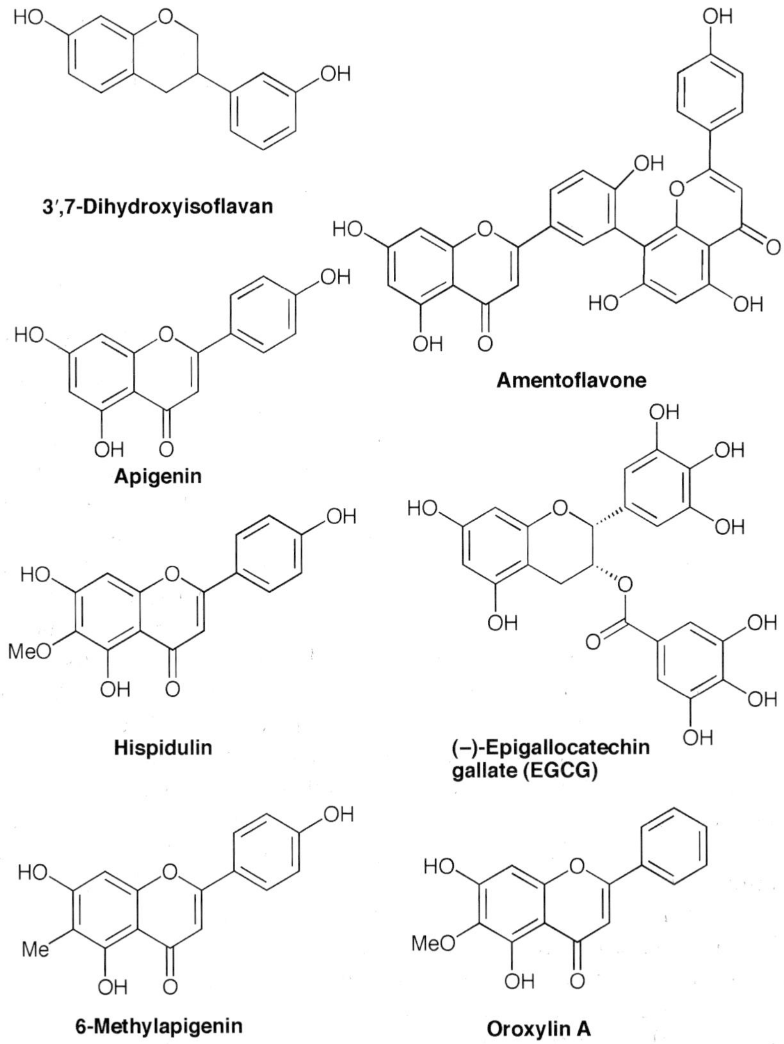

3′,7-Dihydroxyisoflavan

Amentoflavone

Apigenin

Hispidulin

(−)-Epigallocatechin gallate (EGCG)

6-Methylapigenin

Oroxylin A

**FIGURE 1** Some representative flavonoids that have been shown to influence benzodiazepine binding to brain membranes (3′,7-dihyroxyisoflavan, amentoflavone, apigenin, 6-methylapigenin, and oroxylin A), to act at $GABA_A$ receptor as positive modulators (hispidulin) or negative modulators (amentoflavone, apigenin), or at $GABA_C$ receptors as negative modulators (apigenin). In addition, apigenin and (−)-epigallocatechin gallate have been found to have a novel second order modulatory action on the first order modulation of $GABA_A$ receptors by diazepam.

having no effect on the binding of the $GABA_A$ agonist muscimol to $GABA_A$ receptors (Butterweck *et al.*, 2002). Using a functional assay employing recombinant $\alpha1\beta2\gamma2L$ $GABA_A$ receptors expressed in oocytes, amentoflavone has been shown to be a relatively weak ($EC_{50}$ 4 μM) negative allosteric modulator of GABA action acting independently of classical flumazenil-sensitive benzodiazepine modulatory sites (Hanrahan *et al.*, 2003). It may be that amentoflavone has different effects on other $GABA_A$ receptor subtypes.

## B. Apigenin—the Concept of Second Order Positive Modulation

Apigenin (5,7,4′-trihydroxyflavone) (Fig. 1) is a common flavonoid found in a range of plants, including chamomile (*Matricicaria recutita*). The traditional use of chamomile tea as a treatment for insomnia and anxiety led to investigations of its active constituents including apigenin. Apigenin was found to have anxiolytic properties, and it competitively inhibited the binding of flunitrazepam to brain membranes without influencing the binding of muscimol to $GABA_A$ receptors (Viola *et al.*, 1995). Apigenin was described as having "a clear anxiolytic effect in mice in the elevated plus maze without evidencing sedation or muscle relaxation effects at doses similar to those used for classical benzodiazepines" while being devoid of anticonvulsant effects (Viola *et al.*, 1995). These findings are in contrast to a later study in rats where apigenin was shown to reduce the latency of onset of picrotoxin-induced convulsions and to reduce locomotor activity but was devoid of anxiolytic or muscle relaxant activities (Avallone *et al.*, 2000). This later study showed that apigenin could reduce GABA-activated chloride currents in cultured cerebellar granule cells, an action that could be blocked by flumazenil and thus likely to involve classical benzodiazepine allosteric sites on $GABA_A$ receptors. The inhibitory action of apigenin on locomotor behavior, however, could not be blocked by flumazenil and thus could not "be ascribed to an interaction with $GABA_A$-benzodiazepine receptors but to other neurotransmitter systems" (Avallone *et al.*, 2000). Another study from the same group reported that apigenin exerted sedative effects on locomotor activity in rats in a flumazenil-insensitive manner, whereas chrysin, a structurally related flavonoid lacking the 4′-hydroxy substituent of apigenin, showed a clear flumazenil-sensitive anxiolytic effect in addition to the flumazenil-insensitive sedation (Zanoli *et al.*, 2000). The apparent discrepancy between the behavioral effects of apigenin on mice (Viola *et al.*, 1995) and rats (Avallone *et al.*, 2000) may be due to mice having higher baseline levels of anxiety. Flumazenil-insensitive effects of flavonoids on $GABA_A$ receptors have been extensively described (Hall *et al.*, 2004).

Studies on human recombinant receptors in oocytes have shown that apigenin inhibited the activation of $\alpha1\beta1\gamma2S$ $GABA_A$ receptors in a flumazenil-insensitive manner and had a similar effect on $\rho1$ $GABA_C$ receptors (Goutman *et al.*, 2003). Other studies on recombinant $\alpha1\beta2\gamma2L$ $GABA_A$ receptors also found an inhibitory effect of apigenin on GABA responses and, in addition an enhancement of the diazepam-induced positive allosteric modulation of GABA responses by lower concentrations of apigenin, described as a second order modulation by apigenin of the first order modulation by diazepam (Campbell *et al.*, 2004).

The novel second order modulation by apigenin of the maximum first order modulatory action of diazepam of the activation by GABA of $GABA_A$ receptors observed in these studies may result from apigenin altering the coupling of the benzodiazepine allosteric sites with the orthosteric GABA sites on $GABA_A$ receptors (Campbell *et al.*, 2004). There is evidence from binding studies that the nexus between the benzodiazepine and GABA sites on $GABA_A$ receptors is complex and involves other factors, such as phospholipids, that can be removed from brain membranes by detergent extraction (Skerritt *et al.*, 1982).

The flumazenil-sensitive anxiolytic effects of apigenin may be the result of apigenin enhancing a subthreshold effect of an endogenous benzodiazepine system (Baraldi *et al.*, 2000). Evidence for physiologically relevant endozepines has come from the discovery of a mutant $GABA_A$ receptor in childhood absence epilepsy and febrile seizures that has diminished sensitivity to benzodiazepines with no other apparent alteration in functioning (Wallace *et al.*, 2001).

Overall, it seems that the effects of apigenin on $GABA_A$ receptors are complex and involve both flumazenil-sensitive and flumazenil-insensitive components and that other receptors could be involved in the behavioral effects of apigenin. Like most flavonoids, apigenin is known to have a wide variety of biological actions including effects on adenosine receptors (Jacobson *et al.*, 2002) and progestational activity (Zand *et al.*, 2000). Of particular interest are the findings that apigenin at concentrations at which it inhibits $GABA_A$ and $GABA_C$ receptors also inhibits NMDA receptors (Losi *et al.*, 2004); such an action could contribute to flumazenil-insensitive sedative actions of apigenin.

## C. Hispidulin and Related Flavonoids

Hispidulin (4′,5,7-trihydroxy-6-methoxyflavone, i.e., the 6-methoxy derivative of apigenin) (Fig. 1) was isolated together with apigenin from *Salvia officinalis* (sage) using a benzodiazepine binding assay-guided fractionation (Kavvadias *et al.*, 2003). Hispidulin was some 30 times more potent than apigenin in displacing flumazenil binding. Preparations of sage have been used in herbal medicine to assist memory (Perry *et al.*, 1999a, 2000), and an extract of *Salvia lavandulaefolia* (Spanish sage) has been shown to enhance memory in healthy young volunteers (Tildesley *et al.*, 2003). Unlike apigenin, hispidulin has been shown to act as a positive allosteric modulator of $\alpha1,3,5,6\beta2\gamma2S$ $GABA_A$ receptor subtypes showing little subtype selectivity, although being a little more potent at $\alpha1,2,5\beta2\gamma2S$

subtypes than at $\alpha3,6\beta2\gamma2S$ subtypes (Kavvadias *et al.*, 2004). The positive modulatory action of 10-μM hispidulin at $\alpha1\beta2\gamma2S$ receptors was reduced from 47% to 17% by flumazenil, indicating that sites other than classical flumazenil-sensitive benzodiazepine sites were involved in the action of hispidulin. As hispidulin did not influence the action of GABA on $\alpha1\beta2$ $GABA_A$ receptors, this indicates that it does not interact with low-affinity flumazenil-insensitive benzodiazepine sites (Walters *et al.*, 2000) in contrast to other flavonoids such as 6-methylflavone (Hall *et al.*, 2004). Of significance is the ability of hispidulin to act as a positive modulator at $\alpha6\beta2\gamma2L$ $GABA_A$ receptors unlike diazepam; 10-μM hispidulin enhanced the action of GABA at these receptors by 65%, this action being reduced by 1-μM flumazenil to 37% (Kavvadias *et al.*, 2004). Hispidulin was shown to have an anticonvulsant action in seizure prone Mongolian gerbils and to pass the blood–brain barrier (Kavvadias *et al.*, 2004).

Flavonoids structurally related to hispidulin that influence benzodiazepine binding have been isolated from *Scutellaria baicalensis*, an important herb in traditional Chinese medicine (Wang *et al.*, 2002). Oroxylin A (5,7-dihydroxy-6-methoxyflavone, i.e., hispidulin lacking the 4′-hydroxy group) (Fig. 1) inhibits flunitrazepam binding at 1 μM and on oral administration acts as a neutralizing allosteric modulator blocking the anxiolytic, myorelaxant, and motor incoordination effects but not the sedative and anticonvulsant effects elicited by diazepam (Huen *et al.*, 2003b). 6-Methylapigenin (4′,5,7-dihydroxy-6-methylflavone) (Fig. 1) isolated from *Valeriana wallichii*, a known sedative herb, influences benzodiazepine binding at 0.5 μM in manner suggesting it may be a positive modulator of $GABA_A$ receptors (Wasowski *et al.*, 2002). 6-Methylapigenin has anxiolytic properties and is able to potentiate the sleep-enhancing properties of hespiridin, a flavanone glycoside also isolated from *Valeriana officinalis* (Marder *et al.*, 2003).

Thus, flavones substituted in the 6-position with a methoxy or methyl substituent have interesting effects on $GABA_A$ receptor function and may contribute to the properties of some herbal preparations. Natural and synthetic 2′-hydroxy–substituted flavones are also of interest (Huen *et al.*, 2003a). Several flavonoid glycosides including goodyerin (Du *et al.*, 2002), linarin, and hesperidin (Fig. 2) (Fernandez *et al.*, 2004) are also being studied as sedative and anticonvulsant agents likely to interact with $GABA_A$ receptors.

### D. (−)-Epigallocatechin Gallate—a Potent Second Order Modulator

Green tea polyphenols are being considered as therapeutic agents in well-controlled epidemiological studies, aimed to alter brain aging processes and to serve as possible neuroprotective agents in progressive neurodegenerative

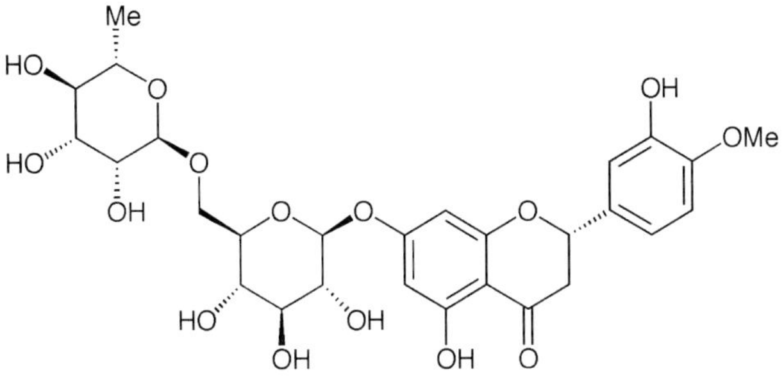

**Hesperidin**

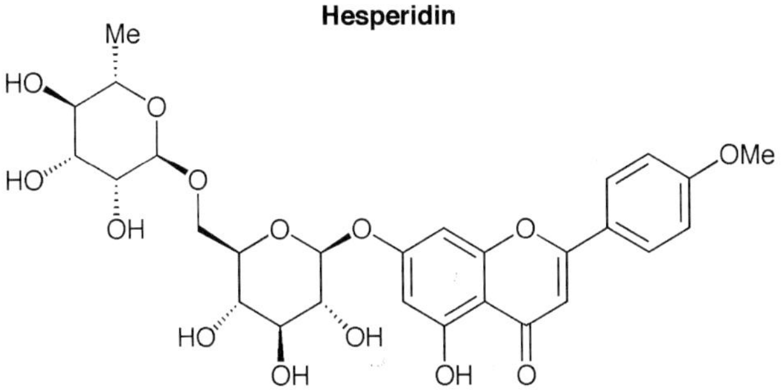

**Linarin**

**FIGURE 2** Two flavonoid glycosides found in *Valeriana officinalis* that show synergistic effects with other positive modulators of $GABA_A$ receptor function.

disorders such as Parkinson's and Alzheimer's diseases (Weinreb *et al.*, 2004).

(−)-Epigallocatechin-3-gallate (EGCG) (Fig. 1) is the major polyphenol in green tea (*Camellia sinensis*). EGCG was found to have an inhibitory action on the activation by GABA of bovine recombinant $\alpha1\beta1$ $GABA_A$ (Hossain *et al.*, 2002b). However, in studies on $\alpha1\beta2\gamma2L$ $GABA_A$ receptors, apigenin at low concentrations (0.1 μM) showed a potent second order modulatory action on the first order modulation by diazepam, while inhibiting the action of GABA at higher concentrations (>1 μM) (Campbell *et al.*, 2004). EGCG was thus an order of magnitude more potent than apigenin in acting as a second order modulator. EGCG and apigenin may serve as lead compounds for the development of more selective agents for the second order modulation of benzodiazepine enhancement of the action of GABA on $GABA_A$ receptors (Campbell *et al.*, 2004).

There is much interest in the anticancer and antitumor properties of EGCG associated with the consumption of green tea (Lambert and Yang, 2003). EGCG has anticancer effects on ovarian carcinoma cell lines (Huh *et al.*, 2004), is a selective inhibitor of COX-2 expression (Hussain *et al.*, 2005), and induces apoptosis in monocytes (Kawai *et al.*, 2005). Little is known about the CNS actions of this flavan, but it is found in the brain after gastric administration to mice (Suganuma *et al.*, 1998) and is neuroprotective in rats on i.p. injection after focal ischemia (Choi *et al.*, 2004) and in a mouse model of Parkinson's disease (Levites *et al.*, 2002). This neuroprotective action may be associated with its antioxidant properties, but enhancement of $GABA_A$ mediated synaptic inhibition could also contribute (Campbell *et al.*, 2004). In addition, EGCG is known to reduce glutamate-induced cytotoxicity via intracellular calcium ion modulation suggesting that other neurotransmitters systems may be involved (Lee *et al.*, 2004).

## V. Terpenoids

Terpenoids are widespread in plants, especially in what are known as essential oils that can be extracted from plants, and have a wide range of uses from perfume constituents to paint thinners. Terpenoids are oxygenated products formally derived from C5 isoprene units and are classified by the number of C5 units in their structure. Thus, monoterpenoids have 2 × C5 units, sesquiterpenoids 3 × C5 units, diterpenoids 4 × C5 units, and triterpenoids 6 × C5 units. The most widely used terpenoid in studies on $GABA_A$ receptors is the sesquiterpenoid lactone picrotoxinin (Fig. 4), a noncompetitive antagonist at $GABA_A$ receptors (Chebib and Johnston, 2000). A number of other terpenoids, however, are of interest for their actions on $GABA_A$ receptors.

### A. Monoterpenoids—α-Thujone, Thymol, Thymoquinone, Borneol

The monoterpenoid α-thujone (Fig. 3) is a psychoactive component of absinthe, a liqueur popular in France in the nineteenth and early twentieth centuries. It is found in extracts of wormwood (*Artemisia absinthium*) and some other herbal medicines and beverages since ancient Egyptian times (Deiml *et al.*, 2004). α-Thujone is a convulsant that acts as a negative allosteric modulator of $GABA_A$ receptors (Hold *et al.*, 2000). It also acts as an antagonist of $5HT_3$ receptors by influencing agonist-induced desensitization (Deiml *et al.*, 2004).

The structurally related substance thymol (Fig. 3), a constituent of thyme essential oil, is a flumazenil-insensitive positive allosteric modulator of $GABA_A$ receptors (Priestley *et al.*, 2003). At higher concentrations, thymol had a direct action on $GABA_A$ receptors similar to that of the anesthetic propofol and other phenols (Mohammadi *et al.*, 2001). The anticonvulsant effects of thymoquinone (Fig. 3), the major constituent of *Nigella sativa* seeds, may be due to positive modulation of $GABA_A$ receptors (Hosseinzadeh and Parvardeh, 2004).

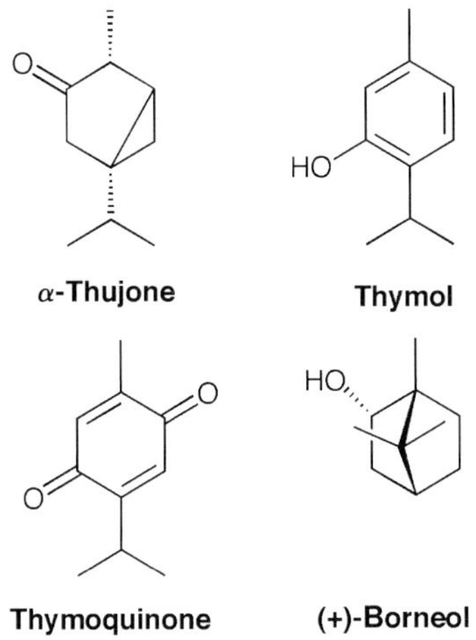

**FIGURE 3** Monoterpenoids (α-thujone, thymol, thymoquinone, and (+)-borneol) that act as positive modulators of $GABA_A$ receptor function.

(+)-Borneol (Fig. 3), a monoterpenoid found in many essential oils, is a flumazenil-insensitive positive allosteric modulator of human recombinant $\alpha 1\beta 2\gamma 2L$ $GABA_A$ receptors of low affinity ($EC_{50}$ 250 μM) but very high efficacy producing a 10-fold enhancement of the action of 10-μM GABA at a concentration of 450 μM (Granger *et al.*, 2005). (−)-Borneol showed similar positive modulatory properties to (+)-borneol, while isoborneol, (−)-bornyl acetate, and camphor (a known convulsant) were much less active. The relatively rigid cage structure of these bicyclic monoterpenes and their high efficacy may aid in a greater understanding of the molecular aspects of positive modulation. (+)-Borneol is found in high concentrations in extracts of *Valeriana officinalis* that are widely used to reduce the latency of sleep onset, the depth of sleep, and the perception of well-being. Extracts of *Valeriana* are known to contain a large number of constituents including flavonoids and terpenoids, many of which are considered to be active at $GABA_A$ receptors.

## B. Sesquiterpenoids—Bilobalide, Picrotoxinin, Valerenic Acid, and Isocurcumenol

Bilobalide (Fig. 4), a sesquiterpenoid lactone from *Ginkgo biloba* that bears some structural similarities to picrotoxinin, including a lipophilic side chain and a hydrophilic cage, is an antagonist at $GABA_A$ receptors (Huang *et al.*, 2003). Both bilobalide and picrotoxinin appear to act at sites in the chloride channel of $GABA_A$ receptors and are thus negative allosteric modulators, although their mode of action is complex. They also

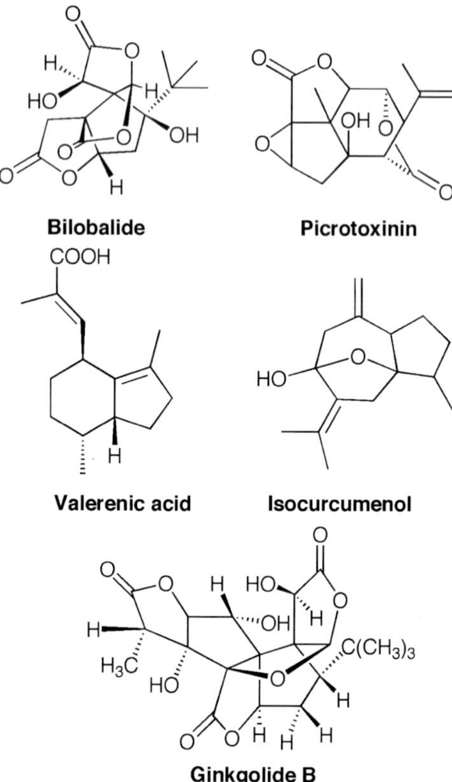


**FIGURE 4** Sesquiterpenoids and a related compound that act as negative modulators of $GABA_A$ and $GABA_C$ receptor function (bilobalide, picrotoxinin, and ginkgolide B) or as positive modulators of $GABA_A$ receptor function (valerenic acid, isocurcumenol).

act similarly on $\rho 1$ $GABA_C$ receptors (Huang *et al.*, 2006; Qian *et al.*, 2005).

The cognition-enhancing effects of *Ginkgo* extracts may be partly mediated by bilobalide acting to enhance hippocampal pyridamidal neuronal excitability (Sasaki *et al.*, 1999b). While picrotoxinin is a convulsant, bilobalide is an anticonvulsant (Sasaki *et al.*, 1999a,b). The lack of convulsant action in an agent that reduces GABA action may be important for enhancement of cognition. The lack of convulsant action of bilobalide may result from inhibition of glutamate release (Jones *et al.*, 2002). Bilobalide has a neuroprotective action in a variety of models (DeFeudis, 2002). The structurally related ginkgolides, especially ginkgolide B (Fig. 4), also act as negative modulators at $GABA_A$ receptors (Huang *et al.*, 2004; Ivic *et al.*, 2003). They also inhibit strychnine-sensitive glycine receptors and platelet activating factor (Chatterjee *et al.*, 2003; Ivic *et al.*, 2003). Bilobalide and the ginkgolides reduce barbiturate-induced sleeping time in mice, an effect perhaps relevant to the clinically observed "vigilance-enhancing" and antidepressant-like actions of *Ginkgo* extracts (Brochet *et al.*, 1999).

The sesquiterpenoid valerenic acid (Fig. 4) has a direct partial agonist action on $GABA_A$ receptors (Yuan *et al.*, 2004). Valerian extract and valerenic acid are partial agonists of the $5\text{-}HT_{5a}$ receptor *in vitro* (Dietz *et al.*, 2005). Valerenic acid is often assumed to be the most important active component of valerian extracts used in herbal medicine, but valerenic acid is only present in *Valeriana officinalis* and not in other active species widely used like *V. wallichii* and *V. edulis* (Fernandez *et al.*, 2004). The sedating and sleep-inducing effects of valerenic acid are dramatically potentiated when co-administered with the flavonoid glycoside linarin (Fig. 2) that is also found in *Valeriana officinalis* (Fernandez *et al.*, 2004).

Isocurcumenol (Fig. 4), a sesquiterpenoid from *Cyperus rotundus*, was found to inhibit flumazenil binding and enhance flunitrazepam binding in the presence of GABA in a manner consistent with it acting as a positive allosteric modulator (Ha *et al.*, 2002).

## C. Diterpenoids

The diterpenoid quinone miltirone (Fig. 5), from the Chinese medicinal herb *Salvia miltriorrhiza*, inhibited flunitrazepam binding at 0.3 μM and was orally active in animal models as a tranquilliser without muscle relaxant properties (Lee *et al.*, 1991). Structure–activity studies on miltirone led to the development of a synthetic compound that was much more potent than miltirone on flunitrazepam binding ($IC_{50}$ 0.05 μM) (Chang *et al.*, 1991). The diterpenoid lactone galdosol (Fig. 5) from the common sage *Saliva officinalis*, inhibited flumazenil binding at 0.8 μM (Kavvadias *et al.*, 2003).

The structurally related diterpenoids carnosic acid and carnosol (Fig. 5) extracted from *Salvia officinalis*, while not influencing diazepam or muscimol binding, did inhibit TBPS binding (Rutherford *et al.*, 1992). This suggests that, like flavonoids, diterpenoids can influence $GABA_A$ receptors in a manner independent of classical benzodiazepine sites and could be missed in benzodiazepine binding assays. The structures of galdosol, carnosic acid, and carnosol (Fig. 5) contain the *o*-isopropylphenolic moiety that is present in thymol (Fig. 3) and the anesthetic agent propofol.

## D. Triterpenoids

Ginsenosides, triterpenoid glycosides that are the major active constituents of *Panax ginseng*, are known to negatively modulate nicotinic and NMDA receptor activity. Of a series of ginsenosides, ginsenoside Rc

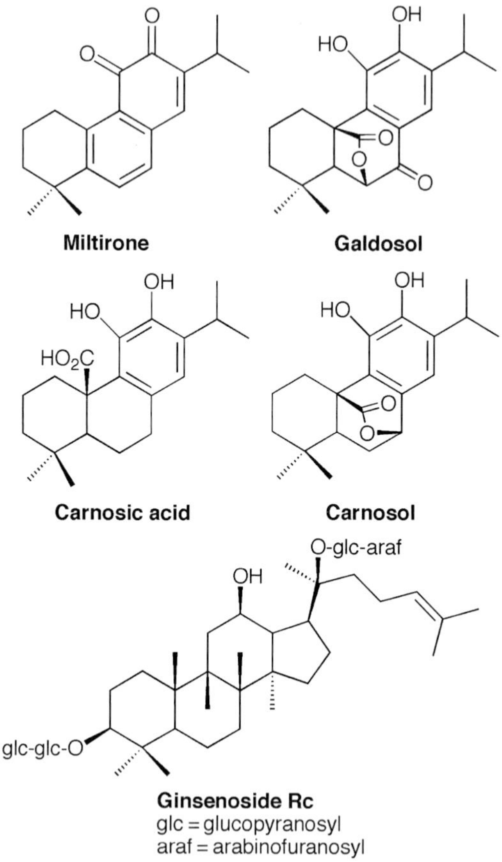

**Miltirone** **Galdosol**

**Carnosic acid** **Carnosol**

**Ginsenoside Rc**
glc = glucopyranosyl
araf = arabinofuranosyl

**FIGURE 5** Diterpenoids and a triterpenoid that inhibit benzodiazepine binding (miltirone, galdosol), act as a positive modulator of $GABA_A$ receptor function (ginsenoside Rc) or inhibit TBPS binding without influencing benzodiazepine binding (carnosic acid, carnosol).

(Fig. 5) was the most potent ($EC_{50}$ 53 μM) in enhancing the action of GABA on recombinant $\alpha1\beta1\gamma2S$ $GABA_A$ receptors expressed in oocytes (Choi *et al.*, 2003).

## VI. Other Phenolic Compounds

### A. Honokiol

The bark of the root and stem of various *Magnolia* species has been used in Traditional Chinese Medicine to treat a variety of disorders including anxiety. The CNS muscle relaxant and depressant actions of the

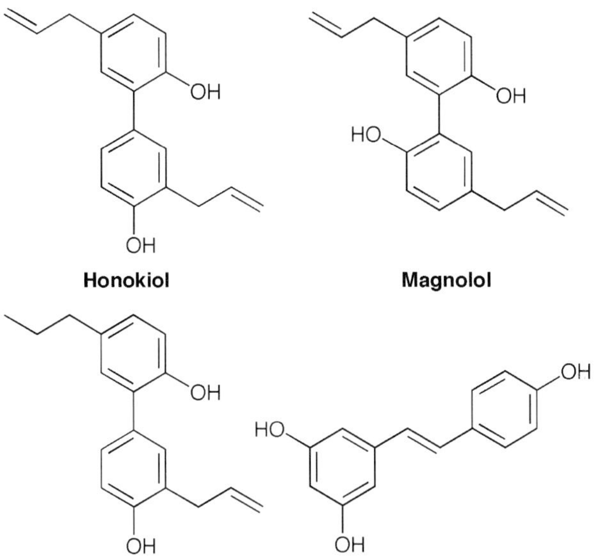

**FIGURE 6** Phenolic compounds that act as positive modulators of $GABA_A$ receptor function particularly those that contain $\alpha2$ subunits (honokiol, magnolol), or at $GABA_C$ receptors as positive (dihydrohonokiol-B) or negative modulators (resveratrol).

biphenols, honokiol and magnolol (Fig. 6), and related compounds extracted from *Magnolia officinalis* have been known for sometime (Watanabe *et al.*, 1975, 1983). Of these compounds honokiol was the most potent. At much lower doses than those that produce sedation, honokiol shows anxiolytic activity in mice in the elevated plus maze (Kuribara *et al.*, 1999). The anxiolytic effect of honokiol was inhibited by the benzodiazepine antagonist flumazenil and by the $GABA_A$ receptor antagonist bicuculline. In contrast to diazepam, honokiol selectively induces an anxiolytic effect with less liability of eliciting motor dysfunction or sedation suggesting that honokiol may act selectively on a subset of $GABA_A$ receptors. At anxiolytic doses, honokiol was less likely than diazepam to induce physical dependence, central depression, and amnesia (Kuribara *et al.*, 1999).

Studies with recombinant $GABA_A$ receptors expressed in the Sf-9/baculovirus system showed that honokiol potently enhanced the binding of muscimol to recombinant receptors containing the $\alpha2$ subunit producing a fourfold enhancement (Ai *et al.*, 2001). This resulted from an increase in the number of muscimol binding sites. Honokiol preferentially increased muscimol binding to rat brain membranes prepared from hippocampus compared to those from cortex or cerebellum. The apparent increase in the number of muscimol binding sites may be due to honokiol allosterically increasing the affinities of low-affinity muscimol binding sites (Squires *et al.*, 1999). The preferential effect of honokiol on $\alpha 2$ subunit-containing $GABA_A$ receptors is consistent with such receptors being associated with the anxiolytic rather than the sedative actions of diazepam (McKernan *et al.*, 2000).

Honokiol protects rat brain from focal cerebral ischemia-reperfusion injury by inhibiting neutrophil infiltration and the production of reactive oxygen species (Liou *et al.*, 2003b), consistent with its antiplatelet aggregation, anti-inflammatory, and antioxidant properties (Liou *et al.*, 2003a). Honokiol has been described as having anticancer properties inducing apoptosis through activating caspase cascades (Watanabe *et al.*, 1975) and as acting on calcium channels to inhibit muscle contraction (Lu *et al.*, 2003). Furthermore, it has been found to have neurotrophic activity in promoting neurite outgrowth in fetal rat cortical neuronal cultures (Fukuyama *et al.*, 2002).

Dihydrohonokiol-B (Fig. 6) was significantly more effective than honokiol in producing anxiolysis (Kuribara *et al.*, 2000). While the anxiolytic activity of dihydrohonokiol-B could be blocked by flumazenil, it was insensitive to bicuculline suggesting that it acted differently to honokiol (Kuribara *et al.*, 2000). Further studies on dihydrohonokiol-B showed that it inhibited ammonia-induced increases in intracellular chloride ion concentration in hippocampal neuronal cultures and that this action was insensitive to bicuculline but was inhibited by the $GABA_C$ receptor antagonist TPMPA (Irie *et al.*, 2001). This study suggests a possible role of $GABA_C$ receptors in protection against potentially pathological accumulations of chloride ions in neurons. Subsequent studies on amyloid $\beta$ protein-induced neurotoxicity in hippocampal neuronal cultures showed that dihydrohonokiol-B protected against amyloid $\beta$-induced elevation of intracellular chloride ions in a TPMPA-sensitive manner indicating the involvement of $GABA_C$ receptors (Liu *et al.*, 2005). The authors suggest that dihydrohonokiol-B and $GABA_C$ receptor agonists can be one of the therapeutic and/or preventative strategies in Alzheimer's disease patients.

The exact role of $GABA_C$ receptors in the neuroprotective action of dihydrohonokiol-B is unclear. The presence of $\rho 1$, $\rho 2$, and $\rho 3$ $GABA_C$ receptor subunits has been demonstrated in rat hippocampus by RT-PCR, and the $GABA_C$ agonist *cis*-4-aminocrotonic acid has been shown to suppress ammonia-induced apoptosis in hippocampal neurons in a TPMPA-sensitive manner (Yang *et al.*, 2003). It is not known whether or not dihydrohonokiol-B, or honokiol, have a positive modulatory action on $GABA_C$ receptors. Furthermore, in other tissues it has been shown that $GABA_A$ and $GABA_C$ receptors have opposing roles (Gibbs and Johnston, 2005) and the interplay between $GABA_A$ and $GABA_C$ receptors may be important in the actions of dihydrohonokiol-B and honokiol.

## B. Resveratrol

The relatively low incidence of coronary heart diseases in France, despite intake of a high-fat diet—the "French Paradox"—has been attributed to the consumption of red wine containing high levels of polyphenolic compounds (Mojzisova and Kuchta, 2001; Sun *et al.*, 2002). Resveratrol (3,4′,5-trihydroxystilbene) (Fig. 6) is one of the most interesting polyphenolic compounds found in red wine. It has been shown to have estrogenic (Turner *et al.*, 1999) and neuroprotective effects (Bastianetto *et al.*, 2000). Resveratrol and related compounds are found in a variety of plants and herbs. Major dietary sources include grapes, wine, peanuts, and soy (Burns *et al.*, 2002). These compounds are also found in Itadori tea, which has long been used in Japan and China as a traditional remedy for heart disease and stroke (Burns *et al.*, 2002).

Resveratrol (Fig. 6) shows some structural similarity to apigenin (Fig. 1). It acts as a noncompetitive inhibitor of the effects of GABA (1 μM) at human $\rho 1$ recombinant $GABA_C$ receptors with an $IC_{50}$ of 72 μM, while having no significant effect at doses up to 100 μM on the effects of GABA (40 μM) at $\alpha 1\beta 2\gamma 2L$ $GABA_A$ receptors (Campbell and Johnston, 2003). Resveratrol did not influence the positive modulation of $GABA_A$ receptors by diazepam, unlike apigenin (Campbell *et al.*, 2004). Resveratrol has been patented for the treatment of mild cognitive impairment based on its ability to increase the expression of soluble amyloid precursor protein (Wurtman and Lee, 2002). The $GABA_C$ antagonist effect of resveratrol may contribute to its effects on memory as other known $GABA_C$ antagonists have been shown to influence memory (Gibbs and Johnston, 2005; Johnston *et al.*, 2003). This is interesting in view of the evidence for an association between the neurotoxic effects of amyloid $\beta$ protein and $GABA_C$ receptors (Liu *et al.*, 2005).

# VII. Polyacetylenic Alcohols

The polyacetylene compounds that occur in plants are generally toxic. Cunaniol (Fig. 7), from the leaves of *Clibadium sylvestre* used as a fish poison by South American Indians (Clark, 1969), is a potent convulsant (Quilliam and Stables, 1969) that acts as a $GABA_A$ receptor antagonist (Curtis and Johnston, 1974). Water hemlock, *Cicuta virosa*, is well known as a toxic plant responsible for lethal poisonings in humans as well as animals, causing tonic and clonic convulsions and respiratory paralysis. The active constituent is the C(17) polyacetylene cicutoxin (Fig. 7), which was shown to be a potent inhibitor of the binding of the GABA channel blocker EBOB to ionotropic GABA receptors in rat brain cortex consistent with cicutoxin acting as a GABA antagonist and a convulsant (Uwai *et al.*,

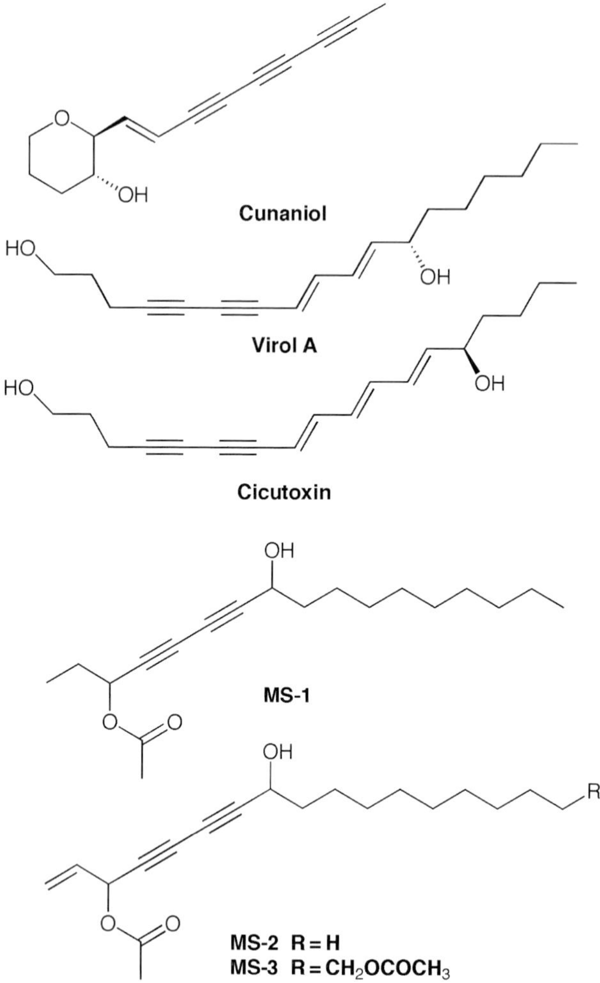


**FIGURE 7** Polyacetylenic alcohols that may act as negative modulators of $GABA_A$ receptor function (cunaniol, cicutoxin, virol A) or as positive modulators of $GABA_A$ receptor function particularly those that contain $\beta 2$ subunits.

2000). A structurally related toxic polyacetylenic alcohol, virol A (Fig. 7), has been shown to inhibit GABA-induced chloride currents in acutely dissociated rat hippocampal CA1 neurons (Uwai *et al.*, 2001).

In contrast to these polyacetylenic alcohols that act as GABA receptor antagonists, some new polyacetylenic alcohols have been described that act as positive modulators of $GABA_A$ receptors that show novel subtypes specificity (Baur *et al.*, 2005). These substances (MS-1, MS-2, and MS-3) (Fig. 7) were isolated from the East African medicinal plant *Cussonia zimmermannii*, which is used in Kenya and Tanzania to treat epilepsy and as a remedy for labor pain. They act independently of the classical benzodiazepine modulatory sites on $GABA_A$ receptors in that their actions are insensitive to flumazenil and are observed in the absence of the $\gamma$ subunit. Half maximum stimulation was observed at 1–2 μM, and the maximum enhancement ranged from 110% to 450% depending on the subunit composition of the $GABA_A$ receptors. The positive modulation by MS-1 was dependent on the presence of the $\beta2$ subunit and varied with the nature of the $\alpha$ subunit. The three substances differed in their relative subunit specificity. These substances represent a new lead structure for the development of subunit selective positive modulators of $GABA_A$ receptors.

## VIII. Alcoholic Beverages Containing GABA Receptor Modulators

Alcoholic beverages are widely consumed. Ethanol has long been known to influence the activation of ionotropic GABA receptors, along with receptors for other neurotransmitters and ion channels (Narahashi *et al.*, 2001; see also Koob and Boehn *et al.*, this volume). $GABA_A$ receptors containing a $\delta$ subunit are particularly susceptible to the positive modulating effects of ethanol (Wallner *et al.*, 2003). Reproducible ethanol enhancement of GABA responses occurred at 3 mM, that is, concentrations that are reached with moderate ethanol consumption producing blood-ethanol levels well below the legal limit for driving in most countries. Ethanol influences the functioning of a variety of other receptors at concentrations in excess of 50 mM. This had been true for recombinant $GABA_A$ receptors (Harris, 1996) until studies on $\delta$ subunit containing receptors. The $\delta$ subunits appear to associate almost exclusively with $\alpha4$ and $\alpha5$ subunits forming functional receptors that are 50-fold more sensitive to GABA and desensitise more slowly than receptor subtypes that do not contain $\delta$ subunits (Jones *et al.*, 1997; Sur *et al.*, 1999). The $\delta$ subunit protein is expressed in brain regions expressing $\alpha4$ (high in thalamus, dentate gyrus, striatum and outer cortical layers and low in hippocampus) and $\alpha6$ subunit proteins (cerebellum) and appears to be associated with extrasynaptic rather than synaptic $GABA_A$ receptors (Hanchar *et al.*, 2004; Peng *et al.*, 2002). Knocking out the $\delta$ subunit gene in mice reduces their sensitivity to neurosteroids (Mihalek *et al.*, 1999) and increases their susceptibility to seizures (Spigelman *et al.*, 2003). As discussed previously, red wine contains the polyphenol resveratrol that acts as a noncompetitive inhibitor of the effects of GABA at human $\rho1$ recombinant $GABA_C$ receptors (Campbell and Johnston, 2003).

Volatile components of alcoholic drinks, such as whiskey, wine, sake, brandy, and shochu potentiate GABA responses to varying degrees (Hossain *et al.*, 2002a). Although these fragrant components are present in alcoholic

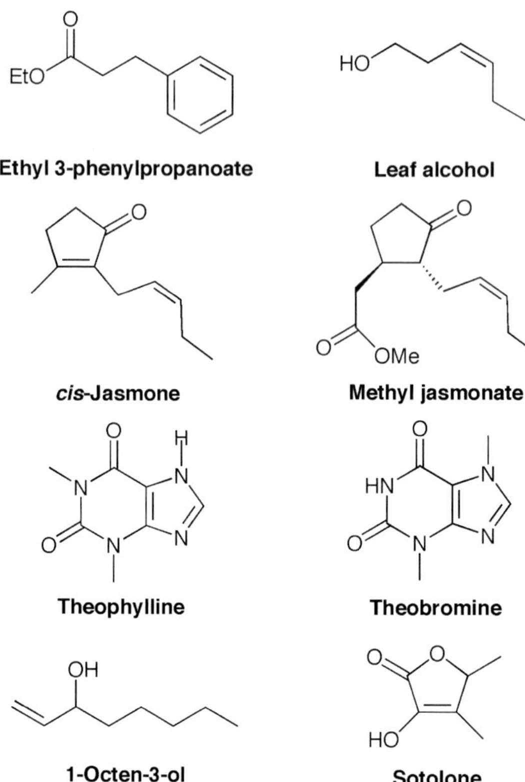


**FIGURE 8** Positive (ethyl 3-phenylpropanoate, leaf alcohol, *cis*-jasmone, methyl jasmonate, 1-octen-3-ol, and sotolone) and negative (theophylline, theobromine) modulators of $GABA_A$ receptor function found in a variety of beverages.

drinks at low concentrations (extremely small quantities compared with ethanol), they may also modulate the mood or consciousness through the potentiation of $GABA_A$ responses after absorption into the brain, because these hydrophobic fragrant compounds are easily absorbed into the brain through the blood–brain barrier and are several thousands times as potent as ethanol in the potentiation of $GABA_A$ receptor-mediated responses (Hossain *et al.*, 2002a).

Many components in the fragrance of whiskey, in particular ethyl 3-phenylpropanoate (Fig. 8), strongly enhanced $\alpha 1\beta 1$ $GABA_A$ receptor responses (Hossain *et al.*, 2002a). When applied to mice through respiration, ethyl 3-phenylpropanoate delayed the onset of convulsions induced by pentylenetetrazole. The aging of whiskey results in enhanced potency of the fragrance in potentiating $GABA_A$ responses and in prolonging pentobarbitone-induced sleeping time in mice (Koda *et al.*, 2003). Sotolone (Fig. 8) is a key component in the "nutty" and "spicy-like" aroma of oxidative aged port wine (Ferreira *et al.*, 2003) that enhances $GABA_A$ responses (Hossain *et al.*, 2003).

## IX. GABA Receptor Modulators in Tea and Coffee

Tea and coffee contain a range of chemicals in addition to GABA that have been shown to influence recombinant bovine $\alpha 1\beta 1$ $GABA_A$ receptors. Extracts of green, oolong, or black tea contained catechins, especially (−)-epicatechin gallate and (−)-epigallocatechin gallate, that inhibited GABA responses and alcohols, such as leaf alcohol and linalool (Fig. 6), that enhanced GABA responses at concentrations of 1 mM (Hossain *et al.*, 2002b). Major components of green ((−)-epigallocatechin gallate) and chamomile teas (apigenin) have been shown to have an additional second order modulatory action on $\alpha 1\beta 2\gamma 2L$ $GABA_A$ receptors that may contribute to the sedative properties of these teas (Campbell *et al.*, 2004). Fragrances of oolong tea have been shown to enhance the responses of recombinant bovine $\alpha 1\beta 1$ $GABA_A$ receptors to GABA, the most active constituents being *cis*-jasmone and methyl jasmonate (Fig. 8) (Hossain *et al.*, 2004). Leaf alcohol (Fig. 8) is one of a number of 6-carbon aliphatic alcohols and aldehydes found in the so-called "green odor" emanating from green leaves and which has been associated with attenuation of a variety of stress-induced effects such as elevation in plasma ACTH levels (Nakashima *et al.*, 2004); as stress is known to induce changes in GABA receptors (Akinci and Johnston, 1997), GABA mechanisms may contribute to the effects of "green odor." Coffee extracts contained theophylline (Fig. 8), which inhibited GABA responses in a noncompetitive mechanism (Ki 0.55 mM), and theobromine (Fig. 8), which inhibited in a competitive manner (Ki 3.8 mM), while a number of compounds including 1-octen-3-ol and sotolone (Fig. 8) enhanced GABA responses (Hossain *et al.*, 2003). When 1-octen-3-ol (100 mg/kg) was orally administered to mice prior to intraperitoneal administration of pentobarbitone, the sleeping time of mice induced by pentobarbital increased significantly (Hossain *et al.*, 2003).

## X. Plant Sources of GABA Receptor Modulating Substances: Implications for Herbal Medicines

The widespread occurrence in plants of agents that are capable of modulating the function of ionotropic GABA receptors in the brain means that most plant extracts will contain a number of active substances. The assessment of the likely effects of such mixtures on brain function is a difficult task especially given the known interactions between many of these substances and the variation in the relative proportions of the active substances in such plant extracts. Ideally such assessment should involve quantitative analytical data on the active constituents and functional assays of the effects of the extract on the biological targets of interest, in the present case ionotropic GABA receptors. This has important implications for the quality control of herbal medicines.

Sage is a good example of the complexity concerning active ingredients. It has been used widely to treat memory deficits and extracts of *Salvia lavandulaefolia* (Spanish sage) have been shown to enhance memory in healthy young volunteers (Tildesley *et al.*, 2003). $GABA_A$ and $GABA_C$ receptors are known to be important in many aspects of memory (Gibbs and Johnston, 2005), and there is a variety of agents found in sage that are known to influence these receptors. Such agents include the flavonoids apigenin, hispidulin, and linarin (Figs. 1 and 2) (Campbell *et al.*, 2004; Fernandez *et al.*, 2004; Kavvadias *et al.*, 2003) and the terpenoids galdosol, miltirone, carnosic acid, and carnosol (Fig. 5) (Chang *et al.*, 1991; Kavvadias *et al.*, 2003; Lee *et al.*, 1991).

Sage also contains α-thujone (Fig. 3), a known $GABA_A$ receptor antagonist as noted previously, which may influence the GABA enhancing effects of the other agents in sage extracts (Johnston and Beart, 2004). The levels of α-thujone in individual sage plants are known to vary considerably (Perry *et al.*, 1999b).

The interactions between active constituents in herbal preparations is a further complicating factor but of great interest with respect to our understanding of the modulation of GABA receptor activation. In addition to agents that are positive modulators of the action of GABA on $GABA_A$ receptors, that is, first order modulators, we now have second order modulators like apigenin and (−)-epigallocatechin gallate (Fig. 1) than modulate only in the presence of a first order modulator (Campbell *et al.*, 2004). Furthermore, we now have examples of positive modulators that appear to enhance the activity of other positive modulators, for example, ethanol and neurosteroids (Akk and Steinbach, 2003). The synergistic action of some positive modulators in herbal preparations is best illustrated with some active substances from *Valeriana officinalis*. The sleep-inducing effects of hesperidin (Fig. 2) are potentiated by 6-methylapigenin (Fig. 1) (Marder *et al.*, 2003), while the sedating and sleep-inducing effects of valerenic acid (Fig. 4) are dramatically potentiated when co-administered with the flavonoid glycoside linarin (Fig. 2) (Fernandez *et al.*, 2004). The specificity of these synergistic actions is particularly interesting. In addition, there are other powerful positive modulators that are found in valerian extract, such as (+)-borneol (Fig. 3), that have yet to be examined for possible synergistic effects with other agents (Granger *et al.*, 2005). We have much to learn as to the key substances in valerian extracts that are used in herbal medicines.

## Acknowledgments

The authors are grateful to their many colleagues who have contributed to their studies on ionotropic GABA receptors including Robin Allan, Erica Campbell, Gary Cutting, Sebastian Fernandez, Renee Granger, Belinda Hall, Shelley Huang, Alejandro Paladini, Keiko Sasaki, Hue Tran, George Uhl, Keiji Wada, and Paul Whiting and to the Australian National Health and Medical Research Council and Polychip Pharmaceuticals for financial support.

## References

Aherne, S. A., and O'Brien, N. M. (2002). Dietary flavonols: Chemistry, food content, and metabolism. *Nutrition* **18**, 75–81.

Ai, J., Wang, X., and Nielsen, M. (2001). Honokiol and magnolol selectively interact with $GABA_A$ receptor subtypes *in vitro*. *Pharmacology* **63**, 34–41.

Akinci, M. K., and Johnston, G. A. R. (1997). Sex differences in the effects of gonadectomy and acute swim stress on $GABA_A$ receptor binding in mouse forebrain membranes. *Neurochem. Int.* **31**, 1–10.

Akk, G., and Steinbach, J. H. (2003). Low doses of ethanol and a neuroactive steroid positively interact to modulate rat $GABA_A$ receptor function. *J. Physiol.* **546**, 641–646.

Avallone, R., Zanoli, P., Puia, G., Kleinschnitz, M., Schreier, P., and Baraldi, M. (2000). Pharmacological profile of apigenin, a flavonoid isolated from Matricaria chamomilla. *Biochem. Pharmacol.* **59**, 1387–1394.

Baraldi, M., Avallone, R., Corsi, L., Venturini, I., Baraldi, C., and Zeneroli, M. L. (2000). Endogenous benzodiazepines. *Therapie* **55**, 143–146.

Bastianetto, S., Zheng, W. H., and Quirion, R. (2000). Neuroprotective abilities of resveratrol and other red wine constituents against nitric oxide-related toxicity in cultured hippocampal neurons. *Br. J. Pharmacol.* **131**, 711–720.

Baur, R., Simmen, U., Senn, M., Sequin, U., and Sigel, E. (2005). Novel plant substances acting as beta subunit isoform-selective positive allosteric modulators of $GABA_A$ receptors. *Mol. Pharmacol.* **68**, 787–792.

Baureithel, K. H., Büter, K. B., Engesser, A., Burkard, W., and Schaffer, W. (1997). Inhibition of benzodiazepine binding *in vitro* by amentoflavone, a constituent of various species of *Hypericum*. *Pharm. Acta Helv.* **72**, 153–157.

Bouche, N., and Fromm, H. (2004). GABA in plants: Just a metabolite? *Trends Plant Sci.* **9**, 110–115.

Bouche, N., Lacombe, B., and Fromm, H. (2003). GABA signaling: A conserved and ubiquitous mechanism. *Trends Cell Biol.* **13**, 607–610.

Brochet, D., Chermat, R., DeFeudis, F. V., and Drieu, K. (1999). Effects of single intraperitoneal injections of an extract of Ginkgo biloba (EGb 761) and its terpene trilactone constituents on barbital-induced narcosis in the mouse. *Gen. Pharmacol.* **33**, 249–256.

Burns, J., Yokota, T., Ashihara, H., Lean, M. E. J., and Crozier, A. (2002). Plant foods and herbal sources of resveratrol. *J. Agric. Food Chem.* **50**, 3337–3340.

Butterweck, V., Nahrstedt, A., Evans, J., Hufeisen, S., Rauser, L., Savage, J., Poedak, B., Ernsberger, P., and Roth, B. L. (2002). *In vitro* receptor screening of pure constitutents of St. John's wort reveals novel interactions with a number of GPCRs. *Psychopharmacology* **162**, 193–202.

Campbell, E. L., and Johnston, G. A. R. (2003). Resveratrol is a $GABA_C$ receptor antagonist. *Proc. Aust. Neurosci. Soc.* **14**, P136.

Campbell, E. L., Chebib, M., and Johnston, G. A. R. (2004). The dietary flavonoids apigenin and (−)-epigallocatechin gallate enhance the positive modulation by diazepam of the activation by GABA of recombinant $GABA_A$ receptors. *Biochem. Pharmacol.* **68**, 1631–1638.

Chang, H. M., Chui, K. Y., Tan, F. W., Zhong, Z. P., Lee, C. M., Sham, H. L., and Wong, H. N. (1991). Structure-activity relationship of miltirone, an active central benzodiazepine ligand isolated from *Salvia miltiorrhiza* Bunge (Danshen). *J. Med. Chem.* **34**, 1675–1692.

Chatterjee, S. S., Kondratskaya, E. L., and Krishtal, O. A. (2003). Structure-activity studies with Ginkgo biloba extract constituents as receptor-gated chloride channel blockers and modulators. *Pharmacopsychiatry* **36**, S68–S77.

Chebib, M., and Johnston, G. A. R. (2000). GABA-activated ligand gated ion channels: Medicinal chemistry and molecular biology. *J. Med. Chem.* **43**, 1427–1447.

Choi, S. E., Choi, S., Lee, J. H., Whiting, P. J., Lee, S. M., and Nah, S. Y. (2003). Effects of ginsenosides on $GABA_A$ receptor channels expressed in *Xenopus* oocytes. *Arch. Pharm. Res.* **26**, 28–33.

Choi, Y. B., Kim, Y. I., Lee, K. S., Kim, B. S., and Kim, D. J. (2004). Protective effect of epigallocatechin gallate on brain damage after transient middle cerebral artery occlusion in rats. *Brain Res.* **1019**, 47–54.

Christopoulos, A. (2002). Allosteric binding sites on cell-surface receptors: Novel targets for drug discovery. *Nature Rev. Drug Discov.* **1**, 198–210.

Clark, J. B. (1969). Effect of a polyacetylenic fish poison on the oxidative phosphorylation of rat liver. *Biochem. Pharmacol.* **18**, 73–83.

Curtis, D. R., and Johnston, G. A. R. (1974). Convulsant alkaloids. *Neuropoisons* **2**, 207–248.

Curtis, D. R., Duggan, A. W., Felix, D., and Johnston, G. A. R. (1970). Bicuculline and central GABA receptors. *Nature* **228**, 676–677.

DeFeudis, F. V. (2002). Bilobalide and neuroprotection. *Pharmacol. Res.* **46**, 565–568.

Deiml, T., Haseneder, R., Zieglgansberger, W., Rammes, G., Eisensamer, B., Rupprecht, R., and Hapfelmeier, G. (2004). $\alpha$-Thujone reduces $5\text{-}HT_3$ receptor activity by an effect on the agonist-induced desensitization. *Neuropharmacology* **46**, 192–201.

Dietz, B. M., Mahady, G. B., Pauli, G. F., and Farnsworth, N. R. (2005). Valerian extract and valerenic acid are partial agonists of the $5\text{-}HT_{5a}$ receptor *in vitro*. *Brain Res. Mol. Brain Res.* **138**, 191–197.

Du, X. M., Sun, N. Y., Takizawa, N., Guo, Y. T., and Shoyama, Y. (2002). Sedative and anticonvulsant activities of goodyerin, a flavonol glycoside from *Goodyera schlechtendaliana*. *Phytother. Res.* **16**, 261–263.

Fernandez, S., Wasowski, C., Paladini, A. C., and Marder, M. (2004). Sedative and sleep-enhancing properties of linarin, a flavonoid-isolated from *Valeriana officinalis*. *Pharmacol. Biochem. Behav.* **77**, 399–404.

Ferreira, A. C. S., Barbe, J.-C., and Bertrand, A. (2003). 3-Hydroxy-4,5-dimethyl-2(5H)-furanone: A key odorant of the typical aroma of oxidative aged port wine. *J. Agric. Food Chem.* **51**, 4356–4363.

Froestl, W., Markstein, R., Schmid, K. L., and Trendelenburg, A.-U. (2004). $GABA_C$ antagonists for the treatment of myopia. *PCT Int. Appl.* 20030627, 8 pp.

Fukuyama, Y., Nakade, K., Minoshima, Y., Yokoyama, R., Zhai, H., and Mitsumoto, Y. (2002). Neurotrophic activity of honokiol on the cultures of fetal rat cortical neurons. *Bioorg. Med. Chem. Lett.* **12**, 1163–1166.

Gibbs, M. E., and Johnston, G. A. R. (2005). Opposing roles for $GABA_A$ and $GABA_C$ receptors in short-term memory formation in young chicks. *Neuroscience* **131**, 567–576.

Gottesmann, C. (2002). GABA mechanisms and sleep. *Neuroscience* **111**, 231–239.

Goutman, J. D., Waxemberg, M. D., Donate-Oliver, F., Pomata, P. E., and Calvo, D. J. (2003). Flavonoid modulation of ionic currents mediated by $GABA_A$ and $GABA_C$ receptors. *Eur. J. Pharmacol.* **461**, 79–87.

Granger, R. E., Campbell, E. L., and Johnston, G. A. R. (2005). (+)- and (−)-borneol: Efficacious positive modulators of GABA action at human recombinant alpha1beta2-gamma2L $GABA_A$ receptors. *Biochem. Pharmacol.* **69**, 1101–1111.

Gutmann, H., Bruggisser, R., Schaffner, W., Bogman, K., Botomino, A., and Drewe, J. (2002). Transport of amentoflavone across the blood-brain barrier *in vitro*. *Planta Med.* **68**, 804–807.

Ha, J. H., Lee, K. Y., Choi, H. C., Cho, J., Kang, L. S., Lim, J. C., and Lee, D. U. (2002). Modulation of radioligand binding to the $GABA_A$-benzodiazepine receptor complex by a new component from *Cyperus rotundus*. *Biol. Pharm. Bull.* **25**, 128–130.

Hall, B. J., Chebib, M., Hanrahan, J. R., and Johnston, G. A. R. (2004). Flumazenil-independent positive modulation of $\gamma$-aminobutyric acid by 6-methylflavone at human recombinant $\alpha1\beta2\gamma2L$ and $\alpha1\beta2$ $GABA_A$ receptors. *Eur. J. Pharmacol.* **491**, 1–8.

Hanchar, H. J., Wallner, M., and Olsen, R. W. (2004). Alcohol effects on gamma-aminobutyric acid type A receptors: Are extrasynaptic receptors the answer? *Life Sci.* **76**, 1–8.

Hanrahan, J. R., Chebib, M., Davucheron, N. M., Hall, B. J., and Johnston, G. A. R. (2003). Semisynthetic preparation of amentoflavone: A negative modulator at $GABA_A$ receptors. *Bioorg. Med. Chem. Lett.* **13**, 2281–2284.

Harris, R. A. (1996). Transfected cells for study of alcohol actions on GABA(a) receptors. *Addict. Biol.* **1**, 157–163.

Havsteen, B. H. (2002). The biochemistry and medical significance of the flavonoids. *Pharmacol. Ther.* **96**, 67–202.

Heim, K. E., Tagliaferro, A. R., and Bobilya, D. J. (2002). Flavonoid antioxidants: Chemistry, metabolism and structure-activity relationships. *J. Nutr. Biochem.* **13**, 572–584.

Hold, K. M., Sirisoma, N. S., Ikeda, T., Narahashi, T., and Casida, J. E. (2000). $\alpha$-Thujone (the active component of absinthe): $\gamma$-Aminobutyric acid type A receptor modulation and metabolic detoxification. *Proc. Natl. Acad. Sci. USA* **97**, 3826–3831.

Holopainen, I. E., Metsahonkala, E. L., Kokkonen, H., Parkkola, R. K., Manner, T. E., Nagren, K., and Korpi, E. R. (2001). Decreased binding of $[^{11}C]$flumazenil in Angelman syndrome patients with $GABA_A$ receptor $\beta3$ subunit deletions. *Ann. Neurol.* **49**, 110–113.

Hossain, S. J., Aoshima, H., Koda, H., and Kiso, Y. (2002a). Potentiation of the ionotropic GABA receptor response by whiskey fragrance. *J. Agric. Food Chem.* **50**, 6828–6834.

Hossain, S. J., Hamamoto, K., Aoshima, H., and Hara, Y. (2002b). Effects of tea components on the response of $GABA_A$ receptors expressed in *Xenopus* oocytes. *J. Agric. Food Chem.* **50**, 3954–3960.

Hossain, S. J., Aoshima, H., Koda, H., and Kiso, Y. (2003). Effects of coffee components on the response of $GABA_A$ receptors expressed in *Xenopus* oocytes. *J. Agric. Food Chem.* **51**, 7568–7575.

Hossain, S. J., Aoshima, H., Koda, H., and Kiso, Y. (2004). Fragrances in oolong tea that enhance the response of $GABA_A$ receptors. *Biosci. Biotechnol. Biochem.* **68**, 1842–1848.

Hosseinzadeh, H., and Parvardeh, S. (2004). Anticonvulsant effects of thymoquinone, the major constituent of *Nigella sativa* seeds, in mice. *Phytomedicine* **11**, 56–64.

Huang, S. H., Duke, R. K., Chebib, M., Sasaki, K., Wada, K., and Johnston, G. A. R. (2003). Bilobalide, a sesquiterpene trilactone from *Ginkgo biloba*, is an antagonist at recombinant alpha(1)beta(2)gamma(2L) $GABA_A$ receptors. *Eur. J. Pharmacol.* **464**, 1–8.

Huang, S. H., Duke, R. K., Chebib, M., Sasaki, K., Wada, K., and Johnston, G. A. (2004). Ginkgolides, diterpene trilactones of *Ginkgo biloba*, as antagonists at recombinant alpha1beta2gamma2L $GABA_A$ receptors. *Eur. J. Pharmacol.* **494**, 131–138.

Huang, S. H., Duke, R. K., Chebib, M., Sasaki, K., Wada, K., and Johnston, G. A. R. (2006). Mixed antagonistic effects of bilobalide at $\rho1$ $GABA_C$ receptors. *Neuroscience* **137**, 607–617.

Huen, M. S., Hui, K. M., Leung, J. W., Sigel, E., Baur, R., Wong, J. T., and Xue, H. (2003a). Naturally occurring 2′-hydroxyl-substituted flavonoids as high-affinity benzodiazepine site ligands. *Biochem. Pharmacol.* **66**, 2397–2407.

Huen, M. S., Leung, J. W., Ng, W., Lui, W. S., Chan, M. N., Wong, J. T., and Xue, H. (2003b). 5,7-Dihydroxy-6-methoxyflavone, a benzodiazepine site ligand isolated from *Scutellaria baicalensis* Georgi, with selective antagonistic properties. *Biochem. Pharmacol.* **66**, 125–132.

Huh, S. W., Bae, S. M., Kim, Y. W., Lee, J. M., Namkoong, S. E., Lee, I. P., Kim, S. H., Kim, C. K., and Ahn, W. S. (2004). Anticancer effects of (−)-epigallocatechin-3-gallate on ovarian carcinoma cell lines. *Gynacol. Oncol.* **94**, 760–768.

Hussain, T., Gupta, S., Adhami, V. M., and Mukhtar, H. (2005). Green tea constituent epigallocatechin-3-gallate selectively inhibits COX-2 without affecting COX-1 expression in human prostate carcinoma cells. *Int. J. Cancer* **113**, 660–669.

Irie, T., Miyamoto, E., Kitagawa, K., Maruyama, Y., Inoue, K., and Inagaki, C. (2001). An anxiolytic agent, dihydrohonokiol-B, inhibits ammonia-induced increases in the intracellular $Cl^-$ of cultured rat hippocampal neurons via $GABA_C$ receptors. *Neurosci. Lett.* **312**, 121–123.

Ivic, L., Sands, T. T., Fishkin, N., Nakanishi, K., Kriegstein, A. R., and Stromgaard, K. (2003). Terpene trilactones from *Ginkgo biloba* are antagonists of cortical glycine and $GABA_A$ receptors. *J. Biol. Chem.* **278**, 49279–49285.

Jacobson, K. A., Moro, S., Manthey, J. A., West, P. L., and Ji, X. D. (2002). Interactions of flavones and other phytochemicals with adenosine receptors. *Adv. Exp. Med. Biol.* **505**, 163–171.

Jarboe, C. H., Porter, L. A., and Buckler, R. T. (1968). Structural aspects of picrotoxinin action. *J. Med. Chem.* **2**, 729–731.

Johnston, G. A. R. (1996). $GABA_A$ receptor pharmacology. *Pharmacol. Ther.* **69**, 173–198.

Johnston, G. A. R. (2005). $GABA_A$ receptor channel pharmacology. *Curr. Pharm. Design* **11**, 1867–1885.

Johnston, G. A. R., and Beart, P. M. (2004). Flavonoids: Some of the wisdom of sage? *Br. J. Pharmacol.* **142**, 809–810.

Johnston, G. A. R., Curtis, D. R., De Groat, W. C., and Duggan, A. W. (1968). Central actions of ibotenic acid and muscimol. *Biochem. Pharmacol.* **17**, 2488–2489.

Johnston, G. A. R., Chebib, M., Hanrahan, J. R., and Mewett, K. N. (2003). $GABA_C$ receptors as drug targets. *Curr. Drug Targets CNS Neurol. Disord.* **2**, 260–268.

Jones, A., Korpi, E. R., Mckernan, R. M., Pelz, R., Nusser, Z., Makela, R., Mellor, J. R., Pollard, S., Bahn, S., Stephenson, F. A., Randall, A. D., Sieghart, W., *et al.* (1997). Ligand-gated ion channel subunit partnerships - $GABA_A$ receptor alpha(6) subunit gene inactivation inhibits delta subunit expression. *J. Neurosci.* **17**, 1350–1362.

Jones, F. A., Chatterjee, S. S., and Davies, J. A. (2002). Effects of bilobalide on amino acid release and electrophysiology of cortical slices. *Amino Acids* **22**, 369–379.

Jones-Davis, D. M., and Macdonald, R. L. (2003). $GABA_A$ receptor function and pharmacology in epilepsy and status epilepticus. *Curr. Opin. Pharmacol.* **3**, 12–18.

Kavvadias, D., Monschein, V., Sand, P., Riederer, P., and Schreier, P. (2003). Constituents of sage (*Salvia officinalis L.*) with *in vitro* affinity to human brain benzodiazepine receptor. *Planta Med.* **69**, 113–117.

Kavvadias, D., Sand, P., Youdim, K. A., Qaiser, M. Z., Rice-Evans, C., Baur, R., Sigel, E., Rausch, W.-D., Riederer, P., and Schreier, P. (2004). The flavone hispidulin, a benzodiazepine receptor ligand with positive allosteric properties, traverses the blood-brain barrier and exhibits anti-convulsive effects. *Br. J. Pharmacol.* **142**, 811–820.

Kawai, K., Tsuno, N. H., Kitayama, J., Okaji, Y., Yazawa, K., Asakage, M., Sasaki, S., Watanabe, T., Takahashi, K., and Nagawa, H. (2005). Epigallocatechin gallate induces apoptosis of monocytes. *J. Allergy Clin. Immunol.* **115**, 186–191.

Koda, H., Hossain, S. J., Kiso, Y., and Aoshima, H. (2003). Aging of whiskey increases the potentiation of $GABA_A$ receptor response. *J. Agric. Food Chem.* **51**, 5238–5244.

Kuribara, H., Stavinoha, W. B., and Maruyama, Y. (1999). Honokiol, a putative anxiolytic agent extracted from magnolia bark, has no diazepam-like side-effects in mice. *J. Pharm. Pharmacol.* **51**, 97–103.

Kuribara, H., Kishi, E., Kimura, M., Weintraub, S. T., and Maruyama, Y. (2000). Comparative assessment of the anxiolytic-like activities of honokiol and derivatives. *Pharmacol. Biochem. Behav.* **67**, 597–601.

Lambert, J. D., and Yang, C. S. (2003). Mechanisms of cancer prevention by tea constituents. *J. Nutr.* **133**, 3262S–3267S.

Le Marchand, L. (2002). Cancer preventive effects of flavonoids: A review. *Biomed. Pharmacother.* **56**, 296–301.

Le Novere, N., and Changeux, J. P. (2001). The ligand gated ion channel database: An example of a sequence database in neuroscience. *Philos. Trans. R. Soc. Lond. B Biol. Sci.* **356**, 1121–1130.

Lee, C. M., Wong, H. N., Chui, K. Y., Choang, T. F., Hon, P. M., and Chang, H. M. (1991). Miltirone, a central benzodiazepine receptor partial agonist from a Chinese medicinal herb *Salvia miltiorrhiza*. *Neurosci. Lett.* **127**, 237–241.

Lee, J. H., Song, D. K., Jung, C. H., Shin, D. H., Park, J., Kwon, T. K., Jang, B. C., Mun, K. C., Kim, S. P., Suh, S. I., and Bae, J. H. (2004). (−)-Epigallocatechin gallate attenuates glutamate-induced cytotoxicity via intracellular Ca modulation in PC12 cells. *Clin. Exp. Pharmacol. Physiol.* **31**, 530–536.

Levites, Y., Amit, T., Youdim, M. B., and Mandel, S. (2002). Involvement of protein kinase C activation and cell survival/cell cycle genes in green tea polyphenol (−)-epigallocatechin 3-gallate neuroprotective action. *J. Biol. Chem.* **277**, 30574–30580.

Liou, K. T., Lin, S. M., Huang, S. S., Chih, C. L., and Tsai, S. K. (2003a). Honokiol ameliorates cerebral infarction from ischemia-reperfusion injury in rats. *Planta Med.* **69**, 130–134.

Liou, K. T., Shen, Y. C., Chen, C. F., Tsao, C. M., and Tsai, S. K. (2003b). Honokiol protects rat brain from focal cerebral ischemia-reperfusion injury by inhibiting neutrophil infiltration and reactive oxygen species production. *Brain Res.* **992**, 159–166.

Liu, B., Hattori, N., Zhang, N. Y., Wu, B., Yang, L., Kitagawa, K., Xiong, Z. M., Irie, T., and Inagaki, C. (2005). Anxiolytic agent, dihydrohonokiol-B, recovers amyloid beta protein-induced neurotoxicity in cultured rat hippocampal neurons. *Neurosci. Lett.* **384**, 44–47.

Losi, G., Puia, G., Garzon, G., de Vuono, M. C., and Baraldi, M. (2004). Apigenin modulates GABAergic and glutamatergic transmission in cultured cortical neurons. *Eur. J. Pharmacol.* **502**, 41–46.

Lu, Y. C., Chen, H. H., Ko, C. H., Lin, Y. R., and Chan, M. H. (2003). The mechanism of honokiol-induced and magnolol-induced inhibition on muscle contraction and $Ca^{2+}$ mobilization in rat uterus. *Naunyn-Schmiedebergs Arch. Pharmacol.* **368**, 262–269.

Luk, K. C., Stern, L., Weigele, M., O'Brien, R. A., and Spirst, N. (1983). Isolation and identification of "diazepam-like" compounds in bovine brain. *J. Nat. Prod.* **46**, 852–861.

Marder, M., and Paladini, A. C. (2002). $GABA_A$ receptor ligands of flavonoid structure. *Curr. Top. Med. Chem.* **2**, 853–867.

Marder, M., Viola, H., Wasowski, C., Fernandez, S., Medina, J. H., and Paladini, A. C. (2003). 6-Methylapigenin and hesperidin: New valeriana flavonoids with activity on the CNS. *Pharmacol. Biochem. Behav.* **75**, 537–545.

McKernan, R. M., and Whiting, P. J. (1996). Which $GABA_A$-receptor subtypes really occur in the brain? *Trends Neurosci.* **19**, 139–143.

McKernan, R. M., Rosahl, T. W., Reynolds, D. S., Sur, C., Wafford, K. A., Atack, J. R., Farrar, S., Myers, J., Cook, G., Ferris, P., Garrett, L., Bristow, L., *et al.* (2000). Sedative but not anxiolytic properties of benzodiazepines are mediated by the $GABA_A$ receptor alpha(1) subtype. *Nat. Neurosci.* **3**, 587–592.

Medina, J. H., Viola, H., Wolfman, C., Marder, M., Wasowski, C., Calvo, D., and Paladini, A. C. (1997). Overview—flavonoids—a new family of benzodiazepine receptor ligands. *Neurochem. Res.* **22**, 419–425.

Mihalek, R. M., Banerjee, P. K., Korpi, E. R., Quinlan, J. J., Firestone, L. L., Mi, Z. P., Lagenaur, C., Tretter, V., Sieghart, W., Anagnostaras, S. G., Sage, J. R., Fanselow, M. S., *et al.* (1999). Attenuated sensitivity to neuroactive steroids in gamma-aminobutyrate type A receptor delta subunit knockout mice. *Proc. Natl. Acad. Sci. USA* **96**, 12905–12910.

Misra, R. (1998). Modern drug development from traditional medicinal plants using radioligand receptor-binding assays. *Med. Res. Rev.* **18**, 383–402.

Mohammadi, B., Haeseler, G., Leuwer, M., Dengler, R., Krampfl, K., and Bufler, J. (2001). Structural requirements of phenol derivatives for direct activation of chloride currents via $GABA_A$ receptors. *Eur. J. Pharmacol.* **421**, 85–91.

Mojzisova, G., and Kuchta, M. (2001). Dietary flavonoids and risk of coronary heart disease. *Physiol. Res.* **50**, 529–535.

Nakashima, T., Akamatsu, M., Hatanaka, A., and Kiyohara, T. (2004). Attenuation of stress-induced elevations in plasma ACTH level and body temperature in rats by green odor. *Physiol. Behav.* **80**, 481–488.

Narahashi, T., Kuriyama, K., Illes, P., Wirkner, K., Fischer, W., Muhlberg, K., Scheibler, P., Allgaier, C., Minami, K., Lovinger, D., Lallemand, F., Ward, R. J., *et al.* (2001). Neuroreceptors and ion channels as targets of alcohol. *Alcohol. Clin. Exp. Res.* **25**, 182S–188S.

Nielsen, M., Frokjaer, S., and Braestrup, C. (1988). High affinity of the naturally-occurring biflavonoid, amentoflavone, to brain benzodiazepine receptors *in vitro*. *Biochem. Pharmacol.* **37**, 3285–3287.

Peng, Z., Hauer, B., Mihalek, R. M., Homanics, G. E., Sieghart, W., Olsen, R. W., and Houser, C. R. (2002). $GABA_A$ receptor changes in delta subunit-deficient mice: Altered expression of alpha 4 and gamma 2 subunits in the forebrain. *J. Comp. Neurol.* **446**, 179–197.

Perry, E. K., Pickering, A. T., Wang, W. W., Houghton, P. J., and Perry, N. S. (1999a). Medicinal plants and Alzheimer's disease: From ethnobotany to phytotherapy. *J. Pharm. Pharmacol.* **51**, 527–534.

Perry, N. B., Anderson, R. E., Brennan, N. J., Douglas, M. H., Heaney, A. J., McGimpsey, J. A., and Smallfield, B. M. (1999b). Essential oils from Dalmation sage (*Salvia officinalis l.*): Vaiations among individuals, plant parts, seasons, and sites. *J. Agric. Food Chem.* **47**, 2048–2054.

Perry, N. S., Howes, M.-J., Houghton, P., and Perry, E. (2000). Why sage may be a wise memory remedy: Effects of salvia on the nervous system. *Med. Arom. Plants Indust. Profiles* **14**, 207–223.

Priestley, C. M., Williamson, E. M., Wafford, K., and Sattelle, D. B. (2003). Thymol, a constituent of thyme essential oil, is a positive allosteric modulator of human $GABA_A$ receptors and a homo-oligomeric GABA receptor from *Drosophila melanogaster. Br. J. Pharmacol.* **140**, 1363–1372.

Qian, H., Pan, Y., Zhu, Y., and Khalili, P. (2005). Picrotoxin accelerates relaxation of $GABA_C$ receptors. *Mol. Pharmacol.* **67**, 470–479.

Quilliam, J. P., and Stables, R. (1969). Convulsant effects of cunaniol, a polyacetylenic alcohol isolated from the plant *Clibadium sylvestre*, on frogs and mice. *Pharmacol. Res. Comm.* **1**, 7–14.

Rutherford, D. M., Nielsen, M. P. C., Hansen, S. K., Witt, M. R., Bergendorff, O., and Sterner, O. (1992). Isolation from *Salvia officinalis* and indentification of two diterpenes which inhibit t-butylbicyclophosphoro[$^{35}$S]thionate binding to chloride channel of rat cerebrocortical membranes *in vitro*. *Neurosci. Lett.* **135**, 224–226.

Sasaki, K., Hatta, S., Haga, M., and Ohshika, H. (1999a). Effects of bilobalide on gamma-aminobutyric acid levels and glutamic acid decarboxylase in mouse brain. *Eur. J. Pharmacol.* **367**, 165–173.

Sasaki, K., Oota, I., Wada, K., Inomata, K., Ohshika, H., and Haga, M. (1999b). Effects of bilobalide, a sesquiterpene in *Ginkgo biloba* leaves, on population spikes in rat hippocampal slices. *Comp. Biochem. Physiol. C Toxicol. Pharmacol.* **124**, 315–321.

Skerritt, J. H., Willow, M., and Johnston, G. A. R. (1982). Diazepam enhancement of low affinity GABA binding to rat brain membranes. *Neurosci. Lett.* **29**, 63–66.

Spigelman, I., Li, Z., Liang, J., Cagetti, E., Samzadeh, S., Mihalek, R. M., Homanics, G. E., and Olsen, R. W. (2003). Reduced inhibition and sensitivity to neurosteroids in hippocampus of mice lacking the $GABA_A$ receptor delta subunit. *J. Neurophysiol.* **90**, 903–910.

Squires, R. F., Ai, J., Witt, M. R., Kahnberg, P., Saederup, E., Sterner, O., and Nielsen, M. (1999). Honokiol and magnolol increase the number of [$^3$H] muscimol binding sites three-fold in rat forebrain membranes *in vitro* using a filtration assay, by allosterically increasing the affinities of low-affinity sites. *Neurochem. Res.* **24**, 593–602.

Suganuma, M., Okabe, S., Oniyama, M., Tada, Y., Ito, H., and Fujiki, H. (1998). Wide distribution of [$^3$H](−)-epigallocatechin gallate, a cancer preventive tea polyphenol, in mouse tissue. *Carcinogenesis* **19**, 1771–1776.

Sun, A. Y., Simonyi, A., and Sun, G. Y. (2002). The "French paradox" and beyond: Neuroprotective effects of polyphenols. *Free Radic. Biol. Med.* **32**, 314–318.

Sur, C., Farrar, S. J., Kerby, J., Whiting, P. J., Atack, J. R., and McKernan, R. M. (1999). Preferential coassembly of alpha 4 and delta subunits of the gamma-aminobutyric $acid_A$ receptor in rat thalamus. *Mol. Pharmacol.* **56**, 110–115.

Tildesley, N. T., Kennedy, D. O., Perry, E. K., Ballard, C. G., Savelev, S., Wesnes, K. A., and Scholey, A. B. (2003). *Salvia lavandulaefolia* (Spanish sage) enhances memory in healthy young volunteers. *Pharmacol. Biochem. Behav.* **75**, 669–674.

Topliss, J. G., Clark, A. M., Ernst, E., Hufford, C. D., Johnston, G. A. R., Rimoldi, J. M., and Weimann, B. J. (2002). Natural and synthetic substances related to human health - (IUPAC Technical Report). *Pure Appl. Chem.* **74**, 1957–1985.

Turner, R. T., Evans, G. L., Zhang, M. Z., Maran, A., and Sibonga, J. D. (1999). Is resveratrol an estrogen agonist in growing rats? *Endocrinology* **140**, 50–54.

Uwai, K., Ohashi, K., Takaya, Y., Ohta, T., Tadano, T., Kisara, K., Shibusawa, K., Sakakibara, R., and Oshima, Y. (2000). Exploring the structural basis of neurotoxicity in C(17)-polyacetylenes isolated from water hemlock. *J. Med. Chem.* **43**, 4508–4515.

Uwai, K., Ohashi, K., Takaya, Y., Oshima, Y., Furukawa, K., Yamagata, K., Omura, T., and Okuyama, S. (2001). Virol A, a toxic trans-polyacetylenic alcohol of *Cicuta virosa*, selectively inhibits the GABA-induced $Cl^-$ current in acutely dissociated rat hippocampal CA1 neurons. *Brain Res.* **889**, 174–180.

Vafa, B., and Schofield, P. R. (1998). Heritable mutations in the glycine, $GABA_A$, and nicotinic acetylcholine receptors provide new insights into the ligand-gated ion channel superfamily. *Int. Rev. Neurobiol.* **42**, 285–332.

Viola, H., Wasowski, C., Levi de Stein, M., Wolfman, C., Silvera, R., Medina, A. E., and Paladini, A. C. (1995). Apigenin, a component of *Matricaria recutita* flowers, is a central benzodiazepine receptors-ligand with anxiolytic effects. *Planta Med.* **61**, 213–216.

Wallace, R. H., Marini, C., Petrou, S., Harkin, L. A., Bowser, D. N., Panchal, R. G., Williams, D. A., Sutherland, G. R., Mulley, J. C., Scheffer, I. E., and Berkovic, S. F. (2001). Mutant $GABA_A$ receptor gamma 2-subunit in childhood absence epilepsy and febrile seizures. *Nat. Genetics* **28**, 49–52.

Wallner, M., Hanchar, H. J., and Olsen, R. W. (2003). Ethanol enhances alpha 4 beta 3 delta and alpha 6 beta 3 delta gamma-aminobutyric acid type A receptors at low concentrations known to affect humans. *Proc. Natl. Acad. Sci. USA* **100**, 15218–15223.

Walters, R. J., Hadley, S. H., Morris, K. D. W., and Amin, J. (2000). Benzodiazepines act on $GABA_A$ receptors via two distinct and separable mechanisms. *Nat. Neurosci.* **3**, 1274–1281.

Wang, H. Y., Hui, K. M., Chen, Y. J., Xu, S. X., Wong, J. T. F., and Xue, H. (2002). Structure-activity relationships of flavonoids, isolated from *Scutellaria baicalensis*, binding to benzodiazepine site of $GABA_A$ receptor complex. *Planta Med.* **68**, 1059–1062.

Wasowski, C., Marder, M., Viola, H., Medina, J. H., and Paladini, A. C. (2002). Isolation and identification of 6-methylapigenin, a competitive ligand for the brain $GABA_A$ receptors, from Valeriana wallichii. *Planta Med.* **68**, 934–936.

Watanabe, K., Watanabe, H. Y., Goto, Y., Yamamoto, N., and Yoshizaki, M. (1975). Studies on the active principles of magnolia bark. Centrally acting muscle relaxant activity of magnolol and honokiol. *Jpn. J. Pharmacol.* **25**, 605–607.

Watanabe, K., Watanabe, H., Goto, Y., Yamaguchi, M., Yamamoto, N., and Hagino, K. (1983). Pharmacological properties of magnolol and honokiol extracted from *Magnolia officinalis*: Central depressant effects. *Planta Med.* **49**, 103–108.

Weinreb, O., Mandel, S., Amit, T., and Youdim, M. B. (2004). Neurological mechanisms of green tea polyphenols in Alzheimer's and Parkinson's diseases. *J. Nutr. Biochem.* **15**, 506–516.

Whiting, P. J. (2003). $GABA_A$ receptor subtypes in the brain: A paradigm for CNS drug discovery? *Drug Discov. Today* **8**, 445–450.

Woodman, O. L., and Chan, E. C. (2004). Vascular and anti-oxidant actions of flavonols and flavones. *Clin. Exp. Pharmacol. Physiol.* **31**, 786–790.

Wurtman, R. K., and Lee, R. K. K. (2002). Compositions and methods for treatment of mild cognitive impairment. *PCT Int. Appl.* **2002**, WO 02/28141 A2..

Yang, L., Omori, K., Otani, H., Suzukawa, J., and Inagaki, C. (2003). $GABA_C$ receptor agonist suppressed ammonia-induced apoptosis in cultured rat hippocampal neurons by restoring phosphorylated BAD level. *J. Neurochem.* **87**, 791–800.

Yang, Z. (2003). GABA, a new player in the plant mating game. *Devel. Cell* **5**, 185–186.

Yuan, C. S., Mehendale, S., Xiao, Y., Aung, H. H., Xie, J. T., and Ang-Lee, M. K. (2004). The gamma-aminobutyric acidergic effects of valerian and valerenic acid on rat brainstem neuronal activity. *Anesth. Analg.* **98**, 353–358.

Zand, R. S. R., Jenkins, D. J. A., and Diamandis, E. P. (2000). Steroid hormone activity of flavonoids and related compounds. *Breast Cancer Res. Treat.* **62**, 35–49.

Zanoli, P., Avallone, R., and Baraldi, M. (2000). Behavioural characterisation of the flavonoids apigenin and chrysin. *Fitoterapia* **71**, S117–S123.

# Index

# Contents of Previous Volumes

## Volume 40

## Volume 41

## Volume 42



## Volume 43

## Volume 44

## Volume 45



## Volume 46

## Volume 47

## Hormones and Signaling
## Edited by Bert W. O'Malley

## Volume 48

### HIV: Molecular Biology and Pathogenesis: Viral Mechanisms
### Edited by Kuan-Teh Jeang

## Volume 49

**HIV: Molecular Biology and Pathogenesis: Clinical Applications**
**Edited by Kuan-Teh Jeang**

## Volume 50

## Volume 51

### Treatment of Leukemia and Lymphoma
### Edited by David A. Scheinberg and Joseph G. Jurcic

## Volume 52

## Volume 53

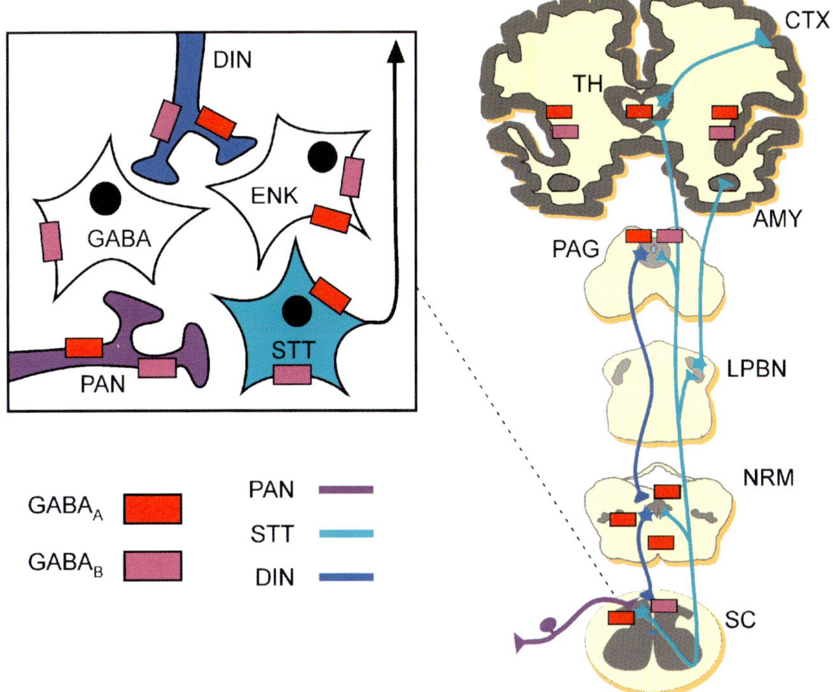


**CHAPTER 1, FIGURE 3** Anatomical localization of GABA receptors in the central and peripheral nervous systems. Depicted in the inset is the circuitry within the dorsal horn of the spinal cord. Abbreviations: CTX, primary sensory cortex; TH, thalamus; AMY, amygdala; PAG, periaqueductal gray; LPBN, lateral parabrachial nucleus; NRM, medullary raphe nucleus; SC, spinal cord; PAN, primary afferent nociceptor C and A-$\delta$ fibers; DIN, descending inhibitory neuron; GABA, GABAergic interneuron; ENK, enkaphalinergic interneuron; STT, spinothalamic tract projection; $GABA_A$, $GABA_A$ receptor; $GABA_B$, $GABA_B$ receptor.

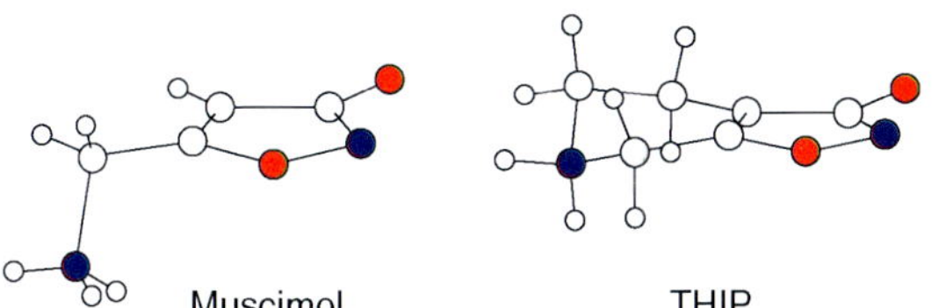


**CHAPTER 3, FIGURE 3** The structures of muscimol and THIP as determined by x-ray crystallographic analyses (from Krogsgaard-Larsen *et al.*, 2002).

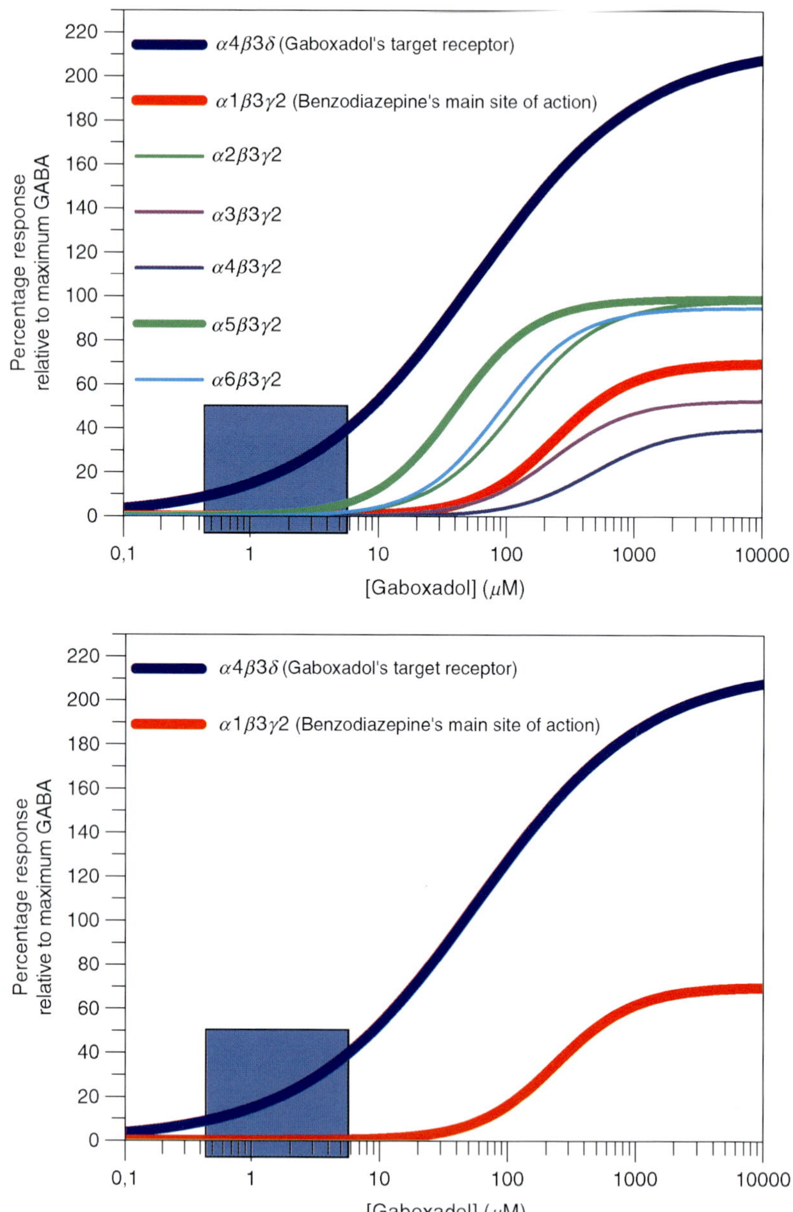


**CHAPTER 3, FIGURE 4** Concentration–response curves for THIP (Gaboxadol) obtained from *Xenopus* oocytes expressing $GABA_A$ receptors of different subunit composition (Ebert *et al.*, 2001). In the lower figure, the effects on α4β3δ and α1β3γ2, the main $GABA_A$ receptor targets for Gaboxadol and the BZDs, respectively, are emphasized. The bar indicates the therapeutically relevant concentration area (Madsen *et al.*, 1983).

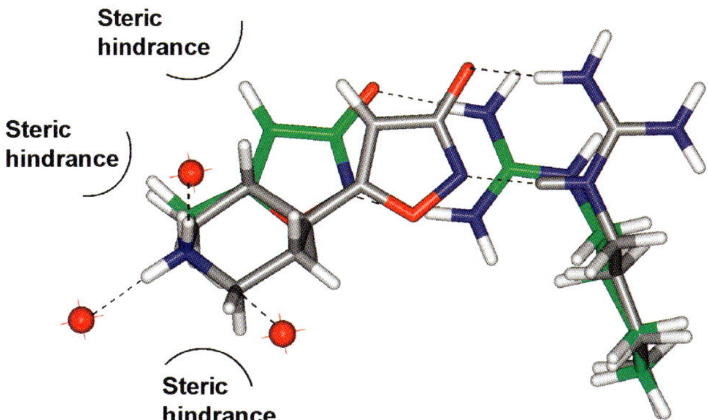


**CHAPTER 3, FIGURE 6** A pharmacophore model for $GABA_A$ receptor agonists showing the proposed binding modes of muscimol (green bonds) and 4-PIOL (light grey bonds) and their interactions with two different conformations of an arginine residue. The red spheres indicate sites to which the ammonium group in muscimol interacts via hydrogen bonds (from Krogsgaard-Larsen *et al.*, 2002).

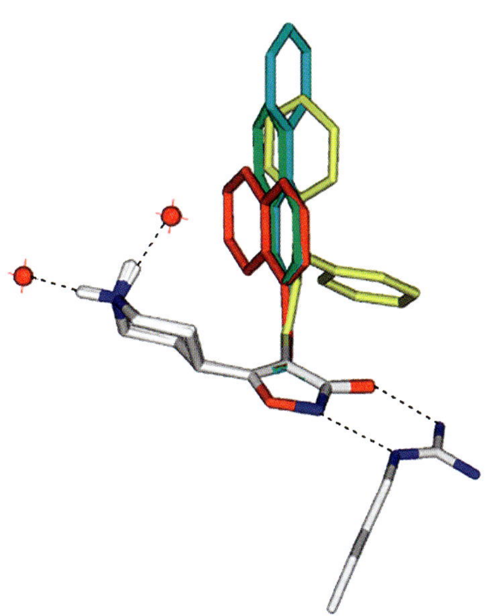

**CHAPTER 3, FIGURE 7** Proposed bioactive conformations for the high-affinity 1-naphtylmethyl, 2-naphthylmethyl, 3,3-diphenylpropyl, and 4-biphenyl analogs of 4-PIOL (from Krogsgaard-Larsen *et al.*, 2002).

The trisynaptic pathway in normals vs schizophrenics

Normal control

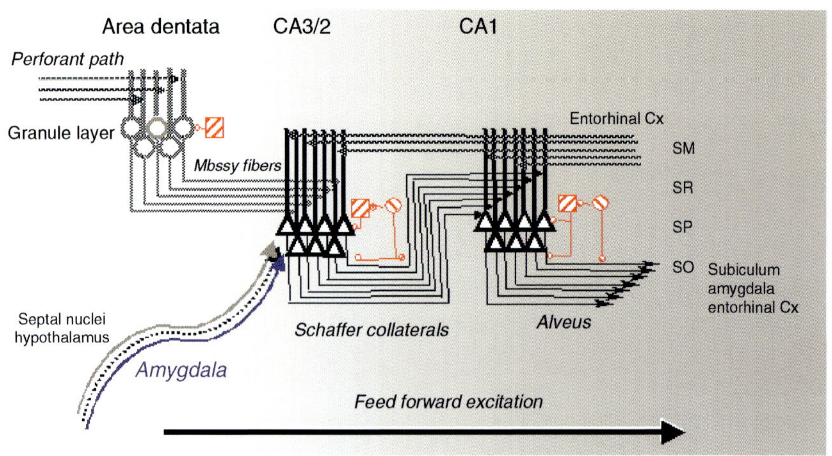


Schizophrenic

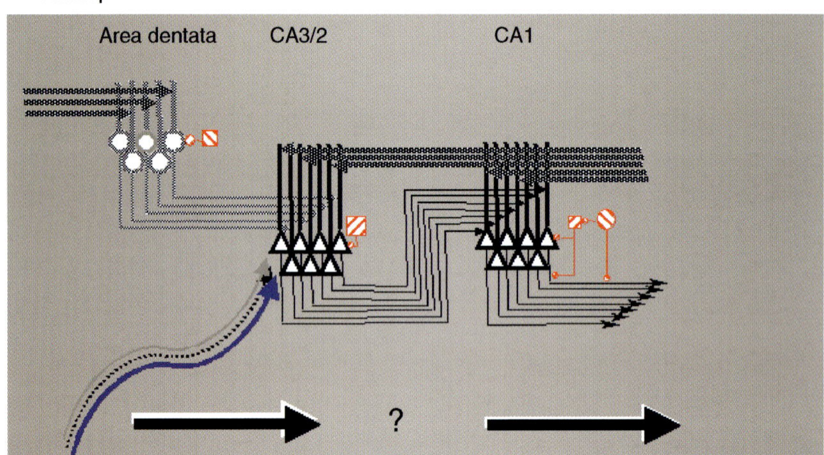


**CHAPTER 4, FIGURE 2** Schematic diagram of the trisynaptic pathway in the hippocampusocampus of a normal control (upper) and schizophrenic (lower) subject. Perforant path fibers provide an excitatory input to dentate gyrus granule cells and the latter, in turn, send an excitatory input to the stratum radiatum-lacunosum of sector CA3. The pyramidal cells in this sector are modulated by both inhibitory and disinhibitory GABAergic interneurons, as excitatory activity is conveyed along Schaffer collater fibers that course toward rad of sector CA1, where they provide an excitatory input to pyramidal neurons of this sector. There is a progressive feed forward increase of excitation as the activity progresses toward CA1, and this is represented by the gradient of background shading. In the schizophrenic circuit, GABA cell dysfunction is present in CA3, and this causes an increase of excitatory activity flowing toward CA1 and a general increase in baseline levels of metabolic activity indicated by the loss of the feed forward gradient. The AMYG is shown sending excitatory afferents directly to CA3 and this is postulated to be increased in schizophrenics and possibly related to the GABA cell dysfunction. This model is consistent with a PET scanning study in which schizophrenics were found to have an increase of baseline metabolic activity in the hippocampusocampus (Heckers *et al.*, 1999).

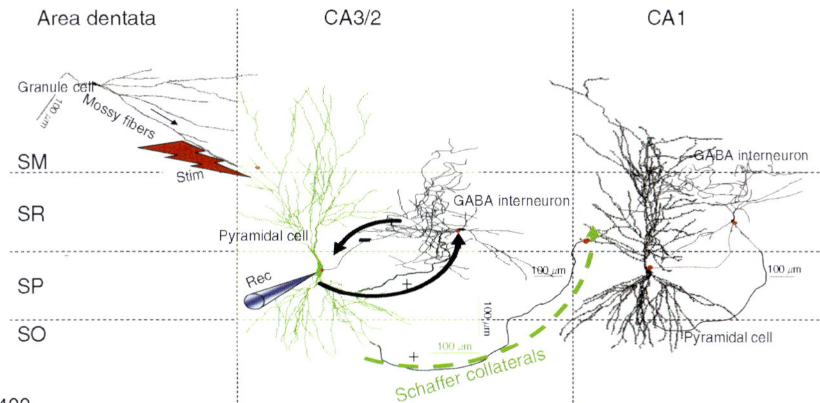


**CHAPTER 4, FIGURE 4** Schematic diagram representing the position of the stimulator (Stim) and recording (Rec) electrodes on a pyramidal neuron stimulated by mossy fibers and inhibited by GABA interneurons. Pyramidal cells, in turn, activate other cells through Schaffer collaterals and their dendrites (Camera lucida drawing of pyramidal neuron and interneurons courtesy of Duke-Southampton archive; see http://www.cns.soton.ac.uk/~iachad/cellArchive).

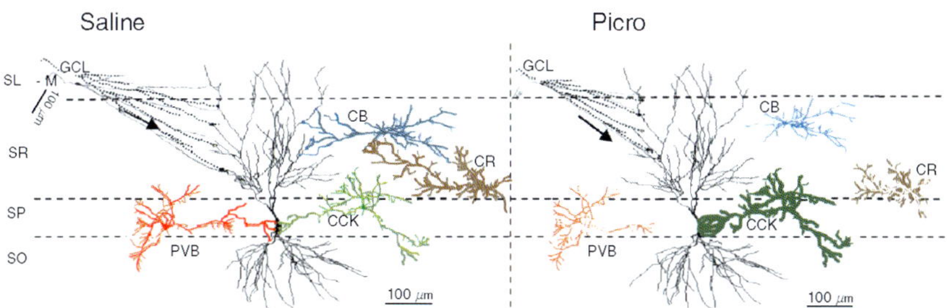


**CHAPTER 4, FIGURE 6** Schematic diagram representing changes in various subtypes of GABAergic interneuron in the hippocampus of rats exposed to amygdalar activation in the rat model. Normally, the hippocampus contains at least four different subtypes of GABA cell defined by the presence of various peptides in the cytoplasm, including parvalbumin (PVB), calbinding (CB), calretinin (CR), and cholecystokinin (CCK). These cells provide inhibitory modulation of pyramidal cells at the level of the cell somata (PVB and CCK) and the dendritic tree (CB and CR). Rats receiving PICRO infusions in the BLa show a significant reduction of PVB-, CB-, and CR-containing interneurons. Those containing CCK show an increase of inhibitory terminals on the somata of pyramidal neurons.

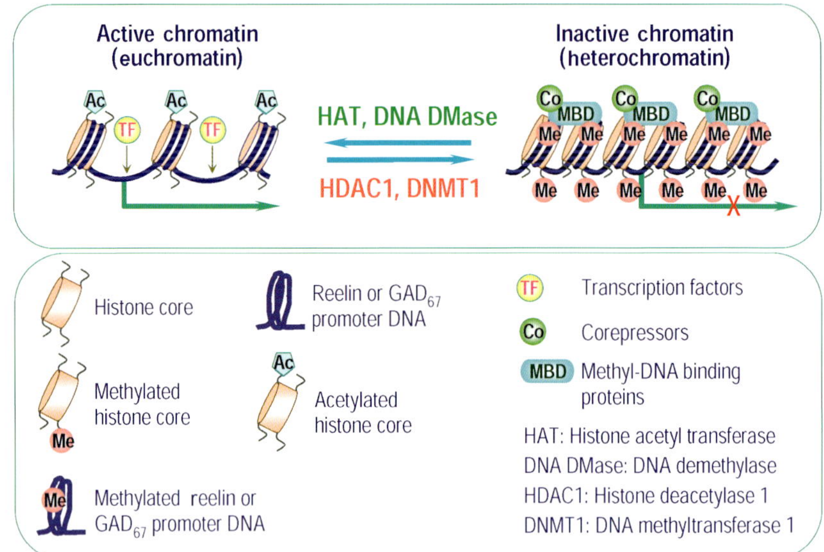


**CHAPTER 5, FIGURE 1** Regulation of *RELN* and $GAD_{67}$ promoter CpG island methylation and transcription. Genes (*RELN*, $GAD_{67}$) expressing CpG islands in their promoters can be reversibly controlled (transcriptional repression or activation) by altered levels of histone acetylation, DNA promoter methylation and the presence or absence of transcription factors and repressors at their promoters. The chromatin structural changes that allow transition from an inactive to an active gene can be schematically represented by a two-conformational state model: (1) Inactive chromatin conformation (heterochromatin) associated with gene transcriptional repression achieved by CpG promoter island methylation, recruitment of MBD proteins, and recruitment of corepressors. This closed conformational state prevents DNA interaction with RNA polymerase II. (2) Active chromatin conformation (euchromatin) associated with gene transcriptional activation achieved by a combination of demethylation of CpG promoter islands, dissociation of MBD proteins from their promoters, covalent histone tail acetylation and recruitment of transcription factors, including recruitment of RNA polymerase II by DNA.

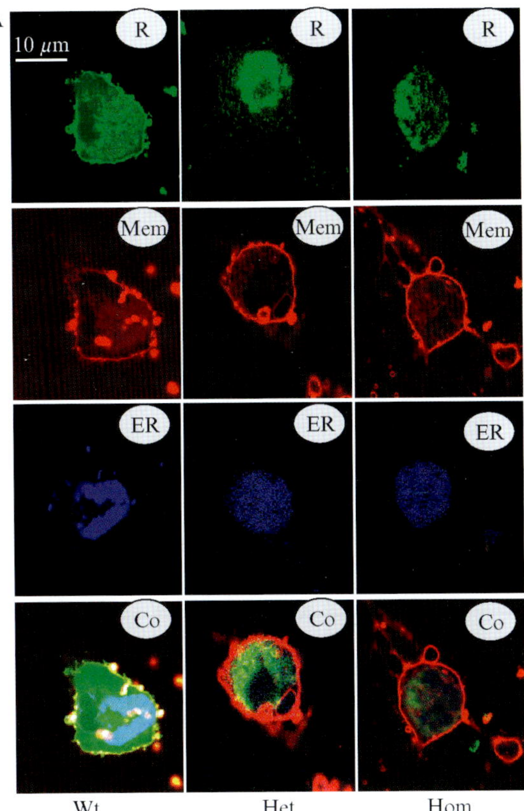


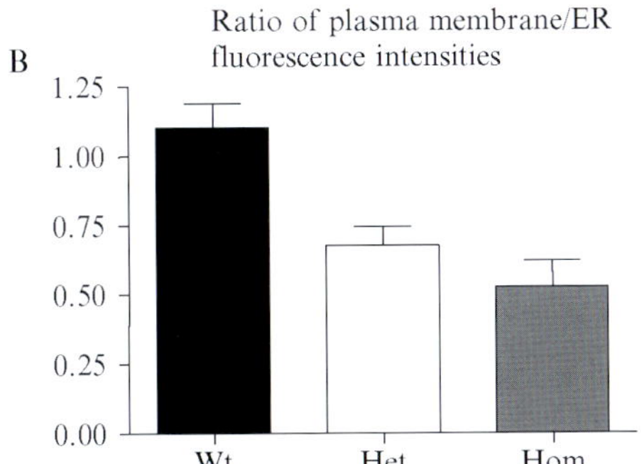


**CHAPTER 7, FIGURE 6** Heterozygous and homozygous α1*b*2γ2S(R43Q) receptors were retained in the ER. (A) COS-7 cells were cotransfected with human α1*b*2γ2S-YFP wild type (Wt) or α1*b*2γ2S(R43Q)-YFP heterozygous (Het) or homozygous (Hom) receptors with enhanced CFP-tagged ER marker and labeled with FM4–64 membrane marker. R, receptor; Mem, membrane; ER, endoplasmic reticulum; and Co, colocalized image. Wt α1*b*2γ2S-YFP receptors were primarily in the cell membrane. Het α1*b*2γ2S(R43Q)-YFP receptors were found in both the membrane and intracellular compartments. Hom α1*b*2γ2S(R43Q)-YFP receptors were primarily found in intracellular compartments with minimal localization on the cell surface. Both Het and Hom receptors had a fluorescence pattern that was similar in distribution to that of the ER fluorescence pattern. (B) The relative membrane/ER fluorescence intensity ratios for Het and Hom receptors were significantly reduced compared with that for the Wt receptors. Modified from Kang and Macdonald (2004).

A

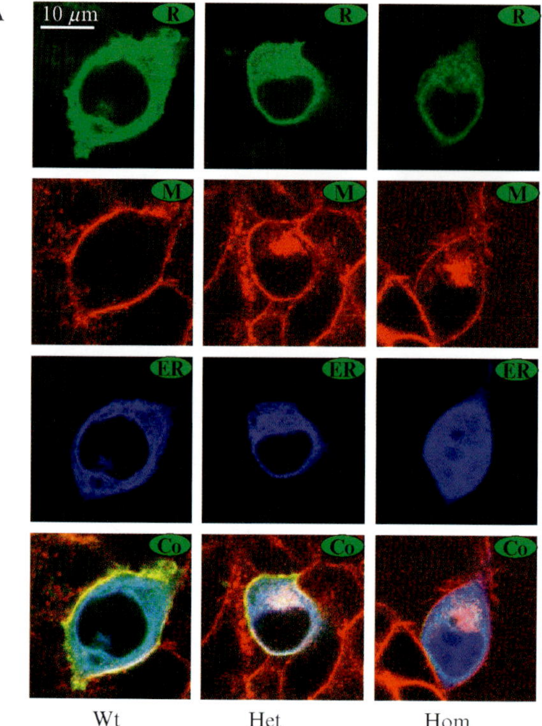


B

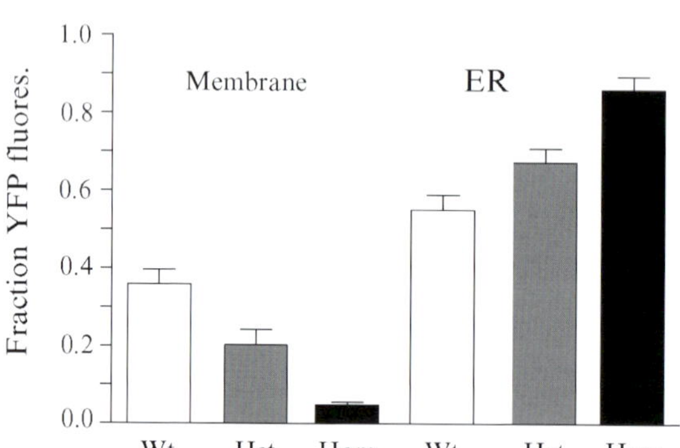


**CHAPTER 7, FIGURE 8** The JME $\alpha 1$(A322D) mutation colocalized to the ER cells were transfected with the ER marker, CFP-ER (ER, blue) and either wild type (Wt, $\alpha 1$-YFP$\beta 2\gamma 2$S), heterozygous (Het, $\alpha 1$-YFP$\alpha 1$(A322D)-YFP$\beta 2\gamma 2$S) or homozygous (Hom, $\alpha 1$(A322D)-YFP$\beta 2\gamma 2$S) receptors (R, green) and stained with the membrane marker, FM 4–64 (M, red). The majority of all receptors colocalized (Co) with the ER (cyan). Only wild-type and heterozygous $\alpha 1$-YFP subunit colocalized with the plasma membrane marker (yellow). The fraction of total wild type, heterozygous, and homozygous $\alpha 1$-YFP that colocalized to the ER or membrane is graphed. Modified from Gallagher *et al.* (2005).

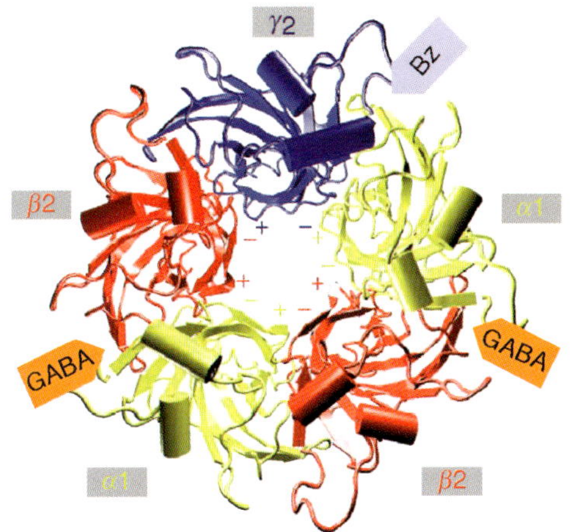


**CHAPTER 10, FIGURE 4** Model structure of $GABA_A$ receptor extracellular domains. The absolute arrangement for $\alpha 1$, $\beta 2$, and $\gamma 2$-containing $GABA_A$ receptors is shown, view is from extracellular. The + and − sides of the subunits are identified on the inner circumference of the channel. Labels indicate the interfaces at which the benzodiazepine binding site or the two GABA binding sites are located. Taken from Ernst *et al.* (2003), with permission.

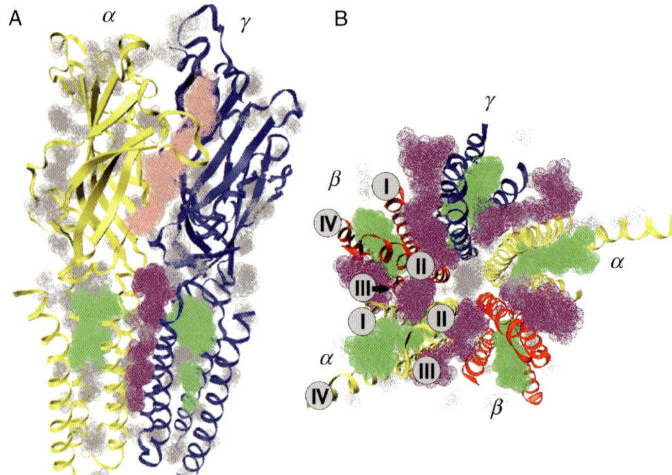


**CHAPTER 10, FIGURE 5** Solvent-accessible space contained in $GABA_A$ receptor models. Two views of a $GABA_A$ receptor model are shown to illustrate the pockets found by pocket-finding algorithms. The left view shows a dimer from the outside of the pore, the right view is from extracellular, with the $\beta$-folded domain invisible. The protein is shown in ribbon representation, the putative pockets identified with PASS are shown in dotted space filling representation. Clusters of connected solvent accessible volumes that may correspond to drug binding pockets are highlighted by colors: pink for the space associated with the subunit-interface of the $\beta$-folded domain, purple for the large cavity present at the subunit interface at the junction between the $\beta$-folded and the helical domain that extends into the interface of the helical domains, and green for the cavity that is present inside each of the four-helix bundles that form the helical domain of each subunit. Additional smaller clusters are shown in pale gray. It should be noted that because of the high uncertainty in side-chain positions, the total volume, shape, and electrostatic prperties of the pockets varies considerably among models; in some models some of the pockets may even be missing. Within the uncertainty of the method, it is also possible that there is significant communication between "pink" and "purple" as well as between "green" and "purple pockets." For this illustration, a representative model was used whose properties correspond to what the majority of models display. Figure was taken from Ernst *et al.*, *Mol. Pharmacol.* e-published ahead of print, August 15 2005, with permission.

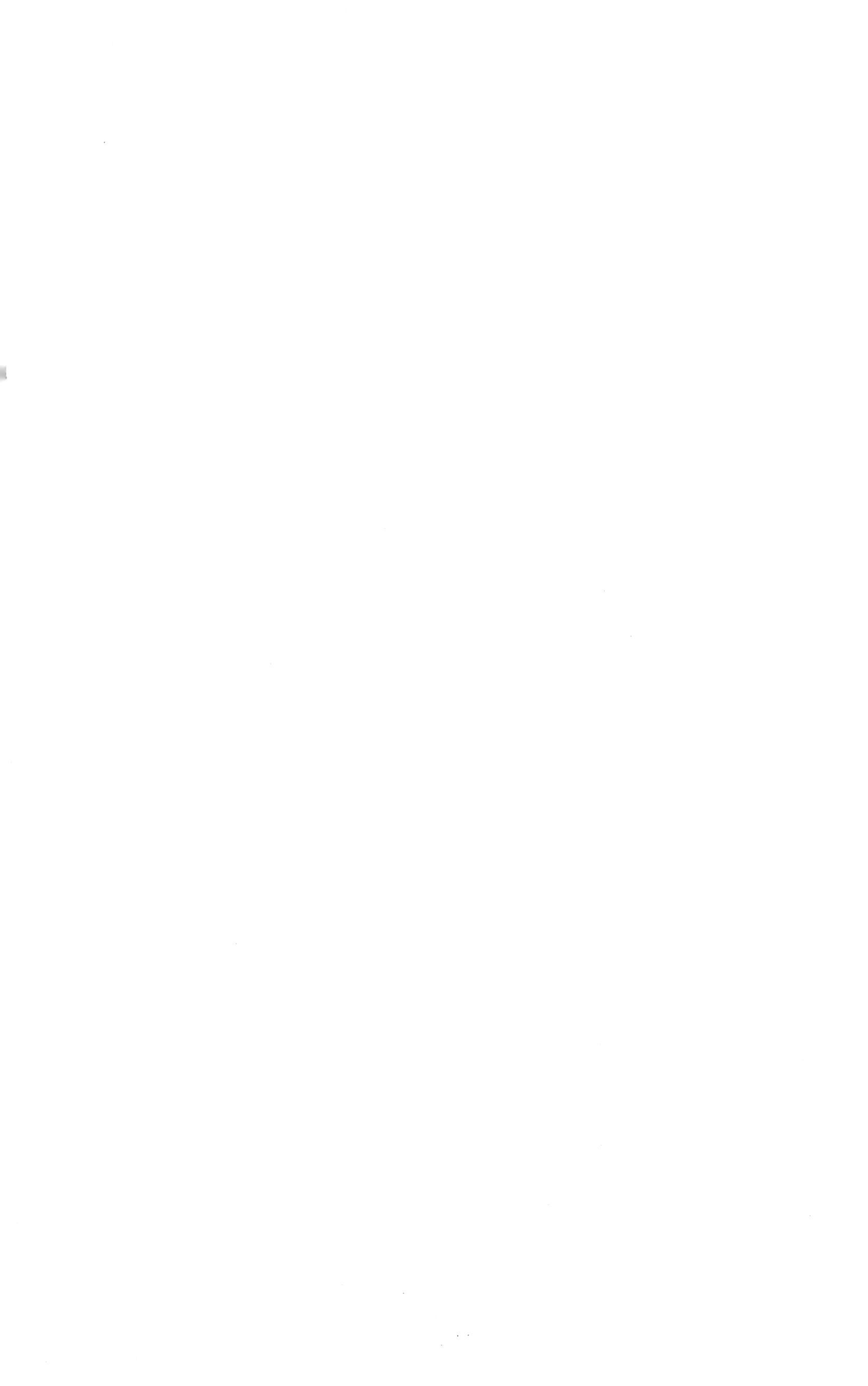